Narcissism and the Psychotherapist

Sheila Rouslin Welt, M.S., received her degree as a clinical specialist in psychiatric nursing from Rutgers—The State University of New Jersey. She is certified for psychotherapy practice in New York and New Jersey, where she is in private practice. In 1963, she coauthored the first book on group psychotherapy by a nurse. Her coauthored books, *Issues in Psychotherapy, A Collection of Classics in Psychiatric Nursing Literature*, and *Interpersonal Theory in Nursing Practice: Selected Works of Hildegard E. Peplau*, received the *American Journal of Nursing* Book of the Year awards. A former Rutgers educator and clinical editor, she has lectured throughout the United States and abroad and is widely published in psychiatric nursing journals. She is on the editorial board of *Archives of Psychiatric Nursing*.

William G. Herron, Ph.D., received his degree in clinical psychology from Fordham University and is a graduate of the Adelphi University postdoctoral program in psychotherapy and psychoanalysis. He is a Fellow of the American Psychological Association and a Diplomate in Clinical Psychology of the American Board of Professional Psychology. He is a professor in the Department of Psychology at St. John's University, Jamaica, New York, and in private practice in Woodcliff Lake, New Jersey. He is an editorial consultant for *Psychotherapy*, and the coauthor of *Reactive and Process Schizophrenia, Contemporary School Psychology*, and *Issues in Psychotherapy*.

Narcissism and the Psychotherapist

Sheila Rouslin Welt
William G. Herron

THE GUILFORD PRESS
New York   London

To Aaron and Jane

© 1990 The Guilford Press
A Division of Guilford Publications, Inc.
72 Spring Street, New York, NY 10012

Printed in the United States of America

This book is printed on acid-free paper.

Last digit is print number: 9 8 7 6 5 4 3 2 1

Library of Congress Cataloging-in-Publication Data

Welt, Sheila Rouslin.
   Narcissism and the psychotherapist / Sheila Rouslin Welt,
William G. Herron.
     p.   cm.
   Includes bibliographical references.
   ISBN 0-89862-398-7
   1. Narcissism.   2. Psychotherapists—Mental health.
3. Psychotherapist and patient.   I. Herron, William G.   II. Title.
RC553.N36W45   1990
616.89′023—dc20   89-27520
                                        CIP

Preface

This book is about the narcissism of therapists, that is, self-interest in and about the therapist–patient relationship. Whereas narcissism has certainly become prominent as an area of concern, most of this interest has concentrated on the narcissism of patients. Since the overall therapeutic interaction is our field of exploration, we will consider that as well; however, our focus in this volume is on the relatively neglected area of therapist narcissism. Too often, the significant impact of such narcissism on the therapeutic process has been overlooked. Yet the need for improving psychotherapeutic effectiveness is constant. Thus, calling attention to the existence and force of therapist narcissism is directed at meeting that need.

In our earlier work (Herron & Rouslin, 1982/1984), we developed a number of previously underemphasized but significant concerns about the inner workings of psychotherapy. In so doing, we were struck by the pivotal nature of the concept of narcissism, especially its development and manifestations in therapists. Thus, in this book we move from our former broader investigative base to a selective emphasis on narcissism as a key concept in understanding previously misunderstood, neglected, or avoided aspects of the psychotherapeutic process.

Why have therapists been less than eager to recognize their narcissism within the therapist–patient relationship? There are a number of understandable reasons. First is that the most desired image of the therapist has been that of the selfless helper. As a result, therapists avoid the recognition of certain personal qualities such as narcissism, which is frequently thought of as emphasizing self-interest as contrasted with the interests of others as well as self-love that uses the love of others. Thus, a social meaning of selfishness that sounds opposed to patient interests has become attached to narcissism (Lasch, 1979) and does not augur well for therapists who think about their own self-interest when working with patients.

A second suppressing factor is the current status of the practice of psychotherapy. Demands for "accountability" and rapid cures are common at this time. Although therapists can recognize the complexity of what is involved and the incongruity between that and pressures to be simplistic, the focus is taken off the art of therapy. This tends to push therapists away from themselves as people and into roles as technocrats with formulae that diminish the personal involvement of all concerned. Psychotherapy becomes viewed as a discipline concerned with symptoms rather than people. Therapists can easily fixate on their own survival and ignore a very basic and creative narcissistic quality of the therapeutic relationship. At times it appears as if the marketing personality may replace the therapeutic personality. Paradoxically such narcissistic exercises are *not* attributed to narcissism.

A third factor is the existing awareness of countertransference, which certainly does get attention but not especially in regard to narcissism. Countertransference emphasizes therapist transferential reactions to patients, and these are usually depicted in object-relations terms. For example, it has been noted that therapists react to a female patient as if she were a seductive mother or to a male patient as if he were a demanding father. Certainly these reactions are related to narcissism, and contain narcissistic elements, but self-interest is not the focus. Because therapists are very concerned about countertransference, in a somewhat paradoxical way, this tends to lessen the possible interest in creative narcissism and heighten interest in apparently transferential aggressive and sexual responses to patients. It is as though by maintaining an ongoing willingness to notice and explore countertransferences therapists have reduced or eliminated the need to do the same for their narcissism. The overlap in these concepts is admitted without sufficient attention to the distinctions being paid.

Throughout this book, these obscuring factors are discussed with suggestions about working with the therapist's image, current psychotherapeutic climates, and the concept of countertransference so that narcissism can be given due recognition. The presence of narcissism necessitates the existence and maintenance of self-esteem. As such, it has many modes, pathological and creative. The former, grandiosity, self-absorption, essentially defensive maneuvers, are better known than the developmental possibilities of subjective experience. Kainer and Gourevitch (1983) suggest distinctions between pathological, malevolent, and benign types of narcissism. Narcissism is not exclusively a pejorative term. Self-interest can be a good, useful, positive, and healthy quality. Therefore, when a therapist listens attentively to a patient, he or she is operating out of the self-interest of being a good therapist that coincides with the patient's need to obtain effective therapy.

Thus, although we certainly discuss the pathological expressions and dimensions of therapist narcissism in this volume, we are ultimately concerned with therapist development of a healthy narcissism. We understand therapist reluctance to engage in potentially negative self-examination. Indeed, writing this book involved a considerable and continual struggle with just that reluctance. Yet we are convinced that exploration and open discussion of therapist narcissism are essential to the effectiveness of the psychotherapies. As practicing psychotherapists for more than 30 years, we are increasingly attuned to the problems all psychotherapists face. Our presentation is an intermingling of personal experience and clinical and research literature and has at its core the conception of narcissism in the personality of every therapist, a quality that may be used positively and creatively or negatively and destructively.

As the book was conceived, we felt its impact would be greatest if we limited ourselves to certain instances of therapist narcissism that struck us as particularly in need of attention. The situations explored are narcissism in the obsessional therapist, occupational demands on the narcissistic self, the therapeutic self in the handling of therapist–patient monetary transactions, the relationship among fantasy, countertransference, and narcissism, the habitual, unexamined narcissistic response, and the intermingling of flexibility and constancy in the therapeutic self. We devote three chapters to illustrating concepts particularly relevant to both the formation and stimulation of narcissism, namely loneliness, envy, and passive–aggressiveness. We stress the importance of theory development and application for therapist self-effectiveness, especially in the areas of contracts and resistance. We discuss the role of narcissism in psychotherapy supervision and conclude with an update on therapist narcissism that portrays the good therapist in the context of an ability to express healthy narcissism.

Although selective, we have tried to be representative and pertinent for therapists of all disciplines and persuasions. Narcissism is often thought of as a psychoanalytic term, but its scope is not limited to any school of therapy. We hope all therapists will read this and think more about how they use themselves most effectively.

Acknowledgments

On completion of this book, I am left with the warm glow of affection for my coauthor, Sheila Rouslin Welt, whom I have known, grown with, and learned from for over 20 years. During that time, we have produced two books that are public reminders of each other, and lived thousands of mutually enjoyable private moments that enliven the present and foretell the future.

I am certainly appreciative of the support of St. John's University, which provided a research leave so that I could write. Among my colleagues there, I am particularly grateful to my friends, Louis Primavera, Chair of the Psychology Department, and Rafael Javier, Director of the Psychological Services Center, for their interest in my work and their unflagging support. I also wish to mention Frank Patalano and Frank Catalano for their contributions to my learning over the many years we have worked together, Jeffrey Nevid, Director of Clinical Training, for encouraging an atmosphere in which psychoanalytic work is treated with respect, and Justin Psaila, a colleague in private practice. There are and have been many other faculty members who have also aided my efforts for many years, and for this they will always have my gratitude.

My experience in the Adelphi University postdoctoral program has had a marked effect on my views, and I thank the many people there who worked with me, particularly Donald Milman, the Program Director, who over the years has continued his unique assistance. I particularly single out my friends and colleagues in my peer supervision group that had its origins in the initial acquaintance of some of us at Adelphi. The group members are Julius Trubowitz, Irwin Sollinger, Thomas Kinter, Mary Jane Herron, and Joan Wolkin.

I am grateful to those who have been, and continue to be, my patients, for they constantly show me what psychotherapy is all about. I have a similar feeling about my students and supervisees, and particularly my daughter Rachel, a social worker, and my brother-in-law, David, a psychiatrist, as they have become a part of the psychotherapy profession. I also want to thank my daughters who are pursuing their careers in other fields, Judith, Lia, and Mara, yet always retain interest in what I am doing and writing. Special thanks go to my younger daughters, Abigail and Allison, who are still around to hear and see the work in progress. Finally, my eternal appreciation to my wife, Mary Jane, who always makes it possible for me to try to make my fondest dreams come true.

William G. Herron

For 25 years, Bill and I have led separate personal and professional lives, yet lives that have been entwined in ways that permeate both our personal lives and professional careers. Although our backgrounds differ, and in recent years our professional communication is largely through our writing, we have developed in pace and tune with each other. It is rare to feel at one with another yet feel separate; to feel competitive with another yet thrilled at the other's success; to feel completely accepted yet encouraged to grow beyond the current measure. I feel all this with Bill and treasure our relationship.

Without my mentor, Hildegard E. Peplau, I would not be the person or professional I am today. I notice her influence daily and feel fortunate to have been her student and colleague. Her scholarly approach to the study of behavioral phenomena has influenced my thinking and my entire career. She continues to stimulate, support, and enlighten me; a clinical/theoretical discussion with her remains a treat. She is one of those rare "parents" who can tolerate and even encourage separation-individuation, one who can survive and move beyond the process to become respectful colleague and genuine friend.

To my year-old son William Philip Rouslin Welt, I am simply Mama. But to me he is a cherished, longed-for child, a child probably happier in his narcissism than I ever was. To be a part of his life and his development is a thrill and a sobering lesson about impingements on one's narcissism. During the later stages of writing this book, he made a little home for himself in my study, perhaps to prevent loneliness, to compete a little with works produced from his hustle and bustle, to aid my resistance, and perhaps, in his therapeutic way, to provide a little dose of healthy narcissism for us both. I am so glad he is here.

My husband Aaron has survived yet another book. When we met, Bill and I were at work on *Issues in Psychotherapy*, and when William arrived to make us a family, Bill and I were once again collaborating. Aaron has had to put aside his needs and precious time to support me in my writing effort. When I needed soothing, he had to be mother and father to both Willy and me, not an easy task. To thank him in print is important. To be with this marvelously intuitive, bright clinician, loving husband, and sensitive father is the best choice I have ever made.

Sheila Rouslin Welt

Contents

I

The Consequences
of Narcissism

*T*his section introduces the concept of therapist narcissism and
its impact on the therapist, the patient, and the integrity of the
therapy process. Here we begin to address those uncomfortable topics
that many therapists have trouble acknowledging, topics that explore
how the therapist's basic narcissistic problems develop, how such a
person then enters a helping profession, and how that person unconsciously stumbles through the therapist–patient relationship.

It is fascinating to note how little is written about the obsessional
patient or therapist. Our speculation is that, in true narcissistic fashion,
should the obsessional therapist write about the obsessional patient, the
act would be akin to looking in a mirror and thus be too intimate and
revelatory to be permitted. Unfortunately, not coming to terms with
one's psychological roots presents drawbacks for the therapist and is in
itself an occupational hazard in work inherently replete with occupational
hazards that impinge on one's narcissistic needs.

How vulnerable is the therapist when dealing with negativistic,
hostile, and often ungrateful patients who try one's skill and spirit? How
much resistance is too much when the therapist's identity as helper is at
stake? And does the therapist's narcissism influence his or her need to be
liked, to be idealized, to have the patient as a friend or companion? Of
course such needs have impact on the therapeutic process, but although
we may stipulate how and why, the explanation often remains elusive.

One narcissistic threat is that an active therapy practice controls the
therapist's time and gratification and leaves little energy for personal life,
which may suffer. Personal dynamics and a sense of self-validation may
also suffer because the therapist cannot quite admit the importance of

being paid for the work done. Indeed, money has not been a popular subject in most therapists' training experience or in therapy literature itself. Somehow, popular wisdom holds that money and altruism do not mix, and this is indeed reflective of a narcissistic problem whereby the therapist sees him- or herself as having an inherent "right" to be "cared for" by the patient and to command respect, regard, and money without having to ask for it. We present reasonable approaches to the money dynamic and stress the need to recognize the psychological impact of charging money for one's knowledge, skill, and time in the real world.

A separate phenomenon that must be acknowledged is that the fantasy world of the therapist is as important as that of the patient. Embedded in the general concept of fantasy is the phenomenon of countertransference, which is explored here as a vehicle that demonstrates the therapist's narcissism. Fantasy is seen both as a route to identifying and understanding the therapist's narcissism as well as a psychological conduit for how therapeutic matters are affected by the need to be a "helper extraordinaire."

1

The Obsessional Therapist

In 1974, Bellak, in writing about the life of a psychotherapist, said: "It is as close a vantage point on the human condition as there is. As you listen to a life history and to the symptomatology, you have a ringside seat all day, every day, to the human drama" (p. 7). He writes, too, of the feeling of competence to intervene, of doing something worthwhile, of intellectual pleasure and "the emotional experience of a sense of a Greek drama unfolding in its inevitability before you" (p. 7). These observations are familiar, yet, although they certainly seem an accurate account of what a therapist experiences, the description feels strangely incomplete. Perhaps this is because it is nearly impossible to describe such an experience succinctly. After all, it is in the process of therapy that there is an intense, often disturbing mixture of therapists' emotional and interpersonal responses to their patients. When these responses are described, the confusion of health and pathology is definitely possible. Words are beggars at describing the mix, but words are what we have to offer here.

It is true indeed that the therapist is an observer, albeit a participant observer. It is true, too, that after the novice's initial grandiosity and subsequent feelings of powerlessness, over time, a therapist does feel an ability to help and make some sort of human contribution. And it is true that there is, over the long haul, a kind of drama unfolding. On the other hand, the rational observations and sentiments expressed by Bellak (1974) unwittingly point up some of the problems that therapists bring to their work: the "need" to help, the conflict about closeness and intimacy, the intellectual operations as a defense against emotional response, all of which fall under the umbrella concept of the therapist's

This chapter was originally published in *Issues in Psychotherapy*, 1982, New York: Brady-Prentice Hall. Copyright 1982 by William G. Herron and Sheila Rouslin Welt.

narcissism, the self-involved use of self with patients—the defensive use of self. In describing such behavior, we use mainly psychoanalytic terminology, since the problem, when addressed, has customarily been couched in these terms. But the problem is by no means restricted to the psychoanalytically oriented. The terms and concepts bear translation to all approaches to the psychotherapies.

Sometimes in the privacy of the therapist's solitude, often in the inner sanctum of the therapist's unconscious, yet rarely in the light of consciousness or in print (Greben, 1975; Lipp, 1978), the therapist asks, "What's in it for me, this business of doing psychotherapy?" Although the question is seldom raised or addressed, its essence repeatedly manifests itself in the therapeutic relationship. The question in fact reflects the importance of understanding the therapist's narcissistic needs—needs that perhaps have drawn him or her to the field, but needs that can work against the best interests of the patients treated and, ultimately, against the therapist. In exploring the therapist's narcissism, our aim is not to indict the therapist. Rather, it is to clarify the dynamics of the narcissism and suggest how the dynamics, in repeating themselves through relationships with patients, impede the relationship through inhibiting the full development of the patient and the therapist.

That the therapist's narcissistic needs arise during the process of therapy is not surprising, for they are always present in one degree or another, ever in seasoned therapists. To paraphrase Sullivan, therapists are, after all, like everybody, more human than otherwise. It is not uncommon, however, to hear it intimated that therapists have more than their share of narcissism. Although to our knowledge therapist narcissism has not been measured on a scale, the phenomenon has been observed repeatedly and is seen by some theorists such as Mehlman (1974) and Sharaf and Levinson (1964) as an inevitable dimension of the therapy situation. This is especially true for the novice therapist, who is relatively helpless, relatively unknowledgeable about him- or herself, patients, and the treatment process, where, unlike most, doing less is doing more. Certain theorists (Ford, 1963; Jones, 1951; Lewin, 1958; Marmor, 1953; Miller, 1979; Sharaf and Levinson, 1964) in one way or another think that the therapist's narcissism is a problem to be reckoned with if the therapy that is engaged in is indeed to prove a therapeutic experience for the patient. Still others, (Miller, 1979; Searles, 1967/ 1979), through a variety of formulations equivalent to the concept of narcissism, hold that the therapist's choice of profession is itself intimately bound up with his or her narcissism.

The point is that in the therapeutic relationship, as in any relationship, the quality and creativity of the relationship are dependent on the ability of the persons to participate through an unencumbered use of self.

By that we mean there is sufficient self-object differentiation and confirmation so the relationship can indeed be a relationship, not a quasi-two-person experience whereby one person is an extension of the other or in the emotional service of the other. At the same time, with the security and self-esteem that come with confirmation and differentiation, there arises the ability for nondefensive or healthy fusion by way of empathy—the automatic, if momentary, experiencing of the other. Obviously, when a patient comes into treatment, he or she is not in a position for such a relationship.The therapist has a responsibility to become aware of how his or her narcissistic stance in the relationship helps determine the course and outcome of the therapeutic process. To this end, we discuss narcissism as a personality feature in general and one of therapists in particular, the obsessional brand of narcissism so prevalent among therapists, and the therapist's need to be a therapist. In the process, through discussion of developmental narcissism and what went wrong and presentation of ways in which the therapist's narcissism manifests itself during treatment, we hope to bring some clarity to the issue of the therapist's narcissism.

NARCISSISM IN PERSONALITY

Narcissism can be seen both as pathology and as an essential part of development. Often a concept difficult to grasp, it has nonetheless captured the imagination and intelligence of major theorists such as Freud (1914/1957), Kernberg (1975), and Mahler (1968), to mention a few. As Blanck and Blanck (1979) imply, the study of pathology will yield greater knowledge of developmental narcissism and vice versa. Normative narcissism and its sometimes pathological vicissitudes, after all, are considered dimensions of the organizing process in personality development.

That narcissism as a feature of personality is of more than one type or level has been postulated by Blanck and Blanck (1979). They theorize five levels of pathological narcissistic formation in a developmental framework (apparently Mahler's, 1968) ranging from the symbiotic phase, through the differentiation, practicing, and rapprochement subphases, to object constancy. Although such a continuum could be useful, at this point the Blancks have not developed the levels sufficiently to make clinical application an easy matter. The idea, however, has a good deal of merit and recalls work done by Bursten (1973, 1977). In his 1973 paper, he postulated that there were four types of narcissism on a continuum ranging from a more primitive end of personality organization to a more advanced end. Further, although initially he classified each type (craving, paranoid, manipulative, and phallic) as narcissistic personality, it was not until the second paper on the subject in 1977 that he modified his view, hinting at but stopping short of actually saying that narcissism is an integral part of various levels of personality organization.

From our work with patients and clinical supervision of therapists, it seems clear that narcissism is part of various personality constellations, some more primitive in their organization than others. In other words, though perhaps there is a theoretically pure "narcissistic personality," there is a developmental, dynamic core of narcissism in all personalities, some more primitively expressed than others, depending at which end of the continuum the personality would be organized and classified.

Although Bursten (1977) implies that the obsessional character has less narcissistic need than other character types, such has not been our observation over the years in our supervisory and treatment work with therapists. First, although we have no hard data on which personality type goes into the therapy field, our observation and that of many colleagues is that the field attracts obsessionals far more than other personality types. This is neither good nor bad; it just seems to be that way. There are a number of possible reasons: what would appear to be thinking operations taking precedence over feelings, the intrigue with "figuring things out," the relative structure of the therapist–patient relationship, and the need for closeness in small doses are several that come to mind. Although we do intend later in the chapter to discuss certain dynamics in the parent–child relationship that exist during developmental narcissism (dynamics we believe result in a personality inclined in a therapist direction), our point here is only that the obsessional personality type seems most prevalent in the field.

In this regard, one of the most striking observations is that the particular brand of narcissism the obsessional has, as well as his or her facility in using it, get the therapist into trouble with patients. Since these obsessional dimensions of a therapist's character do cause a good deal of trouble and severely limit relatedness with patients, it is useful to present the dynamics of the narcissism in the obsessional defense. In so doing, we will point out where in the course of developmental narcissism things go awry and stay that way despite what would appear to be a level of sophistication implying development without such strong narcissistic residual.

Instead of presenting all views, we have tried to use those references that seem to bear relation to certain features of our formulations. In addition, we feel compelled to mention that we are amazed at the obtuse ways theorists have explained various theories of narcissism. Faced with such "autistic" presentations, we cannot guarantee that our formulations have not been recognized before in any way. Further, the writings can certainly make one wonder about therapists (including us) who choose to write about narcissism. All we can say is that we will try to be clear without being simplistic and complex without being convoluted, and to the degree we accomplish that task, we will consider that our interminable analyses have paid off.

NARCISSISM IN THE OBSESSIONAL DEFENSE

A patient, who is also a therapist, reported the following during a session when she had been describing how she finally noticed a gulf between her and her patients:

> As a child I remember feeling perplexed when I heard my uncle say that what he loved best was to have his family all around him. The words seemed inconsistent with his behavior; although he was pleased when he saw us, he never seemed quite "with" us, never quite in touch. The distance between him and us seemed greater than the miles separating his city from ours. I sensed, I guess, that something was missing in the relationship and in him, despite all the words spoken and experiences exchanged when we were together. Actually, he didn't know us very well, nor we him for that matter. The image I consistently had when he'd say all that was, "him" in the center of a circle of "us," his family. I pictured him turning round and round looking at us "out there" surrounding him, there, as distant objects of his pleasure.

Narcissism neatly depicted is our impression.

This therapist had always considered herself quite different from her uncle, until, as a young adult in her first session as a patient in a psychotherapy group, she had an illuminating experience. There she sat, aware of feeling detached, having a fantasy: She was in the center of the circle, turning round and round in her prettiest cool blue lingerie for the group "out there" surrounding, distant objects of her pleasure and she, elusive object of the group's curiosity and pleasure. The experience provides a powerful example of a resurgence of narcissism in case the patient did not see it in herself.

Although narcissism is at the central core of the obsessional defense, it is often well disguised. It is only on deeper acquaintance with the obsessional character structure that it becomes possible to identify the narcissism and understand how it operates for and against the person in human relationships, especially for and against the therapist in relationships with patients. Contrary to the popular notion of narcissism as a focus purely on oneself, and narcissism in some schools of thought as the opposite pole of object relatedness (Freud, 1914/1957), narcissism is not an "one person" phenomenon. As the saying goes, there is no sound to one hand clapping. Narcissism does not in fact occur in a vacuum (Klein, 1952) in its developmental or extended state, although at first glance it would appear to be a solitary experience. We agree with Kernberg (1975) when he concludes that "one cannot analyze narcissism as if it were a drive independent of internalized object relations" (p. 338). Therefore, narcissism manifests itself through one's interpersonal relationships, or, to quote Kernberg (1975), "Normal and pathological narcissism always involves the relationship of the self to object representations and external objects" (p. 341). Developmentally, narcissism arises as the natural tendency of the human infant to fuse, then blend with the mother in such a way that assures getting enough of what is needed eventually to permit separation from this emotional storehouse. Two subphases of the early narcissistic state are postulated. In the first, called normal autism by Mahler (1968), there is perceptual fusion of the infant with the mother. In other words, there is no distinction between self and object; there exists instead what has been termed a self-object; in the infant's world the self and object are one. As the infant matures to the subphase of symbiosis, he or she recognizes a separateness between the mother and the now developing "self." However, the object mother is now considered separate from but existing to serve the self. Thus, the self is still conceived of in relation to another, the self is still a self-object in a sense, a rather powerful one in fact.

In working with obsessional patients, and with obsessional therapists as patients and as supervisees, we have come to think that, developmentally, it is in the phase of symbiosis where their troubles begin. Their difficulties in living, which are considerable, stem from an extraordinary desire to establish relationships where the other person is there in the service of the self. For whatever maternal reasons, during normal symbiosis, the obsessional does not seem to have been in the position of having the object in his or her service. Often, indeed, the positions are reversed, which probably heralds the beginning of what will later be the therapist's "life of service." Although this reversal does not interfere with the development of a self, it noticeably influences the quality of the self that develops. As Balint (1968) might say, the "basic fault" has been lack of fit in the mother–child unit. The mother, unyielding in her emotional position, is unable to bend with the rhythm and child. Furthermore, the dynamics at work turn the child into a mother, a role reluctantly accepted and, although well carried out, a role unconsciously resented.

In fact, at some level, the person who becomes obsessional is forever locked into the struggle to make the mother serve the self. In a sense, life is spent trying to wrench from others what during development was not forthcoming from the mother, not item for item, so much as the state of receiving. The obsessional feels the other should fit into his or her system. Such an attitude is not only determined by the desire to receive in fact what was needed early in life but by a "right" that is now felt due. A sense of righteous indignation develops that regulates self-esteem (Lax, 1975). "Outbursts of righteous indignation enable the child–adult self of these patients to merge again and again with the idealized 'righteous one' (parent), to whose grandeur they had submitted and whose grandeur they still want to attain" (p. 288).

The obsessional has identified with the mother in whose service he or she was as an infant. Consequently, the person is in the difficult position of having identified with the mother without getting from her what was needed, having had only a hint of what it is like to get what one wants. Often this results in a kind of compliant state, in the development of what has been termed by Winnicott (1960/1974) a "false self." With self-feeling not validated, self-esteem remains vulnerable. Aggression becomes directed at the search for and acquisition of the object rather than a tool aiding in separation, individuation, or the development of the self on its own. In other words, the aim of the aggression is to maintain a symbiotic bond by identifying with the mother, whereas, ordinarily, the identification facilitates separation.

Through identifying with the mother, the person tries to right the situation—to right the wrong done, the injustice perpetrated. In the mind's eye, the situation will be redressed by trying to be better to others than the mother was to oneself, a motivation not unfamiliar in the life of a therapist. However, the focus is still on the self—still in effect to prove a point to the mother.

From all this, we might conclude that the person does not feel whole, that a self-object is needed to feel a sense of psychic integrity. In fact, that is not entirely the situation. The object has been internalized; therefore, there is a sense of object constancy, making it possible to function separately from the mother (unlike the schizophrenic personality who cannot function with object loss). The problem is that emotional separation is incomplete because the obsessional lives with the nearly pathological hope that the mother will come through, as seen in relationships with others. Virtually all behavior central to the obsessional way of life bears this out, although (in true obsessional complexity) the meaning and source of the behavior are far from clear. The quest for perfection is directly related to the obsessional's narcissism, for it is not actually for "self"-satisfaction that perfection is sought. In the obsessional mind and heart, the hope never quite dies that if one is perfect, then the parents will show their devotion and give their approval. The corollary is that early in life the obsessional has the idea that the reason for maternal (and, later, paternal) deficiencies lies in himself or herself, not in the parent. To recognize that the mother would not or could not allow the infant's needs to intrude on her own, that is, on her system, would fill the child with rage and anxiety beyond the then current developmental capacity. (This is useful to remember in treatment and supervision, to respect that the obsessional truly feels he or she will surely fall apart in experiencing anger, rage, or anxiety—so much so that secondary anxiety can occur as soon as the feelings break through.)

What is sought as a child and later as an adult is recognition that indeed he or she is a person with a need to be taken seriously, a need for respect of and tolerance for feelings not necessarily shared by the parents. Because there has been little recognition or validation of this "separate-self" concept, what start out as human needs become repressed, then to be distorted through detachment, isolation of affect, and a list of rights due, which all underlie the defensive quest for perfection.

The obsessional's narcissism affects psychic and interpersonal function and makes therapy a lengthy and difficult process. For the obsessional therapist, treating patients creates a situation where there looms a constant threat to his or her narcissism. For example, to acknowledge that there exists an emotional tie, even an emotional reaction to one's patient, may be nearly impossible. Not that the situation does not occur, but to acknowledge it would be admitting that a person has somehow been admitted to the inner sanctum of the therapist's emotional life, that the barrier has been permeated.

Not only have we heard our patients talk about their therapists in the most rational and intellectual terms even after years of contact, but all too often we hear therapists talk about their patients as if someone else were seeing them. We are reminded of such a therapist, who, when referring to the therapist he'd seen for many years, made it clear that the therapist was "bright, perceptive, perhaps not always accurate, but on balance, doing his job well." Clearly, this sounds like a defense against an emotional bond, as though the bond were not growing anyhow, testimony to Kernberg's (1975) point that attachments were originally pure affect cathexes, we think, now being defended against because of the nature of the original affect.

Contrary to what one might expect, that the defense prevents the development of an emotional bond, the intellectual defense allows for the "secret" development of the emotional connection. It acts in the same way as a screen memory; that is, the intellect shields its accompanying or allied feeling just as one memory may shield an allied, emotionally laden memory. In operation, this means that even the therapist with strong obsessional defenses develops an emotional bond with the patient, sometimes quite a surprise to the therapist. It has been noticeable to us that once such a therapist has "discovered" an emotional bond he or she becomes angry. Thus, often the first noticeable and acknowledged genuine countertransference reaction that comes to the therapist's attention is a negative one. But why the defense against the emotional involvement in the first place, and why the anger? We think the defense serves several purposes. It protects the therapist from another taking over, robbing him or her of any autonomy, not respecting his or her existence. The anger is perhaps the first acknowledged countertransferential response is not surprising either, for it is a response to having somehow been caught, if only by oneself, at having dropped one's vigilance and allowed another's entry. In addition, the anger being released is an expression of the rage at having had one's "self-feeling" unconfirmed and self-development thwarted. Further, perhaps it replicates, now in a way distorted by rage, a major dimension of the original emotional attachment, the original narcissistic state, that is, aggression, which shouts, "Look, I exist, damn it; respect that, recognize that!"

Relating on an intellectual level helps protect the feelings of the obsessional, for it does not allow the other access to his or her heart. Further, it does not allow the therapist access to feelings and emotional perceptions that may frighten or threaten, perceptions that for security's sake are not to be noticed. Thus, in a way, the intellectual defense protects, defends, and perpetuates the original parental bond, the original narcissistic state of relations. All this is at great emotional and interpersonal expense personally and great empathic expense professionally. Perception of the therapist's feelings and affectual dimension of cognitive experience are constricted, as is perception of similar patient experience. Such perception would threaten the viability of the intellectual defense as a means of isolating the affectual portion—pleasure or pain—of an experience. Thus, it can be concluded that something is present on one level and missing on another in the therapist–patient relationship. This makes for complicated distortions by both patient and therapist.

MANIFESTATION OF THE THERAPIST'S NARCISSISM

Major features of the therapist's obsessional defense as it arises through the therapist patient relationship have, at their base, narcissistic dynamics. One central feature is *control*. In order to feel in control, the obsessional, by necessity, must control the world around him or her (Freud, 1909/1957; Salzman, 1968). For the therapist with a largely obsessional character structure, this task can reach mammoth proportions, for there are thousands upon thousands of perceptions, thoughts, feelings, and actions of patients to keep in check lest they touch off the therapist's unwanted perceptions, thoughts, feelings, and actions. In other words, because the therapist is not free to experience certain aspects of living, he or she unwittingly imposes a similar restriction on the patient, thereby assuring that the patient will not surpass, threaten, or psychologically leave being in the therapist's "service."

Actually, this is the kind of unconscious control that occurs in subtle ways and, in part, accounts for the many reported incidents of how patient and therapist, each in his or her own therapy, simultaneously deal with the same issues. As the therapist is more free to experience dimensions of self without feeling threatened, "permission" is unwittingly granted to the patient. And although the parallel experience is not happenstance, it is not simply brought about by therapist control. The paradox is that it also occurs because of therapist readiness to lessen control. As Searles (1966/1979) says, "One does not become free from feelings in the course of maturation or in the course of becoming well during psychoanalysis; one becomes, instead, increasingly free to experience feeling of all sorts" (p. 35).

The demands therapists place on patients have both rational and irrational components. For example, the patient is "supposed" to use the therapist as an emotional supplier. That makes sense: After all, the patient needs help and is coming for it. On the other hand, the therapist, in therapeutic zeal, may impose his or her dedication on the patient (Searles, 1967/1979a). An inordinate need to help and the guilt, anger, and anxiety at being rejected by patients who, at certain times, cannot accept help obscure the therapist's ambivalence and self-interest in treating patients in the first place. Further, the need to help distracts the therapists from the mixed mission of contacting yet keeping at a safe distance the projected dimensions of his or her self. Often the therapist foists on the patient the role of his or her own marred parent, who, through the therapist's ministrations, will be made whole or at least well enough to provide the goods needed.

This parent image, flawed though it is, has enormous power. A supervisee told of how anxious he was for months during a period when a patient he was treating would not let him help. Not only did the patient start out with reasons for rejecting the assistance, but in addition, he had sensed the therapist's need of him. This was the need to be needy so the therapist could indentify with him and be taken care of on his terms, something the therapist's mother had been unable to do for him. On another level, it became clear that what the patient sensed was the therapist's narcissistic need to show him up—to be a better mother than he, the patient, was, which of course meant the therapist would be a better mother than his own.

The patient, through letting the therapist help, could at once show the therapist's mother "how to do it right," prove to the therapist's mother that by comparison she was no good at her job, and to boot, get whatever goods were available by being the good, therapeutic child (a theme to be developed in a later section of this chapter). All this power was to be had simply by being the patient to be helped! Little wonder the patient reeled under such a burden of contradictory expectations, and little wonder too that the therapist felt so anxious and feared punishment out of proportion to what the patient was handing out, though admittedly, the patient found expert ways to strangle the therapist with his own needs. It was only when the therapist could extricate himself from the demands he unconsciously made and could allow himself to feel the anger and disappointment with his own mother that he could perceive the patient as just a patient. Far from a disparaging attitude, this perception, in effect, meant the patient was a regular, life-sized person on whom the therapist did not have to lean, one who did not have the giant-sized proportions of a powerful parent in the eyes of a helpless child.

So, then, it is conceivable that the therapist may genuinely want to help, while on another level the desire to help is based on self-interest resulting in the therapist's so-called dedication reaching controlling proportions.

Such dedication was obvious in this example. A therapist was a few minutes late for her supervision appointment. When she arrived she said she had been exhausted lately and seemed inordinately upset about the latest snow. She then reported she was upset, too, and worried about making what seemed to her to be too many interpretations and premature interpretations with her patients. (She had good reason to be upset, according to her supervisor!) She had noticed the problem previously, but that day it seemed worse and in her mind related to her getting to work late the day before. "I felt as if I should have gotten there on time; the snowstorm shouldn't have mattered. I figure if I had left three hours early instead of two I'd have made it on time. I felt so surprised and angry that the snow interfered. It was after that when I noticed how much I was interpreting, as if to make up for lost time."

Actually, the problem went beyond the lost time. It is interesting that it did not occur to her that no matter what time she left she might not have made it. The idea that nothing is predictable, that external events sometimes interfere with reaching a goal, that something could come between goal set and goal achieved was alien to her, though unconsciously she proved to know it only too well. How dare snow, a patient's unconscious, or a mother's unyielding behavior impede simple, human desires such as getting to work, helping a patient become aware, and seeking emotional goods needed for growth. So she, like her mother before her, was trying to force the world to fit into her system, to feel in control by controlling the world around her, and in so doing recapturing the narcissistic experience of childhood in all its intensity. No wonder she was exhausted.

At some point it is necessary for a therapist to recognize the need to control, reaching the point in personal therapy where the need is seen as a defense and reaction-formation against being out of control as well as a need based on a desire for self-confirmation and esteem. One such therapist comes to mind. No sooner had she begun to realize that she feared losing control of herself and others than it became clear why she had been so anxious of late with a particular patient. It seems that the patient had recently "turned" on her. In retrospect, she now understood what was meant in supervision when she had been advised that to be so nice to this particular hard-nosed, contemptuous patient seemed condescending, maybe even hostile, a subject often addressed by Searles (1975/1979) in his writings and in his supervisory demonstrations. Furthermore, she was advised that if she were as ingratiating as she sounded, she would eventually pay for the attitude and its inherent controlling quality.

The therapist came to realize that the value of her controlling behavior was to prevent her from putting herself at the mercy of the patient. Just as the development of self-esteem rests on how the mother responds and reacts to the growing child, the therapist's self-esteem seemed to rise and fall on the patient's reaction to her. Just as the child in effect is at the mercy of the parent, the therapist felt at the mercy of the patient's view of her. She was nice to the patient neither because she liked or valued him, nor was she nice for his benefit at all. Her behavior was self-serving. In the weeks that followed, it became clear that when the patient was accepting of her she felt great about herself, whereas when he rejected her, she would have thoughts of how ugly she was. She would think twice about whether or not she should say something he might not like. Although she fretted that his rejection was because of what she had or hadn't done, she later realized her distress was about the rejection because of what she was or wasn't. She admitted in fact that the main reason she wanted supervision was so she could become perfect, for then she would win the patient over.

Her reaction to the patient appears to be a reflection of the problems in developmental narcissism where the child keeps trying to have an impact on the impenetrable, unyielding mother, who gives what and when she wants. A mother in this god-like position is capable of yielding sufficient power to create or destroy a person; and from a developmental standpoint, this is very pertinent. Little wonder the therapist experienced the patient's rejection as an invalidation of her very being.

Closely akin to the need to control is *power struggling*, which, unfortunately, is a frequent component of therapy. The struggle seems to come out of nowhere, escalating quickly. The issue is of little import, for it can literally be anything ranging from what one might consider benign, such as where the person(s) will sit (or lie—good for prolonged struggling) to a difference of opinion over an interpretation. The struggles occur most with patients who also have the tendency, though a "skillful" therapist can bring the inclination out in almost anyone. In a capsule, what occurs is that each person is trying to place the other in each other's orbits. Obviously, the therapist, with a background of this kind of narcissistic oppression, is not going to like once again being on the receiving end and, in any event, tends to be compelled to start or enter a struggle because of the very history he or she abhors. The "other" gives the "self" life, as in the original symbiotic bond. The aggression, then, is directed at sustaining the struggle (the bond, the life) rather than stopping. If the struggle stopped, the business at hand could proceed, and the aggression could be used productively for the therapist's development, for the development of the relationship, indeed, to do therapy, or whatever. Obviously, however, to stop implies giving in, losing control, as well as the bottom line—emotional separation. And for the person locked in the struggle to bring the other around, to have the other acknowledge one's very being, to stop struggling is a narcissistic impossibility.

Although many power struggles are easy to identify, others are difficult because they are covert and linked to negativistic stances. The following instance is illustrative. A therapist had been distracted for some time with a problem supposedly unrelated to overt power struggles she had been having with her patients. At a university where she taught, she had applied for a sabbatical, and despite the fact that the department chairman was dragging his heels, it looked like she was going to get it. She was pleased, although not without anxiety. Then, suddenly, her department chairman died, after which she felt incredibly guilty about leaving and could not stop thinking that if he were alive she'd not feel so guilty about taking the sabbatical. Although the guilt had no rational basis and could be interpreted on a number of levels, the essence seemed to be that if the chairman were alive and she left on sabbatical she would carry the struggle—thus him—with her through this ostensibly autonomous move. It became clear that taking the step because she wanted to and not in opposition to him implied separation about which she felt guilt and anxiety. Just as the opposition or negativism bind the child to the parent, so the guilt and preoccupation bound this therapist to her chairman.

She was also having trouble with patients, struggling with several, one of whom was a rather smoothly controlling 8-year-old child. One day, they decided to take pictures with two cameras she kept in the office. The child proceeded to take some pictures and then said such things as, "Oh look, that's the kind of thing you like; why don't you take that picture?" The therapist found herself thinking she wouldn't take any pictures he told her to take, then progressed to thinking she wouldn't take any pictures altogether because he wanted her to, and finally she found herself not knowing what she found interesting to photograph. Her rage obliterated the child's presence as she gazed through him.

To this therapist, a suggestion was a command, and since the child probably was issuing a directive, albeit one consonant with the therapist's taste, it was well aimed—namely, at a person who would dig her heels in and become entangled with him in an unending narcissistic struggle for power. Were she to, as she said, "knuckle under" and do what he wanted, even if it were what she wanted, she could not help feeling in his service—an intolerable, yet emotionally familiar position against which she had been well defended most of her life. Consciously, it did not occur to her that to assume a negativistic stance would still put her in his service, though in the guise of standing up for herself. Her unconscious knew better.

Interestingly, it did not occur to her she could do what she wanted even if he did happen to get satisfaction from it. Conversely, at least some of the time it would seem she could do what she wanted (even if it was not what he wanted, and though he might not like it), and so long as she did not make a project of it or do it for hostile reasons, such a show of her "autonomy" would not be such a bad experience for the child. Again, the therapist was locked into a narcissistic system reminiscent of the unyielding parent; in the therapy she felt herself at once her mother, at once her defenseless self, and saw too, both those dimensions in the child she was treating. Her major aim had been to be confirmed, now entreating this child–mother, "Look mother, acknowledge me, consider that I am a person, at least person enough to know what I want to photograph!"

Discussion of power struggling and negativism leads naturally to another problem area for the therapist, what we consider the *fear of being influenced* approached by way of *fear of compliance*, which is the other side of the coin of negativism. Whereas negativism would appear not to bind child to parent, compliance leaves no doubt and is, therefore, willfully defended against. A therapist we know, although bright and scholarly, always resisted trying any new techniques. In a session describing why he was reluctant he said, "I feel like I need to try something new, but if I try the technique and it doesn't work out immediately, I'll feel ridiculous, so I'd rather not try. In fact, it's worse than that. I can't bring myself to try." Obviously negativistic on its face, the declaration indicates that the therapist cannot try something new even if he wants to. He is fighting even his own desire; he is still reacting against complying with his internalized mother who is "pushing him around" so to speak, and against separating from her to do what he alone might want and rationally knows is best. Thus the negativism, in one operation, continues the symbiotic bond, allowing the flavor of autonomy while militating against compliance. Furthermore, when what one independently wants coincides with what the parent would have wanted, there is a dilemma, for the person is surely in a double bind. If he or she does what the parent wants, he or she can't win; if he or she does what he or she wants, there's no winning either. The way out of course is to be able to do what one wants for oneself, neither for nor against the parent, which, however, implies a degree of separation to be aimed for but one not easily attained. With this therapist, there was also an identification with his mother's fear of risk. Therefore, his problem was compounded to the point that indeed if he but tried new techniques, it implied leaving mother.

By this time, it is surely obvious that although fear of influence can permeate a therapist's narcissistic position, it is fueled in operation by interpersonal patterns not immediately associated with such a fear, such as power struggling and fear of compliance. The fear of influence impedes the therapist's ability to let the patient take the lead in setting the pace and determining the direction and flow of the therapy. The therapist, like the mother during developmental narcissism, cannot allow the influence of the child. On the other hand, identifying with the patient's effort and narcissistic need to have a mother there in his or her service gives the therapist an idea once again of the frustration of having no influence. The therapist is now both that child who craves the mother and ideally, the desired mother in the child's (patient's) emotional service. It is little wonder that therapists flee from the emotional paradoxes so reminiscent of their childhood positions, that they seek to influence in concrete ways through advice giving, through overinterpretation, through rigid behavior modification techniques, through prescribing medication, through defensive detachment, through eight-session cures, through having all the answers or none of the answers.

Having all the answers or none of the answers is, as a defense, another feature within the obsessional, narcissistic defense. Actually, they are attitudes reflecting the problem of *certainty versus indecision and doubt*. The certainty is a defense against indecision and doubt and accompanying feelings of powerlessness. Said another way, the sense of certainty is built on a weak base of self-esteem. Yet the indecision is a defense against having identified with the certainty of the unyielding parent. On a dynamic level, this two-sided coin is a replication of the position of the child during narcissistic development: for it is as if "someone"—a parent—will come along and make the "right" decision, have the "right" answer. The child, however, unsatisfied in his or her attempt to influence the parent and angry at imposition of answers, cannot, will not, be sure the answer or decision is right. On the other hand, with such an all-knowing, all-powerful parent, how can the child, short on self-value, be sure his or her own answer or decision is "right." In short, either way, there exists the feeling of fighting the "other," fighting to be recognized and respected, plus the idea that somehow the answer or decision at any minute may be made or snatched away without one's ken or control.

When therapists start their careers, some may have a grandiose sense of what they know and how they can effect a cure. With adequate supervision and therapy this attitude dies, often to be replaced by the feeling that they know nothing and can have no effect on patients. A replication of the original narcissistic position in reverse, this helpless, ignorant phase is acutely uncomfortable. We have heard therapists describe what hot shots they were (or so they thought) when they started out, yet years later, with their grandiosity shattered, they felt they knew nothing and could have no effect on patients.

One therapist felt utterly helpless and ignorant when faced with her first outpatient group, despite years of inpatient group experience and several publications. That she could recognize the group as more ostensibly like her than were the psychotic patients she had been treating was probably the trigger for the discomfort. She became silent in early sessions, shrinking in fear, identifying with the disturbed children these formidable mothers were describing. Although her silence and feelings of stupidity activated how indeed she herself had felt with her mother who was supposed to take care of her yet could not yield her needs to her child's needs, the therapist's immobility was also a defense against her rage—her desire to force the mothers to be influenced, to value her presence, her brilliance, her.

The grandiosity then, is a defense against the helplessness and lack of adequate self-confirmation and self-feeling, but the helplessness and lack of adequate self-feeling are themselves then used as a defense against forcing another to be influenced. This means it is conceivable a therapist starts a career with compensatory grandiosity and feels devalued and impotent when faced with patients beyond his or her capacity to treat. At this level, the helplessness is a rationalized defense—a good one because indeed it reflects the valid feeling of impotence which is a few layers down. This intermediate level of helplessness is used as a defense against the anger and defensive aggression that the grandiosity also served to hide. Once the desire to vent the rage at and "run over," influence, "the mothers" becomes clear, the deepest level of the impotence is felt. It is only then, when the therapist is in touch with his or her own helplessness against parental forces that it becomes possible to entertain the notion that maybe psychotherapeutic work, at its best, is not so gratifying as one might have wished.

A word about the therapist's *anger* seems in order. Although it is not our intention to elaborate on the varied dimensions and defenses against anger, it does seem pertinent to our theme to mention that the therapist is often afraid to experience anger, which instead is rationalized by saying it would not be useful for the patient. The merits or demerits of such revelation aside, it would seem that the main issue is that the therapist is afraid of losing control because the patients may return the anger, thus stirring up the therapist's residual rage. We wonder, though, if the problem does not go beyond the activation of rage, which in itself may have been an unacceptable affect. The more intense problem appears to be that the patient has penetrated, not only stirring up anger but stirring up the memory of a mother–child bond characterized by the mother's emotional intrusiveness, controlling or forcing the child into her orbit. With such memory would come the recollection of an impenetrable mother, a characteristic therapists do not want to notice in their parents, their patients, and certainly not in themselves.

That a therapist's *detachment* can be defensive is best supported by a vignette from the therapist of the group mentioned earlier in the chapter.

> When I felt part of what was going on in the group, the interaction, I couldn't seem to figure out what was happening in the group. But when I could figure it out I felt—and was—so removed that when I pointed anything out or made an "appropriate comment" nobody seemed to hear me. I was like two separate people, two aspects of myself I couldn't put together. They all knew it too; in fact when I finally asked them what it would take for them to listen to me they told me all right. The "spokesman," as I call her, said I seemed to be playing a role, as if from a book, so why should they listen to me when I was obviously an amateur or a dilettante. She couldn't have said it better, and I got so anxious at her "knowledge" of me I thought, "Why in hell am I in this work? If all this anxiety is what being a therapist is all about, who needs it?"

Heretofore, this therapist had rarely felt discomfort with patients, for her detachment provided emotional distance sufficient to ward off feeling intruded on. The earlier detachment had prevented her from feeling involved while being involved; or to put it another way, it allowed her to be involved without knowing or feeling the experience. The progress, yet problem, now that she had had several years of therapy and supervision, meant that she began to take notice when she was involved.

She would become anxious at the recognition only to retreat to a broader, "better" detachment. Since it became clear it was at those times she made her interpretations or interventions, it was unconsciously obvious to the group she was not "with" them. Her clinical comments, accurate as they might be, served her own detachment needs rather than the needs of the patients. Ostensibly, she aimed to be helpful to the patients, but her fear of being overwhelmed by them compelled her to fend them off. In essence, the comments this therapist offered were recognized as emotionally fraudulent and the intent perceived as only helpful to herself. Thus, the whole narcissistic problem was relived in the therapist's eyes: the powerful, unyielding mother (group) to whom the child (therapist) responded with fear and frustration, from which the child (therapist) imperfectly escaped through detachment, surely itself an unyielding state.

Though obviously detachment does occur, it does not work as well as a therapist who needs it may realize. Although it may protect the therapist from uncomfortable self–other perceptions, the result provides only partial protection; that is, it does not necessarily interfere with patients' perception of the therapist, only the therapist's recognition of the process.

We assume at some level that the therapist is "known" to the patient, at least along certain dimensions. Though the therapist may indeed be pathologically detached or may appear "natural," it is a fallacy that the therapist is a blank screen (Goz, 1975). Clinicians such as Searles (1965/1979), in working with schizophrenic patients, have repeatedly noted ways in which the patient's behavior and content often reflect the therapist's unconscious. Not that the patient (or the therapist for that matter) is necessarily aware of the perception or knows what to do with it. But to disclaim that patients and therapists are actually working "unconscious to unconscious," to borrow a Winnicott (1965b) phrase, is to disavow a level of relatedness to which it would seem patients, through the therapeutic process, would aspire. Such denial would indicate the kind of rigidity of roles that is antithetical to emotional mutuality and, in a sense, the complexity of human response and communication. In short, just as it is neither possible nor useful for a therapist to be "uninvolved" with a patient, except at the expense of a detached state of relating (Dorpat, 1977), the patient does perceive more than either therapist or patient may realize. The therapist is revealed to the patient whether or not either chooses to consciously acknowledge it or use the knowledge constructively.

The subject of perception leads us now to a brief discussion of how the therapist's narcissism accounts for problems in *empathy deficit*. Although recent reports (Gomes-Schwartz, 1978) indicate that the function of the therapist's empathic ability as a predictor of therapy outcome has been overrated, it seems to us that empathy is a major component in human interaction (Charny, 1966). As such, it is a vehicle through which one feels understood by another. Empathy, therefore, can be seen as a process and mode of communication, albeit an unconscious one. It is here that we diverge from a major research definition of empathy (Carkhuff, 1969; Rogers, 1961; Rogers and Truax, 1967), although it is clear there is no universal operational definition of the concept. (In fact, the construct validity of a major scale, Carkhuff's Empathic Understanding Scale, has been seriously questioned [Avery, D'Augelli, & Danish, 1976], to add a measurement problem to the conceptual confusion.)

The most frequently used research definition assumes that empathy relates to the therapist's sensitivity to the patient's internal state and not necessarily to the internal state of the therapist. Lewis (1978) amends this concept of "cognitive empathy," to state that what is involved is the therapist's ability for accurate perception of the patient's manifest feelings. Psychoanalytic writers, such as Sullivan (1953b) and Greenson (1960) maintain that empathy relates to the ability to experience the other, the capacity for affective arousal—"affective empathy" (Paul, 1967–68).

Although it is possible for the therapist to appreciate intellectually the patient's manifest feelings and even the patient's internal state without necessarily resonating with the patient, we think it is probably the resonance that is perceived by the patient as most meaningful. Consequently, we see empathy as a combination of cognitive and affective empathy. In other words, empathy is that state that occurs in one person and is "caught" and felt by another as his or her own during any given moment of interaction. Such an experience, then, is automatic, unconscious, and cannot be taught, which is in contrast to cognitive empathy where techniques for its development are taught (Lewis, 1978). In our definition of empathy, the objective of the therapist would be at some point to recognize the state as emanating from the patient and to utilize the empathy—this unconscious emotional communion or bond, as it were—both by simply allowing its occurrence as an end in itself (Havens, 1974) and by recognizing the experience as a subjective clue to objective understanding and analysis of the patient.

Langs (1976a) has described projective and introjective identification, in empathy, referring to the empathic process in both patient and therapist. Our focus of concern is more with an apparent empathy deficit in the therapist. Given a developmental background where, for survival, one has had to be inordinately tuned in to parental emotional states, one would think that such persons who become therapists, would have keen, active, empathic ability. In operation, the reverse seems to be the case, for finely honed obsessional features militate against such skill (Lewis, 1978). Rather, intellectual defenses become the barrier against affectual experience. The empathic experience would be seen as equivalent to being taken over by the mother's needs, in effect to be negated, not confirmed, rendered impotent, to once again be in the mother's emotional service.

The therapist fears losing the control inherent in an empathic process (Katz, 1963), for empathy implies penetration of self by another and another by the self. Control is lost, and the therapist fears no return. Empathy means that at a level beyond the therapist's control, the patient is influencing him or her, not intellectually but emotionally. This implies then, that the therapist is vulnerable, subject to experiencing many feelings, intense feelings, uncomfortable feelings, almost against his or her will. Thus, an empathic experience adds insult to injury in that the therapist comes to the situation troubled about experiencing his or her own feeling states, let alone someone else's. By defending against the ability to empathize, the therapist aims not to recapture the vulnerability of his or her position in the parent–child relationship.

The therapist's developmental narcissistic experience has indeed influenced how readily he or she can empathize and how, through detachment, he or she can escape from what can be seen as a natural ability. As a matter of fact, the therapist probably has more, not less inherent empathic capacity than most persons, but in order to ensure that the original parent–child pattern is not replicated, the growing child, and now the therapist, builds a veiled wall of involvement, a barrier of emotional detachment. So the problem is, whereas the therapist has enormous empathic potential since a significant portion of his or her life's childhood "work" was to be tuned-in, there is not much "available" empathy.

When a therapist reaches a point where he or she is not so afraid of emotional closeness, and is losing a bit of narcissism, the empathic experience may occur but might at first be overwhelming. Sometimes a therapist reacts by taking on the feeling as his or hers in a way to overwhelm and, in a sense, negate the patient, just as the therapist in early life may have been negated. Sometimes, and we hope, eventually, a therapist can "sit" with the feeling and live with its pleasantness or with its disequilibrium or precarious state. Sometimes, and we hope ultimately, the therapist will be pleased that he or she is free enough to allow the empathic process its place in the relationship, and is pleased, too, at the emotional contact if not always comfortable with the particular feeling of the moment.

A word is in order about the discomfort of the empathic experience. Too often, empathy is talked of in glowing, lovely terms as if, through this feeling process, therapist and patient go off together in the sunset. Yes, empathy can be a pleasant experience, but far, far from always. More often, even for a therapist unafraid of experiencing another or of experiencing his or her own or another's feelings, when a patient is full of dread or anxiety or rage, and the therapist feels that feeling, it is not fun. It is decidedly unpleasant. Any therapist could want it to stop. Yes, it may be a sign of real communication, of affectual self–other contact, and indeed, it may be an indispensable quality of a relationship, but those attributes do not make the feeling of the moment necessarily a pleasurable one.

NARCISSISM AS "HELPFULNESS"

As has been indicated throughout this chapter, many persons attracted to the therapy field tend to be those adults who have "served" their parent(s) emotionally. That is, in their development, they have been used in the service of the parental narcissistic needs instead of vice versa. Thus, the kind of selflessness that develops in persons who become therapists is born out of the pathologic hope that by doing perhaps "one more thing" for the parent, the parent will come through. This desire is not based on fantasy alone. Neither is it based alone on the self-interest of making the parents whole in order to identify with them for the sake of maturing, as Searles (1967/1979a) would have it. One can be led to believe the parent will come through because of "good" early caretaking, when the mother's needs were met through fusion with the infant, allowing her then to meet the infant's needs. Later, however, the time comes when she cannot let the infant move on to a point where infant demands no longer meet her needs and in fact exceed her emotional limits.

If, as a growing child, or as an adult, the person for whom being helpful has become a way of life stops being helpful, guilt comes soaring forth; yet when forever helpful, he or she never thoroughly feels satisfaction and security and eventually feels angry and exploited. Such is the case with the "chronic helper."

Chronic helpfulness (Rouslin, 1961, 1963) is a term used to refer to a behavior pattern where the helping behavior has a demand quality to it. That is, instead of the person having a simple desire to help another, there is a driving, compulsive need to help. The behavior was first recognized in state hospital patients, who, through their helpfulness and the hospital's tacit approval of what failed to be consciously recognized as pathology, became indispensable to the psychosocial and economic systems of the hospital. In the process, their pathology was reinforced, and they became chronic. They became the mainstay of the hospital's work force.

When the pattern was first measured, it was recognized that there was a cornerstone of low self-regard and that as soon as a bid for mutuality was made by the helper, the alliance fell apart. The helper would become enormously anxious, then angry, feeling exploited and helpless at the rejection. The way to feel better and in good grace was of course to start all over again. Thus, there was the lack of satisfaction and security and the "chronic" part of the helpfulness. Although the pattern was operationalized, the dynamics were more complex than the original formulation allowed. It became clear, for example, that low self-regard was a function of the more basic lack of self-confirmation, which, developmentally, has its roots in the fusion and symbiotic phases of narcissistic development. That problems in his lack of separate-self-feeling move on a continuum from more (fusion) to less (symbiotic) primitive, accounts for the original observation that the pattern could be found to fall in the framework of any diagnostic category. The expression might be bizarre or highly socialized depending on the depth of ego impairment.

What was observed but not addressed in the original writings was why the chronic helper seeks pseudomutual relationships (Light, 1974). It would appear now that this is related to the lack of separate-self-feeling, causing a rigid structure of helper–helpee relationship to be maintained. Although the chronic helper does at some point seek what would appear to be a more mutual relationship, it is actually a false move. The choice of person (who, too, has some investment in the structure of the relationship) and an unconscious need to be at the mercy of the other while identifying with the person as the one being helped militate against such a shift. The chronic-helper pattern is now seen in a larger context of narcissistic organization where self-feeling and confirmation are sought through the other, with the challenge and hope that the other person will come through being central aims. Interestingly, what was noted but not investigated in the writings on chronic helpfulness was how familiar such a pattern was in helping professionals. Just as the pattern as originally defined is not so simplistic as it appeared, it is also one not confined only to patients. Probably, in fact, every helping professional has at least a touch of it, and it seems to us, because of the nature of the service, therapists lead the list!

The notion that therapists need their patients is not new. Nowadays, Searles is perhaps the most cogent formulator of how the therapist's mother–child dynamics are replicated in the therapist–patient relationship. Although he (Searles, 1975/1979) sees "therapeutic strivings" in all human beings, that is, the aim to make the mother whole in order that she may mother, he considers it of paramount importance for the therapist to "examine personal selfless devotion to complementing the ego incompleteness of the mothering person" (p. 393). Otherwise patient and therapist are engaged in a kind of mutual sustenance and resistance that inhibits growth.

So, we have established that therapists and patients are alike under the skin after all. Each, to one degree or another, at one level or another, has an inordinate need to dedicate his or her life to another for not-so-selfless reasons. Actually, the notion that some children are therapists to their parents has been suggested for years (Ferenczi, 1955; Lichtenstein, 1964). Ferenczi speaks about a premature maturity in children—a developmental phenomenon initiated out of physical or psychic trauma or exploitation. These children give a sage-like impression, often looking older and sounding wiser than their years. They tend to minister to others, mother them, help them. As an example, he reports the "wise baby" dream: The newborn talks to the parents, imparting his wisdom. Such a child early senses the mother's need and meets it, becoming a therapist to the mother and in the process creating a crucial relational bond to be repeated throughout the child's life.

From what adolescents and adults have demonstrated and reported in therapy, it would seem that there is always the hope that through the ministrations the mother will become a mother. As we mentioned earlier, this is probably not based on wish alone but on the fact that early on, some of the child's needs were indeed met, leading him or her to feel tantalized, to continue to hope for more. Lichtenstein (1964) goes so far as to say that the mother creates needs that she then meets, thereby adding fuel to the expectation (and skepticism) that needs will be met. He says that the mother creates and meets the needs for essentially the wrong reasons, for she only creates an instrument for the satisfaction of her own unconscious needs. The child helper becomes mother to the mother then, not out of healthy desire or concern but because there is no choice. Often, this is a therapist's heritage.

Sometimes it does not appear that the child is the mother, as in the instance reported by a therapist. It seems one day she noticed how her mother repeatedly told her 2-year-old grandson that she was going downstairs—interrupted his play in fact to tell him, an action unconsciously designed to help nourish his need for her and feed his anxiety at her absence. When the child finally went looking for her, it would have appeared she was the concerned, missed mother and he the anxious child needing his mother. On a deeper level, however, he was meeting her needs—a projection of her own desire for a mother who wanted her. Further, he helped her to control "nicely," aiding her in her need to appear the good, loving mother, all the while certainly tightening the symbiotic knot.

Some children develop into rather ostensibly mothering persons. Modell (1975) suggests that there occurs precocious separation when such a mother's unreliability or intrusiveness is perceived. A premature sense of self develops, supported by omnipotent and grandiose fantasies. And these are features we often note in those persons who become therapists. However, as Searles (1967/1979a) puts it, "It is our omnipotent self-expectations that more than anything else, pinion us and tend, as well, to stalemate or sever the therapeutic relationship" (p. 73). Surely, the dedication of such a therapist becomes a burden to self and patient, a tedious, unending replay of the therapist's developmental narcissism gone awry.

By this time, you may have concluded that, as Grunberger (1971/ 1979) says, narcissism has a "bad reputation," and if a therapist holds such a strong narcissistic position, better to forget doing therapy altogether. We suggest no such thing. Rather, we think the very hope for the therapist and the therapist–patient relationship lies in the therapist's ability to turn an essentially pathological stance into a therapeutic one, a "narcissistic liberation" as Grunberger would put it. After all, the ability to merge with the unconscious without either compulsion to do so or compulsion to avoid doing so is a narcissistic function, a healthy narcissistic function. And do we not aim for such union as a vehicle for growth in our patients and in ourselves? This is what Searles (1973/1979) is talking about when he writes of therapeutic symbiosis, where there is a genuine degree of selflessness on the part of the therapist, a state as we see it where the therapist has no vested interest in how the patient proceeds in treatment and in life, or in how numerous and lengthy and varied those paths might be.

In this chapter, our point has been that the quality of the therapist's narcissism facilitates, if not compels, him or her into a field where ostensibly the task is to help others. In doing treatment, however, it becomes clear that there is a hidden agenda, namely, that it is the patient who is to help the therapist, simply by being a patient in need of the therapist's help. The therapy situation, then, becomes an arena for the expression of the therapist's narcissism, a dilemma where the therapist's developmental lacks in mothering result in his or her becoming mother to his or her own needy mother, now the patient. The therapist, in a single operation, becomes the competent, all-giving mother *and* through identification, the mother whom the child (patient) must attend.

With this complex "need to be needed," it is, at times, difficult to tell who is therapist and who is patient, a problem that goes beyond the fact that all patients help their therapist's emotional growth. To some degree, the therapist is on a tightrope, trying to balance conscious and unconscious forces, forces where the rational desire to help competes with its unconscious, irrational motivation. The result is a therapist who should take heed of innermost responses and needs, and who, ultimately, will realize that although helping people can be a worthwhile and satisfying pursuit, it is a far cry from the kind of experience providing the special gratification we may have been searching and hoping for.

2

Occupational Hazards

In a recent review of the empirical evidence on the effectiveness of psychotherapy, Lambert, Shapiro, and Bergin (1986) reported that psychotherapies generally were effective, both statistically and clinically. Positive changes exceeded gains occurring in untreated patients and in placebo controls, and changes tended to be lasting. All this is certainly positive news and confirms earlier evaluations of psychotherapies beginning in the 1930s. At the same time, there is a wide range of outcomes, so whereas some therapists are very effective others are not. The therapist factor, in particular, is a major contributor to negative results in the application of all psychotherapies (Beutler, Crago, & Arizmendi, 1986).

The growing awareness of the importance of the psychological well-being of therapists has been accompanied by an increased recognition of the difficulties inherent in psychotherapeutic work (Farber, 1983a; Freudenberger & Richelson, 1980; Kilburg, Nathan, & Thoreson, 1986). Two basic concerns emerge: identification of the stressors and identification of the coping strategies enabling therapists to alleviate these stressors in order to improve the lives of both patients and therapists. Discovering the burnout process in psychotherapists, Farber and Heifetz in 1982 saw the first remedy as greater public exposure of the problem. This has certainly begun to happen and has added an urgency to finding methods of prevention. Our approach is in the service of prevention as we both highlight problems and consider ways to make the impossible profession (Freud, 1937/1964) more possible.

Although psychotherapists are notably positive about their work (Farber, 1983b), there is a growing body of empirical evidence describing the stresses of psychotherapeutic work (Deutsch, 1984; Farber & Heifetz, 1981, 1982; Hellman & Morrison, 1987; Hellman, Morrison, &

Abramowitz, 1986, 1987a, 1987b). For example, Hellman et al. (1986) identified the stress factors of maintaining the therapeutic relationship, scheduling problems, overinvolvement in work, professional doubt, and personal depletion. In our discussion we consider the stresses of psychotherapeutic work as they are manifested in the therapeutic process, the identity of the therapist, and the therapist's personal life.

THE PROCESS OF THERAPY

Psychotherapy is designed to be a progression that depends essentially on the interaction between the therapist and the patient. The major burden for the therapist is to get the patient to change. The manner of doing that can be quite indirect, but there is an inescapable responsibility for at least creating an environment in which any patient would have the opportunity to learn to change. Since success rates for the psychotherapies in general are around 70%, and around 10% of the patients get worse (Lambert et al., 1986), it is clear that failures occur. Thus, a major source of stress is dealing with the probability of inevitable failure part of the time. Some of the reasons for the failures are more the therapist's, some more the patient's, and it is often difficult to assess the proportions accurately. Individual dynamics of therapists promotes exaggerated self-blame in some, denial in others. Also, the individual dynamics of patients allows some therapists room to correct their mistakes, whereas for others there will be rapid and unforgiving rejection.

The major danger for the therapist in the interaction is the seduction of the therapist's narcissism that is repeatedly offered by the events of the therapeutic process. In a broad sense these events are either negative or positive. Negative events include anything that goes against the progress of the therapy as defined by the therapist. These include resistances of the more obvious sort, such as lateness, missed appointments, refusal to verbalize, and repeated lack of insight, as well as more subtle resistances including character traits that just make the therapy a very laborious process. Added to what the patient may do are events in the therapist's life that are not related to characteristics of any particular patient but to working at a particular time or in a particular place, such as sickness, fatigue, and dislike of the working conditions. The narcissistic aspect that is tapped in these situations is the threat to the therapist's competence. Either the patient is getting in the therapist's way, or the therapist is getting in the patient's way. Collusion is still another possibility, and in all of these circumstances the therapist feels the press of inadequacy. A desperation creeps in that has many possible forms. The frustrating patient may become the target of the therapist's hostility and be blamed, disparaged, and ultimately dismissed as unworthy in order to protect the work ego of the therapist.

An example of this type of stress is a patient who externalized, blaming his own depression and rather strong aggressive tendencies on the callousness and disregard by others. The therapist found herself unable to bring about any internal focus by the patient. His problems were always the fault of others. The therapist became frustrated and began essentially attacking the patient, further supporting his contention of being victimized and entrenching his position. The therapist gained some realization of what she was doing and felt guilty about it but then withdrew from the interaction, fearing her own hostility and by this time her dislike of the patient. She missed a few sessions with seemingly plausible reasons, and he retaliated with lateness and forgetting sessions himself. She found herself in pursuit of the patient and very uncomfortable. Although she discussed the progress of the therapy in supervision and gained an understanding of what was happening, everything seemed after the fact and beyond her ability to change it. She hoped the patient would quit, but he did not. This patient was being seen in an outpatient clinic, and instead of his leaving, the therapist took a position elsewhere. The patient was then transfered to a new therapist who immediately took a different tack with the patient. He was very understanding in regard to the numerous complaints and reflective of the feelings involved. He empathized with the patient's paranoid concerns and did not feel frustrated or angry with the patient. After six sessions the patient told the new therapist that he was discontinuing therapy because he was not getting anywhere. His last words to his new therapist were "I wish I had her (the previous therapist) back. At least she understood me."

Here we have two different therapists' styles, and neither appears effective. The patient eluded both therapists and frustrated both of them. The first ended up disliking him, whereas the second felt bewildered. Both were ultimately helpless and left with the possibility that there may have been a way to help this patient, but they were not able to find it. Perhaps there was no way to help the patient. Perhaps he just persisted with the first therapist because he enjoyed upsetting her, perhaps he had come to therapy looking for still another place to express anger based on victimization. When that did not happen with the second therapist, the patient left because therapy no longer met his pathological need. Perhaps, or were both therapists ineffective, whereas someone else could have been successful? It is the failure and the unanswerable question as to the cause that is so stressful for the therapists involved.

Presented continually with emotional pain and suffering, it is indeed difficult to maintain a balance of scrutiny and concern. Some therapists like the struggle, although they also have the issue of accountability. Many therapists do not like the negative aspects of therapy and will go to extraordinary lengths to avoid having hostility directed at them. They feel more competent with the more dependent, conforming patients and less competent with the more challenging, aggressive patients. However, even where they are more comfortable, they are careful not to displease lest the good patients turn hostile. Keeping all this anger in check, in itself certainly of questionable value therapeutically, nonetheless creates a lot of strain for the therapist.

An example of this is a therapist who told his patients that the therapy sessions would be 50 minutes long but always allowed them to go longer. In addition he did not tell this to all his patients but usually only to those who asked about the length of the sessions. For the rest he did not specify a time, although it was always at least an hour. As the number of patients in his practice increased, he developed scheduling problems. He was late for patients because he was running over in preceding sessions, and some patients became annoyed at having to wait. He also had no time to write notes or reports until late in the day when he was tired, so he often did not do routine paperwork. He tried rearranging his schedule to better accommodate his need to give longer sessions, but the more time he provided, the more he used to extend sessions. Whereas he believed in the therapeutic value of a time frame, in particular his original 50-minute sessions, he doubted his ability to satisfy patients during that time. His sense of the situation was that if his adequacy was threatened during a session, as it often was, he must stay with the session until his adequacy had somehow been restored.

This is an extreme example of trying to keep the narcissistic self intact by excluding what may disturb it, and this was not successful. Nonetheless, a lot of that type of maneuvering goes on where boundaries are played with and the patients, to their detriment, control aspects of the therapeutic process that the therapist should handle. Sessions get extended, fees reduced and deferred, sessions are scheduled at inconvenient times for the therapist or at intervals that are by virtue of infrequency of limited value but demanded by the patient, and telephone calls are of great frequency and length. All of this type of behavior is an imposition stressing the therapist and rarely helping the patient, who becomes the omnipotent threatening child who has yet to meet the demands of reality. In order to be exploited in this manner, therapists deny and rationalize and so maintain their white-hat image.

A variation on the need to avoid the patient's hostility by accommodation is to do the opposite and punish the patient. Sessions may be shortened ever so slightly, interruptions such as telephone calls during the sessions may be elongated without any compensatory time, topics that could lead to the expression of the patient's aggression are avoided or given limited attention, and interpretations will take on a flavor of sarcasm and intimidation. The accommodating therapist is usually unaware of the reversals and reaction formations but is vulnerable to considerable guilt if the patient points them out. If this happens, the therapist can feel forced into ever increasing accommodation or cycles of denial and accommodation, either procedure leaving the therapist at the mercy of the patient's aggressive whims. Still another possibility is that the patient feels cowed by the therapist's anger and hides aggression, leaving issues very much both unexpressed and unresolved with both patient and therapist perpetually defensive and therapeutic progress stalled.

For therapists who are combative, the hostile and resistant patient offers considerable opportunity to engage in battle but provides little chance of winning. A protracted struggle is certainly likely, and some therapists may feel exhilarated by it at times, but the therapy becomes unresolved repetition for both therapist and patient. The stress of failure will appear here as well, for now the patient's in-therapy behavior and feelings can justify similar behavior outside of the sessions. The patient will either leave in anger or stay to indulge in the continued expression of rage in its various forms, which will seem quite justified by the therapist's aggressive responsiveness. It is also possible that the omnipotent therapist will seem to win out because an assertive therapist certainly has leverage. After all, it is the patient who is designated as having a problem. Yet for the patient to submit to the therapist is hardly a victory. The therapist may believe for a time that the patient has really changed, but anger and resentment at the therapist will remain and resurface. Certainly the patient's problems with the outside world are not going to be solved by having been outwitted by a therapist, so therapeutic failure remains as a stressor for the therapist who is always right, just as it does for the perpetually inadequate therapist.

The examples cited require considerable narcissistic vulnerability to negative resistance or assertive patient personality styles for the therapist to become very stressed. If the therapist's character structure is stronger in this area, then of course the difficulty is lessened. However, the structure of the therapeutic relationship is such that the patient is to be focused on, and attention is not directed to the therapist regardless of how much or little the therapist may feel the need for it. The relationship is never a mutual one in the sense of a fair and reciprocal exchange of needs. For the therapist, it is akin to having a friend who always has a problem and who always talks about him- or herself. Whereas the patient may have an interest in the therapist, it is not the same type of interest that a close friend would have. The therapeutic relationship is deliberately constructed this way so the patient can project, experience transference, be interpretive and open to interpretations, and change. The therapist is the facilitator of this, and the narcissistic reward is in doing it well. There are other rewards accompanying the process, such as monetary ones, as well as often a rather fascinating window into the richness and variety of how people live. However, having an active psychotherapy practice is not the same as having a social and sexual life. It is a work life that demands a lot of attention, self-scrutiny, and discipline along with an awareness that the therapist's best will not always be good enough.

Developing and keeping a perspective that assures an appropriate amount of self-esteem and inner harmony are essentially the tasks of all therapists. The therapy process threatens the therapist's equilibrium on a regular basis. Is there a psychotherapist who in retrospect can state that he or she never exploited a patient to service some narcissistic need? Of course, such an occurrence is not intentional, but because it can happen and does happen, we have to stay alert to the dangers for the therapist that are inherent in the practice of psychotherapy.

Thus far we have emphasized the stresses involved in dealing with the patient's negativity, hostility, and self-concern. Added to this is the fact that under all circumstances the patient, not the therapist, is the focus of the therapeutic interaction. The latter point needs to be kept in mind even when it does not seem so obvious. Now we are talking about transference that is clearly positive as well as what appears to be the relative absence of resistance. The therapist is placed in an "all good" position, and the stressors now become the need to maintain the therapeutic posture and to avoid the abuse of such power.

The need to be seen positively has been discussed previously in regard to coping with the hostility of patients. Now the hostility is not apparent, and the therapist may well be tempted to keep it that way. A number of possibilities then may occur as the therapist strives to never fall from that state of grace. One is the need to be correct, with just the right interpretations, perfect timing, and complete harmony, all of which are improbables. The therapist is also constricted, and areas of the patient's life that may need to be addressed but could result in the patient seeing the therapist in a less positive light are avoided. Thus, the need to be seen as "good" results in an avoidance of the "bad," stultifying the therapy. The therapist and the patient end up colluding to preserve goodness, peace, and tranquility, while the essence of their concerns, conflict, remains untouched. There is considerable strain in all this, with no ultimate reward.

A second concern is the possible abuse of the power vested in the therapist by the patient. Knowing that the patient will work very hard to construe whatever the therapist does as good for him or her can mean that the range of therapist behaviors is quite large. As a problem area, the therapist has the opportunity to be lazy, indifferent, ignorant, abusive, essentially whimsical, and get away with it. Such behavior does not have to be intentional, and much of it may not be, but the result again is an impaired therapist who, caught up in personal grandiosity, fails to serve the patient. Beyond that, the therapist can now harm the patient, with the positive transference having the paradoxical effect of working against him or her.

The particular example of this misdirection that has gotten the most attention has been therapist–patient sexual intimacy (Pope & Bouhoutos, 1986). In such instances, the therapist has apparently been able to convince him- or herself (more often himself) that the mutual attraction is both real and beneficial to both parties. The narcissism of the therapist voids the existence and impact of transference, and the results have not been good for all concerned. Psychological damage has been found in both patients and therapists, litigation and malpractice risk and rates have all increased, and the public image of psychotherapy and psychotherapists has been defamed.

Although this is an issue that is by no means resolved, the professions involved in psychotherapy practice are now well aware of it and are working toward remedies for both patients and therapists (Pope, 1987). However, narcissistic exploitation of patients may well be more prevalent in less obvious areas. The work of the therapist is experienced as a strain for the therapist when there is just effort, no reward. Thus, the relative balance of effort and satisfaction, always shifting, even within a session, is very important in determining the therapist's objectivity and professionalism. The positive transferential situation presents the temptation for the therapist to bask in it and thereby stall the therapeutic process. Such a setting also provides the opportunity to express hostility displaced from other patients who may arouse it but threaten the therapist. A belief in omnipotence takes over so that the therapist begins to believe that whatever is going on is essentially terrific. The therapist maintains this stance not so much out of fear of its absence but because of a misguided belief in the enlightened accuracy of the patient's positive perception of the therapist. The therapist gets lazy, trolls along, plays, and enjoys, and the patient is as unaware as the therapist that something is indeed amiss. Undoubtedly, it is a relief to see certain patients after struggling with some others. The respite may even be needed, but it cannot dominate. It is too easy and self-satisfying to negate the critical patient and emotionally embrace the rewarding one. Patient reactions and perceptions can be both accurate and inaccurate, but they are always purposive. The therapist has to remain focused on the meaning for the patient, with the meaning for the therapist used in the service of that focus. The task appears more obviously difficult under negative conditions, but it really does not change when the patient is emphasizing positive transference. In fact, it may even feel harder to carry out because the therapist in the process may shift from "good" to "bad" for the patient. The parent–child and child–parent disillusionments ought to be reenacted in the transference, but they do take some getting used to for therapists. The patient's associations trip the therapist's, and the fragility of self-esteem can be painfully apparent.

In discussing the uses of disillusionment, Pontalis (1983) said, "Mirrors would do well to reflect a little more before sending back our image" (p. 287). He meant this as a possible patient-to-therapist message, but it is certainly understandable that therapists may desire the reverse at times as well.

IDENTITY OF THE THERAPIST

In the psychotherapeutic world, identity is a word that is used often, but primarily in reference to patients, whereas the exploration of the therapist's identity has been relatively neglected. Identity can be thought of as a relatively stable self-representation that would appear to emerge as a psychic structure around the age of 2 and to coalesce as a sense of identity toward the end of adolescence; but throughout life, it may retain both the possibilities of flexibility and consistency. As Grinberg (1983) has pointed out, the formation of identity begins as the infant struggles to contain the limits of its body and goes on to introject the function of containment. Pleasurable bodily contact, particularly with the mother, serves a key function in joining the unintegrated and carving the beginnings of an identity. Then, there is spatial integration in which relations with the different parts of the self are understood, and the self is contrasted with others to establish a concept of being an individual. With time, there are different self-representations and bonds established between them to establish a sense of continuity and reliability of the self. Also, there is a need to establish the self in relation to others, using selective identifications, and identity is often described as a social concept set in the context of relationship to the self and others.

Any one of these constructs—spatial, temporal, social, or all—may be threatened in the course of psychotherapy. For example, the desire for physical intimacy on the therapist's part may occur when there is a threat to containment that stimulates regression and the need for pleasurable contact for the therapist to feel like a whole person. The physical contact desired may not even be sexual, though it may take that form, but there are also a number of therapies that routinely involve some physical contact, such as hugging, and their appeal to therapists may be rooted in a need for spatial integration. The converse may also be true, that therapies with the relative absence of any physical contact may have a particular appeal to therapists whose initial containments were tinged with or even dominated by noxious bodily contacts. On this side of the ledger, what a patient might see as a routine handshake could have disturbing associations for the therapist.

The sense of identity has been elaborated by Erikson (1959) as involving uniqueness, sexual gender awareness, stable object relations, vocational identity, and societal recognition. These more obvious social characteristics also have their vulnerability levels in terms of therapeutic interactions. The patient who decries the therapist with "You don't understand me. You're just like all the rest," pokes at the therapist's uniqueness. Every resistive patient who uses various types of unreliabilities to flavor the therapy process also can open wounds around the qualities of the therapist's interpersonal relationships.

Professional identity is particularly nebulous because there is no true profession of psychotherapy in the same sense that there is a medical or legal profession. Instead, people from a variety of disciplines, such as medicine, psychology, nursing, social work, counseling, and other less familiar specialities, occupy positions in society as psychotherapists. Sometimes they are regulated by law, sometimes not. When they are licensed, it is in their discipline, so that psychiatrists are licensed as physicians to practice medicine, psychologists to practice psychology, social workers to do social work, nurses to do nursing, etc. In all these cases psychotherapy is included as a function of each discipline. Since each discipline can do some things the others cannot, yet all do therapy despite differences in training and ultimate overall competencies, the identity as a psychotherapist is hard to define with precision. Attempts to clarify the confusion by developing a profession of psychotherapy with agreed-on training and practice standards have not been successful. The definition of psychotherapy is not universal, with practitioners delineating specifics yet adopting the generic psychotherapist classification. Even within subdivisions, such as psychoanalysis, there is disagreement as to who is really a psychoanalyst. All this confusion is not supportive in terms of fostering a stable identity.

Furthermore, consumers and potential consumers, as well as the media, are confused about the identity of the psychotherapist and not infrequently believe and portray negative images and impressions. Although the mental health needs of our society keep increasing, psychotherapists do not command much respect. The belief that most psychotherapists are crazy themselves and, if they have children, their children are sure to be disturbed is fairly prevalent despite a lack of foundation in fact. In addition to attacks from outside, the infighting between and among therapeutic disciplines adds to the problem. For example, in a society where physicians are treated with a considerable amount of awe, psychiatrists as a specialty receive the least of this, and psychiatry is not a popular specialty among physicians themselves, who often are dubious as to whether it is "really medicine."

The fluidity of the professional and social identity is not appealing because of the misunderstandings involved, but it is a reality that has to be integrated by any psychotherapist. This in turn rests on a personal identity foundation of variable firmness. Certainly if a therapist has a confused and uncertain sense of self, there is plenty of space within the field to wander around. There are also numerous opportunities to contain insecurities by developing strong to fanatic allegiances to a particular school of psychotherapy. However, since our field has a plethora of unanswered questions, a more stable personal identity that can combine a consistent sense of purpose with an equally constant willingness to learn is certainly more the ideal. Such an achievement is not easily had, however. In addition to the slings and arrows already discussed, questions are raised about identity in still another way, namely, personal experience. Thus, we have feminist therapy, gay therapy, radical therapy, black therapy, and other possibilities in that vein. All of these require that to treat the patient the therapist has to be, or have been, like the patient in some general categorical way. For example, only women can treat other women, thereby excluding males from the treatment of females without the converse being true. Sometimes it does seem that whoever one believes himself or herself to be as a therapist, someone is trying to indict those qualities as reason for exclusion from the field. In the history of psychotherapy, this practice has even included questioning the value of the professionally trained psychotherapist.

As demands for accountability have grown, we are increasingly required to prove our value. This is complicated by being in a field where change and improvement can certainly be demonstrated, but cure is another matter. Since insurance carriers have been the major force in this issue, and often have used a rather narrow definitive model in their expectations, we have had to struggle to explain what we do. In turn, we have also had to explain who we are, and in that process some arbitrary decisions have been made. Insurance carriers have actually decided who is or is not a psychotherapist for purposes of patient reimbursement. For years psychiatrists were the only therapists as far as insurance carriers were concerned, and then psychologists became so identified, and subsequently some other disciplines have been included. Thus, there have been instances in which patients were forced to tell their current therapist that based on third-party designation he or she was not a psychotherapist. A more sophisticated version of this tale appears when a psychoanalyst who graduated from one institute is analyzing a person applying to be a candidate in another institute. The second institute may state that the graduate of the first institute is indeed not an analyst, and at least for that candidate, the analyst is disenfranchised by virtue of institute identity. Such challenge to one's professional validity is enough to give anyone castration anxiety. Identity as a psychotherapist is easily come by in one sense, since self-appointment and patients who believe it will supply the identity. However, it is very difficult to keep the identity under anything approaching a sense of universality, and that is a definite stress that shows little indication of vanishing or even being mitigated. As a wizened Mexican picker of California lettuce once said, "for our place in the sun, our struggle may have just begun."

PERSONAL LIFE OF THE THERAPIST

Perhaps the most surprising legacy after practicing psychotherapy for 30 years is the realization that it makes one tired. Yet fatigue is the enemy that cannot be allowed to triumph because attention is so necessary to make the process effective. Yet the repetitive nature of the activity, including the repetition compulsions that are so often packaged in patients' behaviors, is designed to wear one down. It is true that everyone's story in some fashion is unique, but the basic elements of mother, father, child, and ensuing conflict become familiar, as do people's styles. Some of these are naturally tedious, and the process also can take a long time. Particularly if the therapist does psychoanalytic work, one sees the same people much of the time. Some of that time patients tire of the therapist, and some of that time the therapist tires of the patient, and it may even be possible to make the case for termination if patient and therapist get tired of each other at the same time.

In addition to the relative familiarity of the content of sessions and the methods of psychotherapy, there is the even greater constancy of being in the same room and in the same chair and always working within the verbal medium. These may well be offsets to the identity problem in that all this familiarity supports a sense of security, but it can add to the fatigue factor.

The work itself is draining as well. Routine is partially a defense against this, as are objectivity, ambiguity, and anonymity. However, remaining attentive and being appropriately involved means understanding, containing, and interpreting emotional content. There is an affective participation that can mean that every therapy session is an emotional experience. This is the very opposite of being bored, but the emotional demands are high, and the result again can be fatigue. In addition, therapists do not have the same spontaneous outlet for their emotions as patients. Feelings and thoughts have to be processed before they are expressed, and many are never directly expressed. Psychotherapy is not as obviously for the therapist as it is for the patient, so delay of gratifications and sacrifice are fairly usual for therapists.

Patients will ask, "How can you listen to me?" or "Don't you get tired of hearing problems all the time?" or "Wouldn't you like to talk about yourself at least some of the time?" Therapists usually do not answer questions like that. Instead, they will explore the meaning of the question. However, there are answers, and sometimes any therapist will be unable to listen, and will tune out and even go to sleep in the least obvious way. Also, therapists do get tired of hearing problems, particularly from depressed patients who add the burden of affective coloring, and therapists sometimes get out from under this by confrontations about patients' styles. These confrontations look and probably are therapeutic—but not just for the patient. Finally, therapists do like to talk about themselves, and some even find ways to do it in sessions under the rubric of empathic sharing or therapeutic education.

At the same time, most therapists recognize that the patient is meant to be on the stage and the therapist in the audience. The therapist may want to be a player, but that is not the prescribed role. The therapist is in turn left to struggle with the strains of suppression/repression while the patient is urged to cast off these shackles and be free in the very situation where the therapist must remain responsible. It is the therapist who guarantees the holding environment, the snug harbor, the exceptional place that is indeed safe for the patient to say whatever he or she thinks with no recriminations. The therapist has no such privilege but is bound to a rule of relative personal silence, a rule that feels all right only part of the time.

The reliability and in turn durability of the therapist provide another facet of the same problem. Therapists are expected to set boundaries and provide structure for all their patients in a variety of ways, including the previously mentioned insistence on free verbal expression by the patient. Some of the boundaries are experienced as restraints by the patient, even when accepted, such as set times for sessions and a particular duration of sessions. Therapists understand patients will complain about boundaries as well as gain from them, because therapists are also restrained by the very same boundaries that they have created for their patients. The therapist, when locking in a schedule, also develops a self-structure that must be followed to validate its reliability. The therapist must be there, for the attendance expected of the patient is also expected of the therapist. The time commitment can be extensive, and the practice of psychotherapy feeds on itself. Practices grow from the inside, with the once-a-week patient becoming the twice- and thrice-a-week patient, as well as from new referrals. Such growth can certainly be exciting and rewarding, but it is unrelenting in its demand for the therapist's consistent presence. Taking a day off on a whim or when one is feeling tired or somewhat ill is rarely possible. Patients need to be notified in advance, and there is the possibility of an antitherapeutic effect whenever the therapist is absent. Even changing the time of a session may result in this, so it is clear that therapists need to be available in a very reliable way for long periods of time.

Scheduling sessions in such a way that they do not interfere with the rest of the therapist's life is difficult. Because patients come frequently and for some duration, they prefer times that are easily available to them, especially before and after their usual working hours. This usually means early morning, late afternoon, evening, and weekend hours, times when the therapist might prefer to sleep, recreate, and/or socialize. It also leaves the possibility of amounts of in-between times that have the potential for other kinds of productivity but also have the limitations of maintaining preparedness to do therapy and living with the interruption of the task at hand.

The narcissistic threat is that the practice begins to control the therapist. Developing a schedule that allows the therapist sufficient time to have a satisfying extrawork life is a complex process. A certain number of patients are required to meet economic needs, and any therapist has to be willing to give those hours, whenever they may be, which will probably be "prime time." It is true that with experience, relative fame, and success, some therapists are more in demand than others and can in time be more selective about their availability. However, even in such circumstances, patients with whom one is already working have changes in their life circumstances that affect their schedules. To maintain a practice, it is always necessary to have a certain degree of schedule flexibility, which means at times working when one would prefer not to. The acceptance of a context of relative control of one's time is necessary or there will be resentment about what can feel like impingement on the therapist's life. For example, beginning therapists have to face the need to be available at convenient times from the potential patient's point of view in order to develop a practice.

Many therapists also are employed at regular positions in the mental health field and so have a guaranteed income with private practice as a part-time enterprise. However, over the years the lure of independent practice, both with its greater economic potential and the types of freedom offered relative to a structured job, has drawn many new recruits. Some have developed full-time practices, whereas others return to or remain, part-time private practitioners, finding the latter to be less stressful.

Full-time private practice has become a very competitive occupation, since the number of people practicing psychotherapy has sharply increased. New products, meaning new forms of therapy or repackaged old ones, are quickly introduced, and there is a great deal of confusion for the consumer/patient. To be competitive, therapists are now emphasizing the marketing of their services, which requires time, effort, and skills that many therapists lack or do not choose to employ. With third-party payers' emphasis on financial accountability, less insurance coverage is available, meaning higher deductibles, lower percentages of payment per session fee, and shorter terms of coverage. Then, health maintenance organizations are proliferating with prepaid health plans that are not conducive to psychotherapy. Many do not include it, and it is rarely encouraged for any length of time. There is considerable emphasis in our current society on certain psychiatric problems, as drug and alcohol abuse, but still not that much on the general mental health of the people. Any psychotherapy that is primarily preventative or educational will probably fail to qualify for mental health insurance coverage. The focus is on treating relatively obvious symptomatic problems quickly and at the lowest possible cost.

We disagree with the effectiveness of such a rapid-fire approach but recognize its reality. Also, since the true value of psychotherapy is difficult to demonstrate in concise fashion, many practitioners have decided to join the force of current demand as a way to ensure a continuing supply of patients. Rather than continue to educate, they placate to survive. This is understandable, but neither appealing nor necessary. If we believe in what we do, then we ought to work at demonstrating its validity not acquiesce and do something quicker and cheaper because somebody else said that's the thing to do, and they will pay only for that.

The good old days when psychotherapy was the relatively esoteric profession of gentle men and women are behind us, perhaps for the better, although some aspects of a psychotherapist's life were easier then. With changing times, we got insurance funding, and psychotherapy became available to more people. More practitioners appeared and helped meet the increased demand. It became possible to make a comfortable living as a psychotherapist; that, certainly, was appealing. However, results and competencies were challenged, and although this is sometimes appropriate and necessary, it made the profession uncomfortable. Some adjustment has obviously been required, and it has made the mechanics of independent practice more difficult. Added to profession, science, and art is now clearly the word business, and there is a lot of obsessing about it. Psychotherapists have generally not been prepared for business by their training. Past emphasis was on learning how to do psychotherapy because we were convinced of the value and aware of the need. The marketing of our services and proof of their value were not issues of concern, but they are now. In essence, it has become more stressful to become a psychotherapist, and, given the current competitive atmosphere, that stress is likely to remain high.

The present situation is one in which certain sectors of mental health services, such as private practice in metropolitan areas, have increased the number of providers, whereas other sectors, such as large mental health facilities, have decreased their populations and services. The rapid return to the community of the mentally ill has its own problems, however, exemplified in the growth of the homeless and the recidivism rate, so an increase in funding for mental health services may be in the offing as a necessity. The containment of health service costs is also a real issue and will make the health professions a somewhat less attractive career. Already psychiatry and clinical psychology and psychiatric nursing are showing declines in applicants for such training. The reward for the type of training involved is being questioned, and social workers have become the largest number of psychotherapists by discipline. They can reach legitimacy as providers with less training time than those in some of the other disciplines, particularly psychiatry and psychology; but they also tend to be less well paid. The field is once again in a transitional phase, marked by uncertainty about both the present and the future. In our final chapter, we discuss the good therapist and include consideration of optimal training and service systems. Here our concern is stress, and it is clear that there are easier ways to make a living.

In addition to competition increasing, the nature of private practice is such that financial return is variable. Even with the most consistent of fee policies, exceptions will be made, and the result is that from week to week cash flow may be a problem. Added to the probability of some economic insecurity is the rather new specter of malpractice. Psychotherapy by its very nature has a lot of trial and error in the process. For example, interpretations are hypotheses yet to be proven. Thus, it is so easy to make a mistake, as Robertiello and Schoenewolf have aptly illustrated in their 1987 book about therapeutic blunders. Fortunately, the process of psychotherapy provides numerous opportunities to correct errors, and wisely most of us do not hold ourselves out as having the inside track on the patient's truth. Our modality is often uncertainty because that is the reality, but we are getting sued nonetheless, and it is a problem. Goldman and Stricker (1981) point out that although psychotherapists do not guarantee cures, they are responsible for meeting accepted standards of professional practice. These are neither clearly defined nor supported by a substantial body of law, and in the early 1980s there were very few successful malpractice cases involving psychotherapists. That is no longer the case. Suits are increasing, psycho-therapists are being found guilty, and malpractice insurance rates have skyrocketed. The most obvious and persistent issue has been sexual misconduct, but diagnosis, record keeping, and even the manner of collecting delinquent accounts have become ethical issues. Of course, scrutiny and legal and ethical accountability are appropriate and neces-sary for the growth of a healthy profession. Also, compared to most medical specialties, malpractice insurance costs are still low, and the incidence of legal malpractice is also low. However, malpractice is a concern in a way that it was not even 10 years ago.

Then there is the intrusion of all this material about other people's lives into the everyday intrapersonal and interpersonal life of the thera-pist. After spending many hours listening to people's problems, it is often uninviting to listen to anybody else, whether that person has a problem or not. There is a desire to want to be comforted and listened to, rather than to be the comforter and the listener. There is also a need to let down, show feelings, even be irresponsible with people the therapist experiences as being close and trustworthy. The therapist has been under-standing all day, all week, all year; now it is time to be understood. Of course social relationships are rarely that one-sided, and if so, not for long, so the possibility of clashing with significant others is definitely there and may well extend to more incidental others and relatively superficial contacts. Although being a psychotherapist increases one's sensitivity to other people, it also increases one's sensitivity to oneself and one's needs, wants, and flash points. The emotional drain may also result in a feeling of not wanting to be with people, of needing personal time alone to spin fantasies and relax in isolation.

Making the shift from person as a therapist to therapist as a person is a complicated procedure. When we fail in the therapist role, our patients suffer, whereas failing in the personal role causes problems for the rest of our world, of course we suffer with either type of failure, and all therapists do some of both. Being a therapist is no guarantee to the self or others that we will relate to them in a way they will appreciate or that we will be satisfied with them. We can understand almost anything and endure most feelings, including very intense experiences, but we may not want to in our personal lives outside of therapy sessions. When we are not being therapists, we are being patients, meaning that our narcissism is definitely more prominent.

We may or may not be easy or hard to get along with, and the actual practice of psychotherapy influences us in this regard. We are not pleased with ourselves if we are basically unavailable to people we care about, as our partners, children, and relatives, or if we take out our frustration on less significant people in our lives. Yet we will do these things at times, and the fact that we are psychotherapists will not reduce the probability. It may well increase it, sharpening the difference between the personal self and the therapeutic self.

This is not a brief for psychotherapists to feel free to release their feelings on anybody they please as long as the person is not a patient. It is a reminder that because we are psychotherapists we have quite a supply of unreleased thoughts and feelings that other people may not be ready to experience when we have a need to release them. Although being a therapist may provide special stimuli for the need to express in a very self-determined way, the result is not an excuse for such behavior. Rather, we can understand that our occupation presents us with a problem in social and interpersonal situations. Added to the desire to cater indiscriminately to personal needs that can be amply fueled by the justification of deprivation are the techniques of manipulation. We learn how people are moved to change, and we learn ways to help effect that change. We know how we are supposed to use such techniques, namely in the service of our patients. However, when not dealing with patients, we certainly can be tempted to use technical methods to get what we want with little concern for the needs of others. The role of psychotherapist provides the tools of abstinence and indulgence, and we have to be careful about our use of these tools in our personal lives.

There is also the issue of deficits in our lives outside of therapy that we may then try to make up through the work of being a therapist. For example, a lack of socialization can be countered by making therapy into more of a social experience than its purpose should warrant. Therapy can be turned into a way to obtain love, or rage, or punishment, or adulation in service of what we feel is missing for us; by indulging such needs, we turn the therapeutic process into something that helps us more than our patients. Although therapists often see many patients in the course of even one day, psychotherapy is nonetheless a lonely profession because of the limits and boundaries of the interpersonal exchanges. Whereas some therapists are disturbed by their loneliness (Guy, 1987), others, conversely, exaggerate the therapeutic frame to maintain distance because they feel uncomfortable with intimacy. We can easily bring too much or too little of ourselves to therapy sessions, and if the balance is lost, we are no longer who we need to be to make psychotherapy effective.

REMEDIES

We have divided occupational hazards into the three broad and certainly related categories of therapy process, identity, and personal life. The possible solutions will be considered in the same categorical order. First, in order to cope with the stresses of the patient–therapist relationship, it is necessary to understand and accept what psychotherapy is and is not. In regard to the latter, it is not life as one usually lives it, but rather a special situation with its own reality. The patient's feelings, thoughts, verbalizations can all be real enough, but they are appropriate only to the therapy session. Essentially, the patient's feelings about the therapist are not about the real person who is the therapist. The feelings are displaced, and the therapist is a substitute for more significant people in the patient's life. Psychotherapy is mostly transference with the therapist as the object of those projected feelings.

This means that what the patient feels about the therapist is not very real as a response to what the patient actually does know about the therapist in the context of therapy sessions. It is even less real as an estimate of what the patient might feel if the therapist were to become an intimate acquaintance. Many therapists understand and believe this if and when patients are negative towards them but are more inclined toward seeing reality in patients' responses when the feelings are positive. That is an easy way to get seduced. Some therapists do not believe in the scope of transference (or even the concept) and so can get hurt by either side of the patient's feelings.

The patient rarely glimpses the real therapist, even if and when the therapist is intent on exposing him- or herself. The therapist has a reality limited to the sessions. The patient can get glimpses of parts beyond the therapeutic self but is interested in doing so only to the degree that such a view fits the patient's needs. Patients can even correctly estimate some of what the therapist may be like outside of sessions, and this may be facilitated by whatever knowledge the patients have of the therapist's public self, such as where the therapist lives, went to school, etc. The patient is interested in the therapist for the sake of the patient, not to meet the therapist's needs. Whatever relationships exist between patients and therapists through the window of psychotherapy, they are not extendable in any intense way to relating outside of therapy. Thus, Levenson comments, "The truth is we are not the patient's friend but his analyst. It is not a lesser category or a less concerned one: it is simply different" (1983, p. 60).

The therapeutic relationship can certainly feel like a problem for the therapist when the patient acts as if he or she does not want to play by the usual rules of therapy. However, there are a variety of technical procedures available to help the patient keep the perspective and the flow of the therapy. The therapist may feel uncomfortable in some of these situations and make mistakes, but if the therapist does want to follow the rules, then it is generally possible to facilitate the patient doing this as well.

A far greater problem occurs when the therapist essentially disregards the boundaries of the therapeutic frame. The fantasies of patient and therapist appear to match, and the therapist decides to translate this apparent congruence into reality. This will not work. The guideline for the therapist then becomes quite simple. Whatever you think or feel you want to do with the patient in or out of therapy sessions that has no ultimate therapeutic purpose for the patient, do not do it. The inevitability of some contacts outside sessions and their consequences (Strean, 1982) does not require or even really invite the therapist's extension of these into nontherapeutic interactions. At the same time, they do not have to be avoided. They will usually be limited, and even if unexpected, their boundaries will be relatively clear.

Our concern here is with the attempt by the therapist to create an intimate extratherapeutic relationship with the patient with the belief that this will have a positive outcome for both therapist and patient. It will not. There may be exceptions to this, but the odds are against any individual therapist being such an exception. The patient's reactions are transferential, not real, and the therapist will end up disappointed, hurt, frustrated, feeling stupid, and in trouble. So, no matter what the therapist's needs of the moment, he or she must continue to make therapy, not love, peace, or war. The most prudent course is to assure that once a person is (or has been) a patient, the only major relationship with that individual that the therapist will ever have is a therapeutic one. Left to their own predilections, that is with no particular encouragement one way or the other from the therapist, most patients will keep a definite amount of distance by keeping contacts outside of therapy to a minimum, as well as avoiding learning personal information about the therapist during sessions.

Keeping the patient–therapist relationship in its special place is much easier if the therapist has his or her personal life in order. When the therapist's needs are well satisfied outside of the therapy situation, then it is relatively simple to concentrate on the business at hand. Assuming the psychotherapist is sufficiently well trained and manifests a strong sense of identity, then the stress of the tilted relationship will be diminished. If certain situations prove difficult, as will happen, further opportunities for learning are certainly readily available, such as advanced training, supervision, and consultation with colleagues, as well as personal therapy. Reducing stress for the therapist and increasing the probabilities of successful therapy rest on the ability to establish appropriate boundaries for the therapy. When the therapist can develop a therapeutic frame that is personally congruent and validated by the frequency of its effectiveness, then the foundation has settled. The therapist then builds on it, develops focus and purpose, and essentially derives narcissistic gratification from doing therapy well.

The stresses of Identity do not have solutions that are as accessible as the methods for aiding therapists in the therapy relationship. Since the existence of a true profession of psychotherapy is not immediately at hand, the establishment and maintainence of professional identity will have only relative stability. Knowing who one is as a person is certainly helpful, and having definite goals for one's professional life is also very useful. However, the competitive nature of today's therapy marketplace means identifying oneself to the world as a psychotherapist in operational terms. There is a greater need for the demonstration of the ingredients of psychotherapy and the probable effects. The selling of psychotherapy, generally termed marketing, is increasing, and that is a major concern of psychotherapists at present. To embrace the public relations mantle and to indicate to potential consumers in a variety of ways how much they need you and that you are better than your competition, are unusual positions for most psychotherapists even to consider. Our emphasis has traditionally been on learning our skills, not marketing them. Most of us have believed that competency would automatically bring a sufficient number of people who would both need and want us. We did some marketing, such as giving talks or writing articles or even contacting potential referral sources, but it was relatively limited and muted and certainly not our focus.

In contrast, McGrath points out, "Right now, you are probably missing at least 10 ethical, reasonable and practical marketing opportunities . . . whether you are new or old to the psychotherapy profession" (1988, p. 8). Her article contains specific suggestions and makes it clear that marketing is becoming both necessary and valuable for psychotherapists.

For therapists who feel no affection for that idea, consider the words of Forman: "Never ever advertise . . . If potential clients want to know you have a private practice then they'll just have to do some work to find out about you. This way you can be sure that the client is motivated enough to work in treatment" (1988, p. 12).

The above, however, are not words of assurance for practicing as one might have in the past. Forman was writing a humorous article on how to fail in private practice. Times change, and a business identity is being added to the psychotherapist's role. Other changes are being suggested as well, such as prescription-writing privileges and hospital admitting privileges for therapists who are not physicians, and the return to a dominant biological model for psychiatry. Adaptation to the demands for changes in the manner of delivering mental health services is a very complex issue. At the moment we believe that the best source of action is to become aware of what is being asked for, what is being suggested, what is being offered, and why. This awareness can then be used to locate one's position in the current situation as well as to make future projections. Organizations representing the various disciplines involved in psychotherapy practice are the major representative voices available to us, so this kind of involvement is both worthwhile and practical.

Major elements in establishing our identity consist of showing the value of what we do and making others aware of this value. For example, for a long time psychodynamic methods dominated psychotherapy with the presumption that they were indeed valid. Behavioral therapies have challenged the assumption, and we know now that most therapies can work in different ways and bring about different results. Although we personally prefer psychoanalytic therapies, at the moment, these are subject to more criticism than cognitive–behavioral methods. Thus, identifying ourselves as psychoanalytic psychotherapists means explaining to people what we do and how it can be effective. We have to prove our worth in an environment that is more open to other approaches, but 10 years from now, it is equally probable that cognitive-behavioral therapists will have to do more of what is now our burden. Psychotherapy is a trendy business, and it will probably continue to be that way. We do not have to go with the trends to survive as therapists, but we do feel their impact, and we have to adapt without diminishing our integrity.

Prospective patients have the right to ask, "What will this do for me?" In one context we could answer accurately by saying, "I don't really know." However, that is not a legitimate answer in the most likely context of the patient's question. For example, in regard to psychoanalytic therapy, we could answer as follows: "This is a method that explores why people behave as they do. It looks for meaning, emphasizes understanding, and can give you the intellectual and emotional knowledge to make better decisions. You can become a more independent, competent person with less disabling feelings and thoughts. However, we cannot guarantee your cooperation or involvement. If we do our best, and you do your best, the chances are very good that you will feel better."

We do not, of course, promise a cure or guarantee against relapse. We admit there are many other methods that also can make the patient feel better, but ours has its relatively unique aspects, including the fact that we are the therapists. We believe we offer something special, but we know we need a certain type and level of patient participation. Thus, we are not for everybody, but no therapist is, nor is there a need to be, given the variety of psychotherapies available. We also indicate that our method will probably take a long time, years rather than weeks or months. Our logic on that is that the complexity of personality structure and expression needs detailed elaboration, and it has taken the person many years to establish him- or herself as he or she is today. Such construction does not submit quickly to either exploration or change. Our experience has taught us that people who stay in therapy until patient and therapist concur that therapy is completed fare the best. We see people who approach all this in a variety of ways, and we know it is important that they be free to pursue their life as they see fit. We always try to make it clear what the possibilities and limitations of therapy are and what is required of the patient as well as what we will do.

In terms of stabilizing one's identity as a psychotherapist, it is important to be able to explain just what one does. If one does not really know, or cannot explain it in such a way that a patient can understand, then something is wrong. It is also important to be specific about one's role, values, possibilities, and limitations and to know what is or is not true about psychotherapists and psychotherapies.

In regard to the stresses on the personal life of the psychotherapist, we have a number of strategies to make life easier. The first is that one allows oneself to remain aware of how much one likes the job. We say that because, despite the fact that stresses are being highlighted, most therapists find their work enjoyable. In a recent survey (Guy, Stark, Poelstra, & Souder, 1987) of over 700 therapists with a number of orientations, only 53% reported planning to retire by age 70, and 13.5% intended to continue practicing until they died. Prolonging careers was strongly related to emotional satisfactions experienced in the practices. Although Guy et al. raise valid questions about the possibilities of age-related impairments and associated narcissistic denials by therapists of such limitations, our point is the demonstration of therapists' affinity for their profession. Reminding oneself how good it often is becomes a definite balance for the bad times. In addition, the continuing interest shown by therapists in their work can be reassuring to new therapists. Work and the people doing it shift over time, so that initial stresses may be modified, and with experience, new stresses can be handled more suitably.

Also, there is a clear outlet for personal problems experienced by the therapist, namely, personal therapy. In a recent national survey of over 700 psychotherapists from the three disciplines of psychology, psychiatry, and social work that included a variety of theoretical orientations, more than 70% had had personal therapy (Norcross, Strausser-Kirtland, & Missar, 1988). These therapy experiences were primarily for personal problems, not training, and most people found them helpful.

We are very positive about the value of personal psychotherapy for psychotherapists. However, there is not an impressive body of empirical data to support this value (Herron, 1988). The majority of the favorable evidence is indirect. For example, MacDevitt (1987) sampled 185 psychotherapists with a variety of theoretical orientations, and found that 80% of them had undergone psychotherapy. Of these, none rated it as worthless professionally, and the majority saw it as having helped professional functioning. Although it is possible for some therapists to function effectively without it, there is the possibility that they could function even better with it. The timing of the psychotherapy also seems to be an important consideration. It is usually a training requirement, at least for psychoanalytic therapists who are the most likely to have had it. As such, it does not really take into account the possible disruptive effects that may occur and affect the doing of psychotherapy with others. Although therapists may be better off for having had their own therapy, the working and personal situations at the time of the therapy should also be considered. What has been treated as a rather arbitrary issue, to have therapy or not to have it, should be viewed as a more complex concern. For example, some therapists may be better off with personal therapy before their formal training, others at different times during it, still others after they have been in practice for a while. The same sort of variability may apply to how much psychotherapy is warranted as well as what type. Based on our experience with personal therapy and with training therapists with and without it, as well as supervising practicing psychotherapists, we firmly believe that personal therapy can offer solutions to professional problems as well as personal problems. It is an option that therapists ought to consider and make use of even more than they currently do.

In addition to personal psychotherapy, other helpful possibilities include formal supervision and informal peer supervision. We talk more about formal supervision in a subsequent chapter on the listening process. Peer supervision can also be a very useful approach that combines professional and personal growth. One of us has been involved in such a group for about 15 years and has presented and published material regarding its value (Kinter et al., 1987; Sollinger, Herron, Trubowitz, & Herron, 1985). The group has six members most of whom have had formal psychoanalytic training and all of whom have had personal therapy. There are four men and two women, with a tristate geographic distribution, and all members spend some time in private practice. Meetings are approximately once a month at members' homes. There is no formal agenda for each year, although the general purpose is to promote personal and professional growth. Sometimes the focus is on case material, sometimes on personal issues. The members have organized and made formal presentations as well as published material on a variety of clinical issues. There is also a social aspect to the group, and it continually serves the purpose of providing a supportive environment for sharing one's authenticity with peers who are also friends. Thus, the isolation from peers and the competitiveness with them are both markedly diminished by the use of such a group. We would add here that a similar personal–professional, friend–peer relationship has existed for many years between the authors of this book and is experienced as a very positive force for both of us in our continuing developments.

Finally, there is the very large matter of having a satisfactory personal life. Basically this comes down to working out a life situation that permits the therapist to feel personally fulfilled outside the therapy situation. If one's narcissism is satisfied in a healthy way, and the definition of that has to be very personal but certainly will include getting enough of whatever it is one wants in real life, then the chances are markedly increased that one will be an effective therapist. There is no set formula for doing this, but it does seem clear that one's practice must be kept in perspective. The therapist must control it, and that is harder to do when personal distress impinges. Therapists are neither indestructible nor infinite. Guy (1987) has made the cogent point that therapists should plan how to deal with their patients if the therapists do encounter personal problems, including disability and death. The limits of ability need to be evaluated periodically, and the limits of responsibility adjusted accordingly. The practice of psychotherapy is a very exciting, lively, and challenging occupation. The therapist brings a life to it to meet the patient's. It is much easier if that therapist's life is and continues to be a good one.

As this chapter concludes, we note that we devoted considerably more space to the hazards of psychotherapy than the remedies. That is because the solutions are general principles to which each therapist will apply his or her specifics. We have indicated that the best way to make the patient–therapist relationship work for the therapist is always to keep in mind what the relationship is really about. The therapist contracts to operate in a particular way, has a set role, and tries to do this. Mistakes are possible and probable and can be tolerated, accepted, and understood by both parties. It is the role of therapist that cannot really be altered, or trouble ensues. The results are not always terrible, but the role change is in nobody's best interest. We offer that bit of wisdom; then it is up to the therapist to use it. For example, some therapists may have married their patients and consider themselves happy. We doubt most therapists could do this and have a positive outcome. We would not do it because, based on our view of the patient–therapist relationship, such a change would not work. We try to do only what works, with the hope that the id and superego will keep serving the ego.

The same point can be made in regard to identity and personal relationships. Identity as a therapist is a fluid concept to start with, and the current environment does not contribute to its stabilization. Developing and maintaining professional identity requires ongoing attention as well as an educated conviction about one's services, accountability, the production of quality, and appropriate marketing. It is important to be aware of the trends in supply and demand without being captive to them. Psychoanalysis and psychoanalytic therapies are a case in point. If we want to go on practicing psychoanalytically because we believe in the value of such an approach, and in fact often see it as the best approach for many patients, we will have to prove that. The basic way to do that is to have our patients effect changes, but the marketing of our services is more complex, with a variety of possibilities available. Again, one course depends on what one feels is possible, acceptable, ethical, legal, and necessary. Our marketing efforts are relatively indirect, but we have been psychotherapists for quite a long time so that may be all we need to do. However, we all have to keep our eyes on the marketplace and be attuned to it as service suppliers, so that we can influence the demand by educating the world as to the value of what we do. We are invested in our identities as psychotherapists and expect to do whatever is needed to maintain them. Each therapist can operate from the same general conception by developing his or her own specifics.

In regard to our personal lives, we have learned that the interface between psychotherapy practice and personal living requires periodic evaluation. The job has changed over time, and so have our personal concerns. We have lived through what we consider to be many of the developmental stresses of life and will certainly face more, even though our current personal and professional lives appear stable. We have sensed the impact of personal travail on our practice of psychotherapy and have made use of personal psychotherapy, formal and informal supervision, friends and colleagues to help us when it was needed. We intend to continue to do the same if and when such is needed in the future, and we believe such reevaluation and replenishments are necessary for all psychotherapists. Therapists owe it both to themselves and to their patients to attain and then to keep themselves in the best possible mental and emotional state. Whatever is needed to do this must indeed be done, whenever necessary, which, undoubtedly, will be more than once in a professional lifetime.

3

The Money Dynamic

When psychoanalysis began, two topics were notable as taboos: sex and money (Freud, 1913). In subsequent years therapists and patients have reduced much of the discomfort involved in talking about sex. Money, however, has remained more of a topic to be avoided despite its integral role as a significant factor in the psychotherapies. The problem pervades all therapies, not just the psychoanalytic ones. The too frequent result of this avoidance is that money is ignored in a variety of ways designed to reduce its acknowledged existence as part of the therapeutic process. Such oversight is often calculated and rationalized by the therapist and is derived from distorted views of what good therapy and good therapists are supposed to be.

Our purpose here is to let light shine where darkness too often is. Money should not be and does not have to be an avoided topic, and it is therapists' responsibility to redress the wrongs of the past in this area. Therapists who are not willing to do this shortchange their patients and themselves. Therapy where a significant topic cannot be thoroughly discussed because the therapist limits the discussion is simply not good therapy.

Our emphasis is on what therapists do about the subject of money, although this will involve considering patients' attitudes and behaviors as well. It is understandable that therapists' personal feelings enter into what they are interested in and willing to talk about during sessions. At the same time these feelings often have to be put aside in some fashion in order to provide a safe environment for patients to speak freely. It is expected that patients will have difficulty talking from time to time, withholding that is usually categorized as resistance. The therapist's task is to confront the resistance, but this is difficult to do if the therapist does not want to hear or talk about the withheld material either. In this manner, money gets relatively ignored, as do many of the thoughts, feelings, and behaviors attached to it, and the therapy has a deficit.

A therapist is more likely to ask a patient the details of his or her sex life than to inquire about the particulars of a patient's financial structure, yet the latter can have just as much significance to the patient as sex. In fact, most people spend more time and effort in pursuit of money than in a direct quest for sex. Money and sex are certainly related, and just as sex represents many things and is multifaceted, so is money. For example, in addition to being a designated medium of exchange, money can signify security, the ability to meet basic needs, freedom, status, power, and a host of other possibilities for all people, therapists included.

The essential quality of money as a possible representative of a basic aspect of the self gives it a special character. In the development of the psychoanalytic view of the meaning of money, a libidinal component has always been suggested, the pursuit of money having the same clandestine atmosphere as more direct sexual motivation. The psychosexual stage most related to money has been viewed as primarily anal, money being equated with feces. Preoccupation with money has been depicted as a prominent feature of the anal character, symbolized by the three Ps: parsimony, pedantry, and petulance. Fuqua (1986) summarizes the classical psychoanalytic view of money as unconsciously representing anality with pleasure derived through control as well as release. She points out that the money = feces equation can account for the "dirty" quality of money that makes it an inappropriate subject for customary discussion. Fenichel (1938) had also stressed the societal aspects of money, such as prestige, power, and standard of living. He saw a definite instinct–reality relationship for money, and he added the concept of overdetermination of the meaning of money into essentially anything that one can exchange.

Since the medium of exchange is often felt as giving a part of the self, it can be reflective of how narcissism is operating in an individual. Self-esteem may rest heavily on both acquisition and distribution of wealth. The question is often posed in financial services advertisements, "What are you worth?" Although money is the obvious symbol, the question is certainly attached to valuing the self as a person. The implication is that a person of means is worthwhile, whereas a person of no means is not.

Although people can be and often are secretive about money in a number of ways, they also take pride in what they do about and with money. Some love to amass it, whereas others gain status from poverty. Attitudes about money are rarely "pure." Instead they are usually tinged with ambivalence in some form. It is clear that there are quite a variety of intense attitudes about money, all of which point to the fact that it is and will be an emotionally laden topic for most people.

Patients bring these affective colorings to therapists who have their own sets of feelings about money. One would hope that therapists had worked out their money issues so that they are better prepared than patients to listen and talk about money. However, money has not been the favorite subject of most therapists' training, so they are frequently in an avoidant position. In addition, therapists have an image problem. They want to appear interested primarily in helping, incidentally in fees. The image of altruism gets in their way so that they think the less said about money, the better. This avoidance is most marked when it comes to financial transactions between therapists and patients.

We describe elsewhere in this book a recent emphasis on marketing in the psychotherapy field, but that is not focused on the therapist–patient fee transaction. The recent book edited by Krueger (1986) emphasizes the importance of the problem and urges therapists to take a straightforward approach. This is easier said than done, for the problem remains current. For example, in a case summary Pollak stated: "Therapists have to understand and conquer their personal conflicts. Despite Women's Liberation and the Feminist Movement, I still have my own personal difficulties when I must demand payment for my services. I spent considerable time alone trying to sort out reactions of anger and helplessness at not being paid and held on to the trust that one day . . . would pay me" (1989, p. 5).

PAYMENT PHILOSOPHY

Why should therapists get paid? To answer that question therapists first have to believe they provide a specialized service, which requires a skill for which they were trained and that cannot be provided by people who do not have such preparation. Many therapists do not believe this or have a fainthearted belief. Of course it is true that people other than therapists can be therapeutic, just as someone who is not an attorney can provide accurate legal advice, and the same for other areas of expertise. However, the client's chances of getting the best service in any field are increased by using a trained person. Unfortunately, the quality of psychotherapy with its emphasis on the relationship between the parties often obscures the fact that it is a skill best rendered by the skilled. That skill is the reason therapists should be paid.

Of course if a therapist does not believe that he or she does something special, then getting paid seems a sham. Another mitigating factor is patient remonstrances about therapist inadequacies in the therapy situation. Therapies where the therapists are less active are particularly vulnerable to such attacks, although probably all therapists have been told more than once in their careers that their services were not worthwhile.

Thus, the beginning point is that psychotherapists believe they offer a skill similar in concept to skills offered by other professionals, lawyers, dentists, etc. In our society people get trained and paid to render such services. Therapists are legitimate members of our service economy. Psychotherapy is their work and the way they have chosen to make a living. This is a primary issue that every therapist has to resolve. Being a psychotherapist is an occupation designed to produce income.

Profit is neither the sole nor major motive, which is service, but therapists do want and need to make money from their efforts. However, if one wants to make a great deal of money by being a psychotherapist, one will be disappointed because the structure of the situation makes that impossible. There are definite limits to the number of hours that can be worked as well as the amount per hour that can be charged. It is possible to make a comfortable living, but that is it.

In addition, there are easier ways to make a comparable living, so choosing to be a psychotherapist requires a particular fascination with the work. The stresses and strains are described in our chapter on occupational hazards. Since it is not an easy profession either to train for or to practice, logic dictates a monetary reward in line with that enjoyed by other service professionals. Physicians tend to set the standard for the psychotherapy profession, with other mental health workers charging according to their status as reflected in the marketplace.

An example of the realities is provided in a national survey of psychologists in independent practice (Prochaska, Nash, & Norcross, 1986). The sample consisted of 327 full-time practitioners with a 35-hour average work week. Their dominant theoretical orientation was eclectic, and they were experienced with practices averaging 11 years in operation. Their average hourly fee was $63 as of 1983, which probably would be adjusted to $70 in a current national survey. Thus, it is certainly possible for therapists working full time in private practice to gross more than $100,000 a year but difficult to get beyond $150,000 and close to impossible to surpass $200,000. We are thinking here of psychoanalytic therapists who work 45–50 minute sessions for approximately 35–40 hours per week.

Neither wealth nor hardship appear in this picture, but the problem for therapists is that they do not want patients to know that they have more than a passing interest in monetary matters. As a result, the area in which there is the greatest difficulty for therapists to talk about money has to be their fees. Therapists have such a narcissistic need to have patients see them only as helpers that they dislike, avoid, and minimize fee transactions. Therapists are willing to have patients know they will take money, but they do not like patients thinking therapists want money. The helping, good person image must prevail with exclusionary vigor.

Psychoanalysis provided a cover for therapists with regard to setting fees by promoting the idea that the fee represented a sacrifice by the patient to ensure proper motivation (Freud, 1913). Thus, the fee became necessary for the therapy with its size depending on the patient's economic circumstances. A sliding-scale policy was placed into operation with the therapist setting and collecting the fee primarily to help the patient, secondarily to support the therapist. Such a view effectively took apparent acquisitive motives out of therapists' behavior.

However, as a recent review of the empirical literature on fees has demonstrated (Herron & Sitkowski, 1986), patients will improve with or without paying a fee. At the same time, none of the existing studies had a situation in which therapists' livelihood depended on the fees paid by patients. Whether or not patients in private practice would improve without paying fees has not been tested. The implication is they might not because fees are probably more for therapists' motivation than patients'. Thus, countertransference could be a major problem for therapists who are not getting paid for their work.

Both therapists and patients are motivated by money, but overall, patients will do better without paying than therapists will do without getting paid. Many therapists avoid the issue by creating job situations in which they do not have to get money directly from their patients. One way to do this is to work for a salary so patients' economic status is of no consequence to the therapist. In fact, therapists who work in situations where the fee is of some significance to the agency are notorious for failing to discuss fees with patients and often identify with the patients as victim's of the agency's fiscal policy.

Identification with patients in terms of payment is common in training situations. There the therapists may take an antiestablishment attitude wherein they see the training program as exploiting its trainees who in turn can use the patients to exact revenge. Also, there is a tendency in training therapists to minimize the fee issue so that many trainees are inexperienced in this important area by the design of their supervisors.

Other therapists set up practice settings in which their economic situation does depend directly on patient fees, but a third party, often the secretary/receptionist, actually deals with the patient in terms of collecting fees. This makes it appear as if the third party is the "heavy" who wants money while the therapist remains untainted.

Thus, we see avoidance, guilt, and ambivalence about the acceptance of the profit motive by therapists as well as extraordinary measures taken to avoid having patients recognize its existence. A different and realistic approach is definitely in order. Therapists need to accept whatever degree of interest they may have in making money and openly include that in establishing a fee policy. This means that each therapist should decide on a certain lifestyle and in turn expects his or her patients to be willing to pay for it. Fees are set accordingly. Whereas fees can serve as motivation for patients, fees are primarily there for therapists' wellbeing. This fact is not something to be hidden from patients, nor is it something therapists should be ashamed of or guilty about.

PATIENTS' ATTITUDES

The focus here is on patients' attitudes about fees that can affect therapists and how these may be handled. The first of these is the "barrier effect" (Herron & Sitkowski, 1986), where patients are put off from entering therapy or leave after one or a few sessions, either because there is a fee or because of the size of the fee. Generally patients do not enjoy paying a fee but develop an acceptance of it. However, therapy is often viewed in advance as a kind of empathy–sympathy–direction-giving encounter that ought to be part of ordinary help and kindness among people. The idea that people should pay for that is unappealing to many, and they in turn avoid such a situation despite very real needs for therapy.

The fee also formalizes the process with patients as designated people with problems and therapists as paid problem solvers rather than kind and good new friends. Fees work against patient denial mechanisms, which can be valuable but also threatening because of the variations in patients' readiness to remove such mechanisms from their array of current coping operations.

If therapists recognize that fees may initially appear as obstacles, then they can discuss fees from that viewpoint. An understanding of patients' reluctance to commit to a fee-paying situation can be communicated while at the same time it can be made clear that a fee is going to be a definite part of the process. Also, since the fee highlights the structure of the relationship, it is an opportunity to try to ensure the patient's acceptance of having a problem and getting professional help for it. The therapist can use the fact of the fee to indicate that there is "something wrong" that can be worked on and changed. The fee is charged for that service and in turn can help the patient identify the service.

A related concern is that even if the patient is willing to concede the existence of a personal problem, doubts may exist about the workings and effectiveness of the therapist. The therapist needs to explain what he or she is going to get paid for by the patient. The specificity of this will vary with the type of therapy to be employed, but it is always important to make the process understandable to patients. Again, such awareness by therapists will make fees more acceptable to patients.

Prochaska et al. (1986) indicated that more therapists continue to enter the field, and competition has increased. We discuss this "crowding" issue in our chapter on occupational hazards as part of the increasing tendency for therapists to become proficient in marketing their services. Some marketing is also often needed in the early sessions of a possible course of therapy because therapists may have to help patients see how therapy can be of value.

For example, Shulman (1988) takes the view that since long-term psychotherapies are not popular either with many patients or with most insurance companies, therapists ought to consider brief therapies targeted to patients' apparent problems. He sees the approach as responding to patients' needs rather than therapists', whereas we feel therapists also get paid for diagnostic expertise. Thus, our position is that the therapist ought to tell the patient what he or she thinks would work best rather than to let the patient write the prescription. However, Shulman further points out that patients may want something other than what therapists have in mind to offer. So therapists have to explain what they believe patients need and why, and then patients can make their choices.

This is more of an issue with most psychoanalytic therapies than other types because of the customary length and, in turn, the greater cost. However, we believe psychoanalytic psychotherapies offer patients the best therapeutic opportunities, and we indicate that. There is sufficient range within these therapies to accommodate the range of current psychopathologies. We describe in our chapter on theory and its application the mechanics of the accommodation. Empirical support for this position can be found in the naturalistic study of psychoanalytic psychotherapies described by Wallerstein (1989). In essence, then, what the patient gets for the fee from the beginning is identification, recognition, and understanding of problems, recommendations for treatment, and a description of the treatment procedures.

Another problematic situation occurs when there is a change in a patient's financial circumstances during therapy. The change may be adverse, such as a job loss, or it may be positive, such as a job promotion and increased salary. A reduction in income sometimes contributes to a depressed view, with the patient wanting to leave therapy rather than negotiate a fee change with the therapist. Or, such a happening may cause the patient to feel more dependent on the therapist and in turn limit the expression of the patient's hostility lest the therapist retaliate. Also, such financial restrictions play into the vulnerability of therapists who are eager to demonstrate goodness and have the patient feel grateful for whatever accommodations are made regarding payment.

The therapist's first step should be an exploration of the meaning for the patient of the change in financial circumstances. The therapist needs to be flexible and try to provide an appropriate way for the patient to remain in therapy. However, it is a mistake immediately to offer to take a lower fee or to have payment deferred. Instead, if, for example, there has been a job loss, one should find out what this means to the patient and how it really came about. Since tragedy strikes people for a variety of reasons and people differ in their contributions to inducement, with some deriving satisfaction from difficulties, the understanding of the event and its ramifications are an essential part of the therapy process. This will be curtailed or missed if the therapist is in a hurry to show personal understanding by offering a solution. In contrast, the therapist can find out how the patient would like to solve the problems and work it out from there.

There is no set solution. The guiding principle is what will work for patient and therapist at that time in therapy. Generally an adjustment will be made to keep the therapy active, but the specifics will vary. Sometimes the most therapeutic thing to do is to discontinue therapy until the patient is ready to face the responsibility of the fee. Naturally a therapist would prefer not to be known as someone who stopped seeing a patient because the person lost his or her job and could not pay the therapist. However, if the patient lost the job because he or she wanted the world to take care of him or her, then by cooperating, the therapist could be fostering a delusion and promoting irresponsible behavior. The therapist's choice of what to do about the need for a fee reduction should be therapeutic, not popular. Whereas the choice may often be both, it will not always be, and the therapist is expected to act accordingly.

Some financial difficulties occur over time and seem integral to the patient's pathology, as masochism, depression, or impulsivity. The therapist may have explored and interpreted this trend and its potential liability for treatment. If the patient is not responsive, then when the inevitable disaster strikes, the therapist, as reality's representative, may have to allow treatment to end, since the patient has done nothing to ensure its continuance. This does not mean that "free therapy" cannot work, but in the example given, the original contract is being violated. Such a patient apparently feels the therapist is such a good (or foolish) person that he or she will continue therapy regardless of what the patient does about the fee.

The meaning of financial change is also of interest when patients' financial circumstances improve. Patients may see this as an opportunity to spend money on something that eventually may result in less money being available for therapy. For example, a patient may buy a house or a car or get married or have a baby because the person has more money. Yet the carrying costs of these events may turn out to make it difficult to pay for therapy. Such situations often occur as a patient is improving in therapy and can be reflective of a growing sense of competence. At the same time, the event does not coincide with the "ideal" termination point for therapy. Patient and therapist priorities differ here in terms of timing, yet the patient is not attempting to sabotage therapy. Instead, the patient is indicating that he or she feels good enough now that if other desired expenditures were to preclude therapy, it would be acceptable. The therapist in turn can understand that whereas therapy could continue to benefit the patient, that person on a cost–benefit basis might prefer someone or something else.

Of course an increase in a patient's money supply could be used to interfere with therapy. A patient who has agreed to a fee increase when he or she makes more money and then reneges is one example. Another would be the patient who ignores a real need for continuing therapy and, with an increase in funds, creates a situation as described previously that interferes with continuance. All this highlights the complexity of knowing when money is being used as resistance differentiated from money as a real but unwanted problem for therapy. Also, "reality" can have resistive elements as well.

For example, a patient begins therapy with an income from alimony, gets a job during therapy, but an unexpected problem occurs about the alimony, and it stops. Legal efforts and costs are required to pursue its resumption. At the same time, difficult issues have arisen in therapy for the patient. Because of her new financial difficulty, she cannot afford to continue therapy, nor can she know when she could restart. Although the patient did not anticipate such a problem, she is also relieved at having a way out of dealing with the current subject matter of therapy. Although the therapist is willing to wait for payment until the alimony is restored, the patient indicates that since this will occur at an unknown date, she does not want to incur such a possibly large debt. Therapy is making her anxious, and she wants a way out so she seizes the reality as her possibility.

In that example, the resistance is clear, but such is not always the case. It is difficult for any therapist to tell a patient that he or she can afford what the patient states is not affordable. Occasionally the opposite also occurs where a patient is insistent on more therapy sessions than can be realistically paid for. Here the therapist will have to question the dependency and overvaluing of therapy, but this is rare relative to the first scenario. If the patient's finances have been adequately discussed in therapy, and this assumes the patient has been truthful, then at least the therapist has a better opportunity to judge the element of resistance.

Therapists also have the flexibility to alter their fee structure. Hofling and Rosenbaum (1986) found in a sample of 157 psychoanalytic therapists that about 80% extended credit, usually did it more than once, and that about two-thirds of the patients eventually paid all that they owed. Therapists are usually willing to work something out with patients, so if a patient turns down a credit arrangement, resistance is probable.

If a patient needs therapy, and wants it, then most therapists are open to arranging the fee so the patient can afford it. This may involve referring the patient to other therapists with more time available or lower fees, but patients who need help can generally count on most therapists to do something to help the patients get what they need. Prochaska et al. (1986) reported that about 60% of their sample of therapists provided some free therapy service on a regular basis, and a sliding scale fee arrangement tends to be common. Therapists are more guilty than greedy so the errors that appear are more likely to be to the therapists' financial detriment than to that of the patients.

Although evidence indicates patients can improve with a no-fee or low-fee situation, patients are not impressed with such arrangements (Herron & Sitkowski, 1986). The fee can have motivational consequences for patients, such as more frequent attendance and impressions of therapist competence based on the size of the fee. Such impressions extend to the location and furnishings of therapists' offices as well as anything connected to the therapy that costs money and implies success or failure. By demonstrating an appropriate regard for money, therapists improve the possibility of patients having initial and continuing positive reactions to the probable effectiveness of therapy.

Patients have to be willing to give psychotherapy a monetary priority over a span of time that usually includes emotional ups and downs before there is a consistent feeling of betterment. Essentially patients are agreeing to support therapists' lifestyles, which tend to be middle to upper-middle class, in return for their expertise. This is how private practice functions, and it is part of the conventions of our society. Assuming most therapists accept such conventions, then they certainly do not have to be ashamed of their role in this respect and can certainly explain it to patients.

Of course some therapists may prefer a different societal model, perhaps one that is socialistic, and can approach their economic transactions with patients accordingly. These therapists seem to be in the minority, however, as all the current talk about marketing and financial planning for therapists would suggest. These are just relatively acceptable ways to dance around the topic of "financial getting." Still, accepting capitalism as a definite component of therapist patient transactions is uncomfortable for therapists. Actually, patients are often less ambivalent about the structure than therapists. As Lasky (1984) points out, psychotherapists are often new arrivals to their social class and not so comfortable with its values. Other contributors to therapists' discomfort are the still distasteful aspect of talking about money that carries over from psychotherapy training, and gender and personality differences among therapists in their attitudes toward money.

THERAPISTS' ATTITUDES

As stated above, we see fees as more of a problem for therapists than for patients. The principal cause of this is the therapist's identification with the caregiving role that tends to translate erroneously into service with or without a fee. Women have been found to have more trouble here than men (Burnside, 1986; Lasky, 1984), and this is an increasing problem because more women are entering the profession all the time so that there are now more female than male therapists. Thus, women have to be particularly careful that they do not contribute to society's devaluing their services relative to men, which already tends to occur despite efforts to prevent or correct it.

Considerable difficulty can be avoided if therapists accept the idea that therapy is constructed to be a service for a fee. Although the therapy itself can be effective without the fee, as can other services that are also designed to have a fee, such an outcome involves a change in the structure of the therapeutic contract. This can only happen part of the time and is only expected to happen part of the time, because therapists need to earn a reasonable living. Therapists may accept this premise on the surface, but in practice, guilt often sets in. As we have indicated, some of this guilt is based on doubts about their own competence. Probably because of the elusive nature of the psychotherapy, and the relationship bond forged within it, therapists devalue the technical knowledge base of the therapeutic process. The idea that it is also a job gets hidden or lost, and then, so does the fee.

An intriguing paradox often takes place. Most therapists want to live comfortably and show no interest in being poor, but they can be persuaded on a one-to-one basis to lower their income. They are certainly reluctant to admit to patients that their fees are designed to give them a certain living standard that they want. They prefer patients to believe they are not engaged in this profession for the money *at all*, yet the last part is untrue. The degree of monetary interest varies from therapist to therapist, but it is assuredly there. Furthermore, if therapists work for institutions and get paid salaries, they will be quite vocal about their needs for money because confronting the impersonal is acceptable and even laudable.

Some therapists have taken the route of developing their careers in salaried positions where they are not directly dependent on what the patients pay. As noted earlier, others have created private practice groups where the fee is handled at a distance by a collector, analogous to "paying at the desk" in the dentist's office. Even when these therapists are forced to take up fee issues with patients, they may attribute the confrontation to a request/demand from the "financial people" or the "other partners." Finally, even the tremendous current emphasis on marketing psychotherapeutic services is heavy on getting clients and light on getting paid. Prochaska et al. (1986) point out that part-time practitioners charge less than full timers. This may be that because they have other jobs their need is less, but it also may be a way to avoid conflicts with patients about money.

Tulipan (1986) does not like the fee-for-service concept and proposes replacing it with "patient subsidy." He asserts that a variable fee arrangement can work out well for the therapist, somehow eliminating the more customary unpleasantries that may emerge around fees. The latter assertion is unconvincing, but it is clear that Tulipan's depicted interpersonal therapist is also worried about the fee issue and has designed some way to try to make it less of a personal concern.

So we return to the fact that fees are a problem for many, if not most, therapists. Granted there are times when money talk is most indelicate, yet necessary. Consider the initial session with a patient who tells a personal tale of horror that is obviously distressing. At such a moment it may not seem appropriate even to mention that there is a fee, far less to name a number. This is just one of those times when it is no fun to be a therapist. However, if the fee goes unmentioned at this point, that patient will probably not pay then or have an accurate idea of what therapy will cost. The session is going to end, arrangements are going to be made for the future, the mood is going to be altered, and all this is part of the therapist's job. Of course it needs to be carried out tactfully and with understanding and empathy, but none of that justifies avoidance.

The first few sessions, let us say the first three, may be considered evaluative for both therapist and patient. Both are trying to find out if they are going to work together. It is necessary to indicate a fee for these sessions, which may even be stated in advance since most initial contacts are made over the telephone. Then, if both parties agree, policies related to fees should be explained. As Tulipan has stated, "A better atmosphere is generated through . . . congruence of practice and its roots in personal style and theoretical orientation. The resultant overall consistency will prove most salubrious to both patient and therapist alike" (1906, p. 87).

Thus, the therapist's fee policy ought to make sense, emotionally and intellectually, to both parties in the transaction. The therapist needs to avoid excessive narcissistic pulls to be anything other than a therapist in setting the fee, which is primarily designed to meet the economic needs of the therapist, rather than his or her status needs, or hoarding needs, or denigrating needs, or charitable needs, or manipulative needs, or seductive needs, and so forth. Also, the therapist's economic needs have to be reasonable or there will be few consumers, so a probable fee range is available formed by market structure. Within the perspective of the therapist's monetary needs, he or she makes the decision as to how much free or low-cost service can be given.

Beginning therapists often charge as much as experienced therapists, which can annoy some of the experienced therapists. Also, unless the beginning therapists have quite a patient supply, which is unusual, the high fees may limit the number of patients they will see. An alternative method to build a caseload is to begin more modestly. Higher fees will undoubtedly follow. The real issue for the beginning therapist ought to be, "What am I worth based on what I know and can do right now?" An honest answer to that question ought to produce an appropriate "regular fee."

The issue of one's regular or customary fee deserves some comment. For some therapists this concept is a fantasy. It is a fee they would like to get but rarely do. It is a fee they tell their friends about but infrequently receive. It is their power symbol, and it is used to make patients feel grateful and themselves magnanimous when they accept a lower fee. These ambiguities can be avoided by making the regular fee appropriate in the first place so that it can be the real fee.

In this regard one of us was approached by a relative who is young, relatively inexperienced, and beginning her practice. She wanted to know what she ought to charge. When asked what she would like to receive, she indicated $40, though she said her potential patient had limited means. Certainly $40 is a modest fee by current standards, but in light of the patient's circumstances a lower fee appeared likely if the patient was to go into therapy. Thus, the therapist was asked what was the lowest fee she would accept, and she indicated it was $20, so her fee range became $20–$40. She told the patient she would like to get $40 and could the patient afford that? The patient indicated she could only pay $25 and would that be acceptable? The therapist agreed since it was within her range, and the therapy started. This type of self-negotiation and self-other negotiation appears as one realistic way to begin. Since there was an acceptable fee for both, they could begin without hidden feelings of resentment or gratitude. This was further assured by the therapist indicating that the fee could be reviewed and revised upward depending on improvement in the patient's ability to pay. This provided a future incentive for the therapist in getting closer to her desired fee and left the patient with an awareness of her fee responsibilities so that she would not have to feel indebted to the therapist for being at the lower end of the fee range.

Sliding Fee Scales

A limitation in this arrangement is endemic to all sliding-scale fee situations. If one has no patients, then a low-fee patient is usually more appealing than no patient, so it is acceptable as a beginning. However, with more patients, the therapist may begin to feel more positively about the higher-paying ones. This can result in finding ways to get rid of the lower-paying patients, such as quickly "curing" them or finding them unmotivated or unworkable. Another possibility is a reaction formation to the resentment so that extraordinary efforts go into the lowest-paying patients without recognition of what is really happening.

Low-fee patients also have particular opportunities to be resistive. They may devalue the therapy based on the fee and so be late, miss sessions, waste time in sessions, and be contemptuous of the therapist. In contrast, by feeling gratitude, they may block hostile feelings toward the therapist and look on therapy as something that takes place more for the therapist than the patient. In situations where the patient pays a low fee and the therapist is paid a salary by the treating agent, both patient and therapist may show less regard for the consistency of the therapy. In such situations, the therapist has limited personal concern about the fee. If the patient does not appear, or is late, the therapist has time to do other things and still gets paid. It is a free vacation, whereas in private practice such "vacations" could be costly.

Another issue with sliding scales for fees is how to determine what the patient can really pay. Clinics and therapy service centers have struggled with this problem forever. Patients may balk at providing too much detailed information, and even when they do the possibility of hiding income exists. If simply asked, patients may understate their income. Also, if it is understood that fees will rise and fall with the available funds, there is an inducement for patients to conceal rises and highlight falls. The sliding scale will generally err in favor of the patient.

These concerns need to be recognized if a therapist is to adopt a sliding fee scale. Since this is the most popular method used, more attention needs to be devoted to an awareness of the problems and ways for each therapist to cope with them. At the moment this approach is probably popular because it looks fair rather than because therapists like it that much. It also has the historical tie to the "necessary sacrifice" by the patient that conceals therapist monetary motivations, but we have shown the fallacies existing in that idea. Still, therapists may still lean toward such a cover.

Some therapists may be interested in devoting sufficient scrutiny to the patient's finances to be assured that the fee is indeed fair to both therapist and patient. However, most are not, and it is easy to see that such evaluation could create considerable antagonism between the parties involved. The more likely and acceptable scenario is that therapists have a fee range and that they accept the patient's word regarding his or her ability to pay. They also accept the patient's evaluations as to ability to have an increase or need to be given a decrease. Therapists tend to stay within their range, so they may refer patients to low-cost services if the patient is initially unable to meet their lowest fee. This is more of a problem once the patient has been in therapy for a while and needs a fee below the therapist's minimum. As indicated previously, this may result in a termination or reduction of sessions, or it may mean a different fee arrangement so that the therapy can continue.

A problem with no fee or low-fee situations for the therapist, which can be attested to particularly by therapists undergoing training programs, is that it can lead to resentment. In training programs, the trainee is usually required to treat a certain number of people for long periods of time and receive no fee or a small fee. The people being treated pay a fee, but it goes to the program rather than the therapist, who is supposed to find his or her reward in fulfilling training requirements and having a learning experience. This works all right at the discipline level because most of the work is novel and exciting for the trainee who is in no position to be in private practice anyway. Also, the treatment is customarily for relatively brief periods of time with a variety of patients. This contrasts with a licensed therapist with an ongoing practice who is also in an analytic institute and is required to see a patient three times a week for 2 years without receiving a fee. The situation makes economic sense from the training institute's point of view, but more attention needs to be paid to how trainees feel about it and how these feelings may affect the treatment.

What we have just described tends to be a no-choice situation in regard to a particular patient, the choice having taken place when the therapist enters the program and agrees to the requirements. The situation is better when there is a choice about treating a specific person for a low fee or no fee. The reasons for making such a choice may be that a therapist wants to devote a certain amount of time to this kind of service in keeping with the spirit of being a psychotherapist. Combined with this may be a specific intent in helping a patient for learning purposes, or a match between skill and need. It is important that the therapist have a deliberate reason for giving such service as opposed to feeling manipulated and then rationalizing the action.

Assuming that an appropriate rationale is in place, the therapist should keep in mind the possibility of a shift in his or her feelings about what is happening. For example, a therapist may have some open hours and want to fill them regardless of the fee. Once these hours are filled with low-cost patients, however, the therapist is no longer available for subsequent patients who may be able to pay a higher fee. Then the therapist may begin to wish the current patients would finish the treatment process so they could be replaced.

It appears that patients and therapists are both better off when a fee can be paid that can feel satisfactory to the therapist. Therapists will honor their commitments, but they will do better therapy when they feel adequately compensated. When this cannot be, the therapist can alleviate possible problems by creating a realistic time-limited situation. Therapy will start with a certain fee but be subject to periodic review with regard to the cost structure. In this way, the patients remain attuned to their economic responsibilities to the therapist. However, therapists do have a commitment to patients and should expect to work with a patient for as long as it is needed even if the patient does not arrive at a position to pay a higher fee when the therapist would like it.

Fixed Fees

Another way to deal with the problems inherent in sliding scales is to eliminate them to a large degree by having a fixed fee. Every patient gets charged the same amount, and those who cannot afford the fee are referred to lower-cost therapy services, of which there are a large number of good quality. For example, the previously mentioned psychoanalytic training programs offer low-cost therapy by therapists who are in training but who also are experienced. This uniform-fee approach does not completely eliminate fee variations, as the need to raise fees with existing patients, or lower those for patients who have been seen for a while and have experienced financial problems that require a different fee arrangement for the therapy to continue. However, it does eliminate initial, as well as frequently repeated, assessments of what the patient can really afford as well as preference for patients based on what they pay. Perhaps this system is used by a minority of therapists because of the images of inflexibility and monetary interest that may be suggested. Still, there is nothing to prevent a therapist from lowering the fee in a particular instance, so flexibility is a possibility. Also, the fairness of a sliding fee schedule is questionable because some people may feel that they are being penalized because they are financially successful and consider that unfair. Furthermore, as previously indicated, prospective patients may be deceptive about their income when faced with a sliding scale possibility, and that is fair neither to the therapist nor to the patient, who begins a process of truth by lying. Furthermore, the relatively fixed fee approach is a more direct expression of therapists' interest in their own incomes.

Third-Party Payers

Finally, there is the issue of third-party payment, most prominent in the use of health insurance but also appearing in other instances such as parents paying for a child or one spouse for another. Although such arrangements have certainly increased the availability of therapy, they decrease the responsibility of the patient. It works better when the therapist can deal directly with the patient about payment. Thus, where patients use insurance, it is a useful policy to have the patient pay the therapist directly and have the insurance company reimburse the patient. A similar approach can be used when somebody else is responsible for the patient's bill. Have the patient deal with that person and have the patient pay the therapist. There will be exceptions to this, such with young children, but it is better if exceptions are kept to a minimum.

Also, the way insurance companies are currently operating with repeated and intrusive requests for information and apparent attempts to limit therapy benefits, it is more appealing to have patients who do not use insurance. Confidentiality is weakened when insurance is involved; there is pressure to achieve results quickly via a threat to limit or terminate payment; and there is an ever-increasing amount of paperwork that is questionable both in its form and value in determining the appropriateness and reasonableness of the therapy. Therapists need to make sure that the patient really knows how the insurance policy works so that financial commitments to the therapy are realistic. If a patient plans on a certain course of therapy based on insurance reimbursement, that adds a tenuous element that both patient and therapist need to evaluate before beginning to work together. This is particularly true if the therapy is intended as long term because insurance carriers are negative about such a procedure unless the patient is very disturbed. The value of psychoanalytic therapies for a range of pathologies where the treatment is open-ended is not well received in insurance circles.

Prochaska et al. (1986) indicate that there is a definite move toward briefer therapies, approximating 15 sessions for the average patient. In addition, there has been the proliferation of "alphabet soup"—HMOs (health maintenance organizations), PPOs (preferred provider organizations), IPAs (individual practitioner associations), EAPs (employee assistance programs), and DRGs (diagnostic related groupings). These programs are aimed at cost containment and emphasize both quantity over selectivity and rapidity over lengthy treatment. In the chapter on occupational hazards, we discuss these trends from other viewpoints, but here we want to raise the possibility that an appealing feature to all this is that it reduces a therapist's needs to deal with patients about fees. Although the alphabet groups can really cut a therapist's income, and the quantity of patients required by short-term approaches requires much more extensive marketing, the arrangements and brevity reduce the impact of the fee. Therapists can have security for the price of lesser income, but if the quality of treatment suffers, then therapists will have to rethink their apparent peace of mind. Psychoanalytic therapists already have to challenge these trends because they are in most instances simply at variance with what is considered effective psychoanalytic treatment. In addition to educating third-party payers as to the value of providing for a range of treatment opportunities, it is also necessary to find ways to incorporate existing possibilities within the structure of effective psychotherapy. This is becoming more difficult.

Contract Details

Assuming that a fee structure has been satisfactorily established, there are other concerns related to the therapist's income. Essentially the therapist and patient establish a contract that states that the patient will pay the therapist, first for making a certain amount of time available during which direct service can be provided. Then, assuming the patient uses the time with the therapist, the patient's payment is also for the service given during that time. Additional service is rendered outside of the time as well, including theoretical and technical formulations designed to help the patient when therapist and patient have contact, telephone calls, and paperwork with respect to the patient. It is a package, and the patient can make use of all or some of the parts. Regardless, the patient pays the fee. Thus, there is reason to charge patients for all scheduled sessions since the therapist's availability aspect of the contract has been carried out.

Such an approach provides a constant structure for all parties concerned. This contract should of course be explicitly explained to the patient, and the therapist should keep in mind that the patient may really not comprehend all details until a problem arises, such as a missed session. Then the contract will have to be invoked, probably with a reexplanation referenced to the original explanation. It is to be expected that patients may have negative feelings about specific applications, and therapists must be willing to deal with these feelings as part of the therapy process. We discuss the rational and irrational aspects of contracts in therapy in a later chapter.

An aim of the contract is to establish comfortable and therefore effective, stable working conditions. Some flexibility is generally required to do this. For example, it is advantageous for the therapy that it have an external structure of fixed appointments, a set amount of time, and policies for payment including when payment is customarily made, as well as arrangements for vacations, cancellations, and missed appointments. The point can be made with a patient that the maximum use is to be made of the time available, so that all appointments need to be kept. What if they are not? There are a variety of ways to handle this. One is to charge for all scheduled appointments so that the patient pays for the time regardless of the reason the session was missed. This certainly observes a constancy principle, and it provides a rather steady flow of income. However, it is a difficult policy to follow without exception. Suppose the patient is pregnant, about to deliver within the week, but naturally does not know exactly when, and wants to keep her appointment during the time when she may have to deliver. If the appointment is scheduled, must she pay? Or to avoid a complication such as this should the therapist not schedule appointments until she delivers even though she then may miss appointments she could actually make?

A more practical and flexible policy is to charge for all scheduled appointments but to offer make-up sessions at no additional charge for ones that may be canceled. These sessions should be within a reasonable time span from the missed sessions and should be at the therapist's convenience. They should be used for canceled sessions, not sessions where the patient just did not appear, and the patient should request the sessions. Sometimes patients cancel because they do not feel like coming and are willing to pay for the time. Patients should also be informed that the therapist will do what he or she can to make up the session but that it is not guaranteed and requires the patient's cooperation. If the therapist offers time possibilities and the patient turns them down, then the patient should pay for the original session without a substitute session.

One way to ensure access to time when time has been lost is to provide for the use of telephone sessions. Thus, even if a patient calls to say there are impossible travel conditions, or the patient is not feeling well enough to go out, the session can still proceed on the phone. Some patients feel uncomfortable doing this, as do some therapists, but other patient–therapist pairs find this a convenient way to work when it is necessary to avoid a missed session. We are not claiming that it is the same as an in-person session, but it is not automatically inferior either, and it is better than no session.

The concept being advanced is to have the patient and therapist in all the sessions contracted for over a given time period, say a year, which with therapist vacations probably amounts to 45 sessions on an once-a-week basis. The policy is designed to be reasonable and fair to both patient and therapist, but it is open to potential manipulative attempts by the patient. Since the feelings about missed sessions should always be explored, the therapist has the opportunity to discuss resistance and to confront it if such is the case. However, the essential idea is to have the patient in the sessions, not to punish the patient for resistance. Paying for cancelled sessions is not automatically a motivator to cancel less, nor is that the main idea inherent in it, even when it may serve as a motivator. With provision of reasonable substitutes, the number of sessions per year can remain the same. Having a cancellation policy that allows for not paying if the notice was within a reasonable time (determined by the therapist) does not convey an impression that the therapy is important. It also puts therapists in the position of having to make frequent decisions that may seem arbitrary to patients. The possibility of an adversional relationship is increased, with the therapist either assuming a "hard line" so that the patient feels victimized or the reverse where the therapist is masochistic.

Tulipan (1986) has described a policy of not usually charging for missed sessions and assuming that a certain number will be canceled over a year so that the therapist's expected income will include the expected loss. He feels this approach reduces therapists' feelings of deprivation and indicates the mutuality of trust. Although Tulipan agrees with the idea of exploring the meaning of missing sessions and at times charging for a missed session, his approach deemphasizes the value of the reliability of the therapy. Also it may still result in controversy between therapist and patient because of possible failures to negotiate a satisfactory solution with patients who are missing sessions.

Vacations

The therapist usually models the therapeutic value of vacations, with the "analyst's August" a stereotype of therapists always taking some vacation time, often at least a month. There are some therapists who rarely take a vacation, but patients are usually surprised by this and question the therapist's motives for constantly working. The same skepticism may occur with therapists who are frequently canceling or changing sessions, with the latter group being suspect in respect to their concern for patients. The former group are more likely to be thought of as really "in it for the money."

Assuming the customary approach of the therapist having designated vacation time that is explained to patients sufficiently in advance so they can be prepared, some therapists go on to insist that the patients' vacations coincide with the therapists'. If not, the patients are expected to pay for their missed sessions. Again, this is a difficult policy to carry out and strikes many people as unreasonable. Certainly patients may be encouraged to take their vacations during the same time period as their therapists because that will simplify the situation, but that is often not possible. Patients take vacation when the time is made available to them or when they need to for personal reasons, and this can be recognized as therapeutic.

Still, the vacations may take away from therapy time. Again, patients should be encouraged to make this time up with the therapist providing acceptable substitute time. Vacations are generally planned well in advance so that make-up sessions can also be planned. It is reasonable for the therapist to require substantial advance notice in order to provide the substitute time. Vacations are in a different category than cancellations and no-show sessions, given their ostensible therapeutic purpose. Thus, the more prudent policy here may be to recommend that they be made up, but not to insist or charge for them if they are not.

It is also true that vacations can be used as resistances in terms of avoiding therapy, so that the intent and meaning for the patient needs to be explored. However, the exploration is not aimed at determining if a resistance exists as proof that the session must be paid for but to diminish or eliminate the resistance. The effectiveness of psychotherapy depends on patients giving it substantial priority and not letting other events interfere. In developing a schedule for therapy sessions, the time pattern needs to be realistic for patients and therapists or resistance will be inherent. For example, it can be particularly difficult to work out a consistent schedule with patients who have jobs requiring a great amount of travel. It is best to use a schedule that guarantees the comfortable presence of both parties. This may limit the patient to fewer times a week than therapist and patient consider ideal, but if there is going to have to be frequent reshuffling, it is better to go with a simpler schedule with the hope that at some point the ideal could become workable. If either patient or therapist has to go to extraordinary lengths to meet a therapy schedule over a lengthy period of time, there will be difficulties around this schedule and in turn around fees.

Therapeutic Fee Arrangement

The usual fee arrangement is whatever works for the individual therapist, which in turn means that enough patients also find it acceptable. By "works for the therapist," we mean that the therapist feels comfortable with his or her approach to fees. The rate of return for the therapist's efforts certifies the therapist's needs symbolized through money. However, particular fee arrangements always bear scrutiny because the needs getting satisfied may not be in the best therapeutic interests of patients. Therapists who are manipulated by patients about fees and pass this off as healthy flexibility or satisfy their "good person" image while promoting irresponsibility are not being therapeutic. At the same, feeding the therapist's grandiosity with excessively high fees or extremely rigid arrangements are ways to manipulate the patients and again are antitherapeutic. Therapists need to address the question of the meaning of money for themselves and how this translates to their interactions with patients. Just as therapists have learned to be more comfortable with how they deal with sexual matters in therapy, the same thing needs to happen with respect to money matters because they remain a difficult issue for patients.

NARCISSISTIC ILLUSIONS IN FEES

Mitchell (1988) has described illusion as a key feature of all theories of narcissism. Thus, the self is constructed through illusions, essentially hope that what one wishes for indeed is or becomes reality. Such illusions are particularly striking when therapists are dealing with fees. The desired image is that of a caregiver with human attributes, including aggressive and sexual feelings although excluding such behavior toward patients. A desire for money, however, which is certainly related to or representative of sex and aggression, tends to be hidden from others and from the self.

Two illusions are prominent here. One is that such a desire can be successfully hidden. It certainly seems true that most psychotherapists have a primary interest in providing help in a special way. Caregiving is a major motivation for entering the profession, and at that time the profit motive might be quite limited and even seem antithetical to being a good helper.

However, as one proceeds in life and acquires responsibilities and new interests and desires, money becomes more important. If one functions as a psychotherapist, then this is the primary way to make the money you feel is needed. Although providing effective service certainly has to be the first consideration, this can be carried out in such a way that therapists have comfortable lives. It is an illusion to think therapists are not interested in making money via seeing patients, and it is an illusion to think that patients do not know this. Making money and providing psychotherapy are compatible concepts.

Well, what about those who cannot afford to support the therapist's desired standard of living? This will always be a cogent question for the profession and the individual therapist. It can neither be ignored nor become the burden of only a few therapists. However, in this chapter we assume the integration of a service obligation with making a profit. Then we emphasize the necessity and mechanics of doing the latter.

The second illusion is connected to the first because the attempted deception about the significance of money leads to the idea that such an approach has no effect on the therapy. This is a fantasy designed to service the therapist's narcissistic image. Actually, there are two faces involved in supporting such an icon.

One group of therapists portray themselves as relatively indifferent to fees. They charge what patients indicate is affordable, and they are casual about cancellations, lateness, and when fees are paid. In essence, they leave fee paying up to the patient, which makes them vulnerable to negative reactions to patients who do not treat them well and overvaluations of patients who do better by their therapists. A lack of structure is also fostered by the approach, which seems designed to make the therapist look good and money a nonissue; this approach is usually unrealistic. There may be some therapists who can be this indifferent to how they will live and who want to provide such a model for their patients, but it is a questionable approach. The therapist is trapped by it in many instances, and patients get a distorted view of the usual importance of money.

The other group of therapists make fees a definite issue with rigid rules but indicate that these are all for the benefit of the patient. Structure and motivation are emphasized as the essence of fee paying, with the implication that if it was not good for the patient, the therapist would have little interest in fees, and no interest in high fees, which these therapists tend to charge. These therapists make more money than the first group, and they also maintain a lofty image, but patients may question the validity of the therapists' views on fees. These therapists treat such questioning as resistance, so it may get some air time, but it cannot persist if the patient remains in treatment. Again we have an unreal approach that hides therapists' motivations and dismisses patients' objections when they sense a profit motive.

There are undoubtedly some therapists who are money hungry and do not disguise this fact as well as some who work for little compensation with patients of limited means and who are content to live modestly themselves, but these two groups are minorities compared to the first groups. What most therapists struggle with is how to feel comfortable with making money and at the same time feel that patients and the world at large see them as helpers.

The good–bad dichotomy is understandable, but it actually serves as an obstacle to effective psychotherapy. In describing the mutative factors of psychoanalytic therapies, Pine (1988) highlights a number of relational factors. The therapist has a consistent presence. The therapist does not condemn, seduce, retaliate. Instead the therapist understands, values the patient, and survives as a person to be trusted in terms of concern and positive intentions. These relational factors can easily be interfered with if therapists have not mastered the basic issue of fee transactions. This means therapists must become honest with themselves about their motives in receiving fees. If their motives are other than being fairly compensated for rendering their services, then a reexamination is in order because avarice, or status, or idealization, or gratitude are not useful emotions for the therapy.

Once the profit motive is faced and put in its appropriate place, namely the therapist's way to survive in a reasonable manner, this should be made clear to patients. Even though there are motivational and structural values of fees, they are not the sole or even primary reasons for the fees, nor is it accurate to present them in this manner. Therapists see patients for a variety of reasons. Earning a living is one of these reasons. Therapists should know this, and patients should know this. Such knowledge will both clarify what psychotherapy is and improve how it works. It will also remove a major overlooked distortion in the therapeutic relationship that inhibits the mutative power of the interaction.

4

The Use and Abuse
of Fantasy

We have previously documented the potential impacts of certain therapist behaviors on patient behaviors, and the reverse, thus alluding to the countertransferential types of responses that are likely to occur, especially through the medium of the therapist's narcissism. These responses are embedded in fantasy and reflected by the therapist's fantasies. For example, not only is it possible for the therapist's narcissism to be manifested through fantasy operations that he or she brings to the therapy situation, but fantasy arises or may be triggered by the assault on the therapist's narcissism once therapy begins. Moreover, the therapist's fantasy picture of what therapy should be and how patient and therapist should act governs much of what goes on in the name of establishing rational and irrational contracts, and contributes to the concept of termination.

It appears that we have the interrelated concepts of fantasy and countertransference, with their associated narcissistic elements, all in need of further exploration. Again as with many of the issues in this book, these have been "thought about" by others but at the same time too much left alone, as though they were really and completely understood, and so, no longer "issues."

If we take fantasy as the first example, purely from the standpoint of normative human behavior, it can be seen as a level of thinking. It is a cognitive operation used to process anecdotal and emotional events. Fantasy is a way of making sense out of unconscious and conscious

This chapter was originally published in *Issues in Psychotherapy*, 1982, New York: Brady-Prentice Hall. Copyright 1982 by William G. Herron and Sheila Rouslin Welt.

observations, of internal and external events and their relationships to each other. It is a vehicle for the expression of a given intellectual aspect of knowledge and its corresponding affect. Clinically, the therapist's fantasy manifests itself through privately thought "stories" or less formalized "images" that occur fleetingly or word or picture associations. At times, fantasy may only be inferred from sudden unexplained breaks in expected or rational behavior.

The interest here is not so much in what the therapist should or should not think about, but with the *fact* of therapist fantasy and how it can be used or abused and, in particular, the function of the therapist's fantasy and its relationship to countertransference. Through elaboration of the concepts of countertransference and fantasy, and through clinical examples and discussion of the concepts as they operate in clinical work, we try to shed some different light on the therapist at work. Throughout the development of this chapter, the intent is that some insight may be found in this complex area, both in regard to the ways in which the therapist's fantasy can work for and against the therapist and for and against the patient.

We begin by considering the value of the availability of fantasy to the therapist and illustrate what can occur when fantsy is held out of reach as opposed to its potential utility for the therapeutic relationship. From here we move to the key role of fantasy in understanding the countertransference response of the therapist. We briefly outline the definition and development of countertransference to show its current conception. We point out the possible "good" use of countertransference, note its problematic aspects, and suggest the need for an accurate perspective on its presence and possible effects. Then we explore the applications of countertransference, its consequences, and the possible ways of dealing with the problems. This exploration leads to a classification scheme for countertransference responses that is designed to expedite their recognition and concurrent management. Following this, we consider the more generalized idea of the function of therapists' fantasies in therapy. The link with countertransference is continued, and the issue of fantasy that therapists "share" by virtue of practicing therapy is illustrated along with the possible problems engendered. We conclude by suggesting an increased recognition of the role of the therapist's fantasy in the therapeutic process.

THE AVAILABILITY AND POTENTIAL VALUE OF THERAPISTS' FANTASY

Whereas fantasy at some level is always active, not all therapists are aware of their own. That can severely limit their therapeutic efforts. Fantasy as a route to understanding countertransference is then not available to the therapist, thereby eliminating a source of data for the understanding of the patient and the interaction. Unfortunately, it is not uncommon that therapists, without assistance, remain unaware of their fantasies. Here is an example:

A young therapist was with a patient in her hospital room where the patient had insisted on being for her session that day. Much to the therapist's conscious dissatisfaction (for "therapeutic" reasons), the patient, who did not need her thinking loosened further, lay down on the bed next to the therapist's chair. She was tired, she said, and anyway got a kick out of "playing psychoanalysis." At one point, the patient reached over to the therapist, touching a pearl necklace she was wearing. The therapist, in reporting the incident to her own therapist, said she remembered stiffening up and "seeing herself" with the patient's hand on "her pearls." It was not that she feared that the patient would hurt her, for she had been seeing the patient in therapy for a few years and knew pretty much that "direct attack" was not really the way the patient operated. The therapist best described her own reaction as feeling vaguely uncomfortable but definitely detached.

Appropriately, to gain a more comprehensive picture of what had happened, the therapist's therapist asked her what fantasies she had had at the time. The patient–therapist, who herself had been in treatment for a few years, answered indignantly, saying didn't he realize she was working after all, so how could she be having a fantasy! Unimpressed, her therapist said it sometimes happened anyway and asked about when she told him about the event. Unreached, she was appalled that he thought she might be so out of touch as to fantasize. When he changed the term to daydream, she did allow that it happened rarely, but yes, once in a while. This therapist was one with tight obsessional defenses that were limiting her contact with her inner self and others. In that respect she was like her schizophrenic patients, in flight beyond where she worried fantasy would take her, although nobody would have usually thought to make the comparison. Ultimately, the therapist became aware just how much she fantasized, and in years to come, just how much of her life was fantasy. And she felt like a freer, more human, more frightened, but better, therapist.

As Searles (1975a) has written, "Analysis is effective insofar as it has given . . . ready access to, rather than somehow effaced, the [therapist's] capacity for primitive feelings of jealousy, fear, rage, symbiotic dependency, and other affective states against which [the] patient's schizophrenia typically is serving to defend the patient from experiencing in awareness" (p. 223). Unconsciously, this therapist held such feeling in check by defending against awareness of the fantasy process whereby the feelings would manifest themselves. For if fantasy occurred and was attended to, then the feelings might be recognized, and they themselves might emerge directly. To her way of seeing things, thought would no longer be pure; rather, it would be adulterated and perhaps influenced by feeling; and thoughts and feelings would be open to influence by others, including patients, with whom the therapist had heretofore felt safe. She would then be vulnerable; instead she unconsciously chose to protect herself at a cost to the development of the therapeutic relationship.

Fantasy is very much a part of therapists' lives as therapists. Part of their business is to figure out the place their fantasy operations hold in their work with patients. Exacly how the therapist's fantasy operations influence treatment on a moment to moment basis is highly individual and hard to pin down, but our experience has shown that indeed the therapist's fantasy operations have clinical effects, that there can be clinical use of the therapist's fantasy through direct or indirect means, and that there can be clinical abuse of the therapist's fantasy through direct and indirect means.

In one respect, the therapist's fantasy can be seen as a "striving to define oneself" (Giovacchini, 1977). Too, it can be seen as an isolating state explained by Winnicott (1971) in his discussion of a patient who used unconscious and later conscious fantasy as a device to withdraw from relating. As with Winnicott's patient, and the one we described, it is possible for the therapist to become so engrossed in fantasy as the whole of an experience that he or she does not in fact perceive all that is happening in the experience. In such a state, the thorough absorbtion in fantasy governs how and what will be perceived. Such a state may mean that realistic hope for relating is implicitly abandoned, and the fantasy becomes the life. The fantasy is lived, the life not quite observed. And though fantasy may have started out unconsciously as a way to find a place for oneself, a place in the universe (Giovacchini, 1977), the result is a kind of distance. The therapist's "place in the universe" becomes one of aloneness—not existential aloneness, but defensive aloneness built on conflict and anxiety about relating.

Accordingly, in the process of psychotherapy, it becomes the therapist's task to examine his or her place in the relationship with the patient. One means for this exploration is looking into the therapist's fantasy operations. To do so requires an understanding of a central contributor to the therapist's fantasy arousal and fantasy content: the countertransference response.

THE COUNTERTRANSFERENCE RESPONSE

Countertransference is an inevitable in psychotherapy as transference is ineludible. Countertransference goes beyond the early classical psychoanalytic narrow model holding that it is a response to the patient's transference (Freud, 1910/1964b). Instead, it involves the therapist's emotional response as transference-object, as projection-object of the patient's personality, as nontransference object (Heinmann, 1950; Kernberg, 1965; Racker, 1953). Further, countertransference can be thought of as the therapist's total emotional response, though that view needs some delineating.

It has been some time now since countertransference was seen simply as an unwelcome impediment to the therapy process (Glover, 1955) to be edited out rather than understood as a reaction emanating from the interaction of patient and therapist (Epstein & Feiner, 1979a). And it would seem useful that the thinking has progressed. Although Freud (1910/1964b) considered countertransference an obstacle to be overcome, he too thought that the unconscious might be used as an instrument (1912/1964). Perhaps it was then that the movement began toward considering it entirely possible and maybe even necessary that the countertransference response be seen as an integral and useful part of treatment rather than simply pathological responses of the therapist to the patient's transference as Freud (1910/1964b) initially conceived it. Theorists such as Winnicott (1947), Heinmann (1950), Racker (1953), and Giovacchini (1989) attest to the growing interest in an expanded view of countertransference in the years that followed.

For many years, it had been one of the field's most enduring beliefs that, with effort, countertransference reactions could be and should be eliminated. The idea was comforting for those looking for a "clean," supposedly "scientific," though perhaps sterile approach, but it was neither practical nor as useful as it seemed. Whereas today, in analytic circles a prevailing attitude is that "countertransference is an instrument for research into the patient's unconscious" (Heinmann, 1950, p. 82), some therapists practice the kind of therapy that tends to ignore the reaction, although it would be impossible to stop its occurrence altogether. In a way, countertransference has probably always been a source and a guide for understanding the patient, albeit an unconscious resource. Indeed countertransference can be a source for the therapist's self-understanding, for it is "intimate self knowledge that is the precondition for the intimate relations with others" (Ehrenberg, 1975, p. 330), and that is, after all, what therapy is about.

One noteworthy feature of the current view of countertransference is that it is practical. In the past, clinicians seemed disdainful of their reactions, or, at least indifferent toward their potential value. "Legitimacy" has helped take some of the sting out of countertransference occurrence while preserving the need for its recognition and facilitating its dynamic understanding. Another important element of the view is that free, unbiased examination of countertransference as a natural and expected phenomenon points the way to a more systematic approach for enhanced understanding of the patient's dynamics: the interpersonal expression of intrapsychic experience. Through the interpersonal experience, it is often possible, in Segal's (1977) words, to "become aware of conscious derivatives" (p. 36) of unconscious, intrapersonal experience. Moreover, it is part of being in touch not only with self, but with the other.

The broadened current view of countertransference is quite reasonable and useful. In addition, even if the therapist were to appear to be "rid" of the reaction, often there is no "quick fix" for the reaction the therapist seeks to end. The danger lies not in the occurrence of the countertransference reaction, but, that the reaction may go unrecognized or worse, when the treatment "technique" is unconsciously or consciously rationalized on the basis of countertransference. Ultimately there are no beneficiaries of such a situation, although for a while either patient or therapist, or both, might feel more comfortable.

Although countertransference reactions have the potential of being helpful *because* the therapist responds (Giovacchini, 1989) and therapist and patient potentially can use that response to promote progress, countertransference problems also account for difficulties in treatment. Even so, difficulties with the treatment do not automatically imply uncontrolled countertransference responses destructive to the patient and to the treatment process.

In that regard, at times it seems countertransference responses are valued beyond their inherent worth, and not simply as a contribution to the therapeutic process. As Singer (1980) says, "While appropriate use of countertransference furthers understanding and dissolution of the pathological system . . . this doesn't mean countertransference is worthy of reification. Countertransference is an important phenomenon, not to be ignored or wishfully treated as if it could be eliminated, but to be recognized not only as part of the solution, but as part of the problem" (p. 264). He cautions that becoming enamored of countertransference is "countertransference at its worst" (p. 265); whereas it is not a "necessary evil," it is a life-sized "inevitable necessity" (p. 264).

Countertransference Applied

There is a notable lack of authoritative (and not so authoritative) agreement as to whether the therapist directly confronts the patient with his or her countertransference-laden response (in the form of fantasy or not), or interprets, or silently processes the response, or bases direction on it. There are, however, some characteristics of countertransference important to recognize whether or not a therapist formally acts.

First, we must remember that at some level the patient is probably sensitive to and influenced by the therapist's countertransference no matter what the therapist "does" with it (Langs, 1976b; Little 1951; Searles, 1958, 1978); second, that countertransference reactions are automatic and often initially out of awareness (Segal, 1977), except for a few fantasy or behavioral hints; third, that countertransference reactions are inevitable because, as Searles (1975a) puts it, the therapist's "own more primitive modes of experience, and of interpersonal relatedness . . . are subject to being revived in the course of his ongoing adult life experience" (p. 223), including work with patients; fourth, that counter-transference is not simply as Heinmann (1950) would have it, the patient's creation and a function or part of the patient's personality. The therapist makes a contribution and that becomes a resource, a kind of measurement of the interpersonal process at hand. In that sense, both therapist and patient have a hand in determining the nature or quality or quantity or intensity of the response. And fifth, we must accept that countertransference is an inner response, an intrapsychic phenomenon reflecting processed interpersonal experience, present or past, touched off, often suddenly, by interpersonal events and at times expressed interpersonally.

So, because countertransference is an automatic response to which the patient is sensitive, because it is an inevitable and spontaneous, often primitive response based in the patient, therapist, or both, it is not always easy to "plan" how to use it and the fantasy that may house it. However, some help is provided by Epstein and Feiner (1979b). They note that it certainly is useful to "distinguish between countertransference as an inner experience, to be *digested*, scrutinized, clarified, understood, and subsequently harnessed for therapeutic understanding, and countertransference as directly, impulsively enacted or discharged" (p. 499). There is a difference. Seen as a discovery, countertransference can be used by therapists to assist patients to examine their contribution to the therapist's response.

Too often we have seen therapists who are too certain of the meaning of their responses, so certain of this never-absolute formulation that they foist it on the patient to the point of absurdity and struggle. If they are indeed right, time will tell and so will the patient if given the freedom. Interpretation is not valuable when used as a hostile device, a device to control or to create distance. Overzealous interpretation creates distance, signaling the patient that the therapist is indeed in charge, that the patient should "go away" to stop making the therapist uncomfortable, or to continue making the therapist comfortable, which is both controlling and distancing in that the patient must be close to the therapist in the way the therapist deems "right."

Too often we have seen "honesty" in the therapist's use of fantasy material as simply a narcissistic exercise, something of which Searles (1975) warns. Also, these "honest" confrontations or presentations of countertransference response are sometimes devious. Their expression, whether directly expressed or presented as a formulation, may certainly instead be hostile, burdening the patient with that which he or she cannot deal, at least in that particular context at that particular moment. Honesty, says Giovacchini (1989), should be thought of as a tool rather than as a general virtue. After all, therapist irrationality, in all of its diversity, can be treated as a discovery rather than used as a weapon.

So then, is seeing countertransference as a helpful occurrence a bit heavy on the side of rationalization? Is it merely seeing a silver lining on a dark horizon? We think not, although that is not to say that much damage cannot be done in the name of "using" one's countertransference response.

There is a fundamental difference between using a countertransference reaction as one indicant of what *might* be going on in a complex field and using it as the complete explanation of what is transpiring. There is a fundamental difference between using a countertransference reaction in an irrational way and in a rational way. Irrational use may not always appear so because it is often disguised to look psychologically presentable, and the reaction itself may have merit. However, even with a gilt-edged theoretical explanation by a therapist forever reacting and "sharing" or "acting out" the response, who can guarantee vindication by a patient grown weary of what could be seen as the "therapist's problems," no matter what the provocation?

Furthermore, some irrational responses look all too rational, or the irrational and rational exist side by side, and it is hard to distinguish whether the therapist is acting on the irrational or the rational response. Indeed, an act such as having to terminate prematurely with a patient can have rational and irrational motives. In fact, we are familiar with a case in which therapy was finally terminated for highly rational reasons, but the therapist could not terminate while knowing he had irrational motives for wanting to stop. He did not want to stop for the wrong reasons. To complicate matters, in the process of figuring out his countertransference, he also came to see that he had irrational motives for continuing, for being afraid to terminate. Here is what happened:

The patient began coming to the sessions full of whatever tranquilizers he could get his hands on. The behavior had been going on for several months, in and out of therapy sessions which were now in their third year. The tranquilizers did anything but calm the patient. Instead, feeling less inhibited, with less felt anxiety about his considerable rage, he was freer in shutting out the therapist and acting out against the therapist.

The patient had no desire to stop "treatment" yet also had no desire to either stop acting out or to analyze what was going on.

The therapist, who had the usual "need" to help, was thwarted in every attempt. An experienced and long-analyzed therapist, he was totally aware of his rage at the patient, not so much for the bulk of the hostile acting out, but for not being allowed entrance. It seemed he could put up with telephone calls from unknown colleagues the patient had "somehow" contacted, who advised him of his misjudgment as to how sick his patient was and who, in bursts of unsolicited supervision, told him he was not really doing his job. And he could put up with rumors circulating "somehow" that the patient was to jump off a 12-story building, which the therapist's building just happened to be. And he could put up with the patient's propositioning a few of the therapist's neighbors, because they were friends and knew about what sometimes happens in therapy from their own treatment experiences. Not that he liked any of it. Not that he ignored it or neglected to take a stand with the patient about all those things. It occurred to him regularly that other therapists might terminate and that maybe he should and that, although he put up with the behavior, he might like living better without it. He clearly entertained the idea of terminating but did not want to do so for irrational reasons. He was not sure yet.

What this therapist could not deal with was his persistent anxiety, his almost literal fear of the patient at times, and a vague feeling of guilt. In supervision he had copious notes, determined to find out what surely he was doing wrong. In each session, it seemed there was nothing he did that could be pointed to as "the culprit." That was the therapist's problem, at least the tip of the iceberg. Here he was doing what was useful, what was therapeutically indicated, and had done relatively the same for the years prior to this period. Yet there continued to be this terrible, seemingly unresolvable acting out by the patient who actively, to be euphemistic, turned a deaf ear to the therapist.

Although both he and his supervisor considered it useful not to terminate with the patient precipitously, to try to ride with the situation for a while, the therapist began to question his persistence, what he came to think must be his masochism, his need to help. It was his sustained anxiety after a time that provided some clues. When he was anxious, he noticed he had a recurring fantasy that the patient would knock on his home door, he'd answer, and the patient would take out a huge knife and kill him. At first the therapist thought the content was reflection of the patient's rage and of his own projected rage, both of which it probably was. As time progressed, however, it became clear that being killed had little to do with rage in itself. Rather, it was seen by the therapist as punishment for not doing his job, not being allowed to help.

Indeed, his need to help filled him with enormous guilt at facing the reality that he, even he, could not help this time. Even though it was better not to terminate at this point, he could not *allow* himself to terminate. Initially, the search for what he was doing wrong was not for the patient's sake alone, it was for his own sake as well, for the therapist's life was compulsively dedicated to making "mother" whole, and in early life he would have truly suffered immeasurably had he not taken on the task. Now, as then, the task meant security as well as satisfaction, and provided a protection against guilt. The powerful mother was still alive and functioning. On some level, the therapist's persistence was reflective of the hope that the patient, his mother, would let him in. This was not the mature hope that Searles (1977/1979) talks about, but the pathological hope that the patient–mother will come around. The fantasy of a reasonably giving mother prevailed far beyond its time for this therapist.

When the therapist was ready to live with the guilt and anxiety of "not doing his job," he could continue to do his job. He then told the patient that he would have to terminate if the patient would not stop acting out without ever trying to analyze it, particularly were he to continue coming "buzzed out" to session after session, and that when the patient wanted *therapy* he would be glad to see him. The patient left immediately, stumbled in front of screeching cars beneath the therapist's window, surviving, but never to return. This represented the death knell of the therapist's fantasy.

In this instance, the rational and irrational existed side by side and at different levels. Early on, were the therapist to have terminated, his response may have seemed rational, but it would not have been. To have terminated would have protected him from coming to grips with his internal state and the process at hand, and it just was not useful for the patient at that point. When termination looked like it might be the necessary, rational approach, he had difficulty with it for the same reasons he felt anxiety and guilt when continuing with the patient.

In retrospect, whereas initially he stayed with the patient for the right reasons and for the wrong reasons, ultimately, when he terminated, he did so with good reason, but suffered anxiety before, during, and after. The fantasy that was dying was that of the chronic helper therapist, the adult–child needing and hoping to fix his mother. The countertransference response inherent in the fantasy roles and the fantasy images, although helpful in explaining what was happening, was terribly distressing.

Did the patient sense the countertransference? It would have been impossible for him not to. In fact, it may have been used by the patient to thwart the therapist. All this seemed to happen when the patient had felt closer to the therapist than he had ever been, and when he could not tolerate the closeness, he reduced the efficiency of the therapist by drawing on needs he saw in the therapist before they became so mani festly obvious to the therapist at this particular time.

Classification of Countertransference

From experiences such as this, several questions may well be raised. Is countertransference always idiosyncratic, that is, is there ever a response to a patient that any therapist is likely to have? Might it then be possible to classify kinds of countertransference? Answers are possible, but complex, as attested to both by the literature on countertransference and our own experiences. Many definitions of the concept exist. Some are similar to others, some bear acknowledged similarity, and some do not. Other definitions are in their own camps, sometimes bringing clarity or adding depth to the concept, sometimes not. It was surely apparent that we had not discovered the concept (that would be a hard fantasy to sustain!), but it was clear that each therapist does have a personal sense of discovery when countertransference occurs. What we did discover was that, as in writings on narcissism, the literature on countertransference is at times written in language so private, so convoluted, that it becomes nearly impossible to follow. Furthermore, many authors seem quite unaware (at least they give no evidence of knowing) that anything on the subject has been written before. They set up their own classification systems that might well be incorporated in or subsumed by others, or at least correlated with other classification systems.

Instead of presenting all major viewpoints or the chronology of the shift away from the "pathology only" viewpoints such as the review done (and so well "translated" in some instances) by Epstein and Feiner (1979b), we chose to abstract and distill consistent ideas, putting them together in such a way as to make sense out of the various, seemingly close pieces that are rarely seen in relation to one another. To this end, we introduce a system of classifying countertransference data, categories we think represent the essence of what many authors say. Our intention is not to add still another definition of countertransference but to bring order and classification to those that exist. Where particular existing terminology would seem helpful to include, we include it.

In the old days, countertransference had one meaning. Now that there are more, there is a danger of promulgating meaningless classifications and nitpicking distinctions of what is and what is not countertransference and in what microcategory the data belong. There continue to be "disputes in the literature over whether countertransference should include all of the analyst's emotional reactions in the treatment situation or only those specifically in response to the patient's transference" (Firestein, 1978, p. 230). So, that is one problem. Furthermore, there are disputes as to whether countertransference should include any emotional reaction of the therapist or only those that interfere with treatment. And then, where does positive countertransference fit in? Can positive countertransference become an impediment to treatment, and if so, how is it to be classified?

To limit drastically the scope of countertransference definition is too simplistic and is probably a carryover of the negative connotation countertransference has had. But with all the problems of comprehending its origins and manifestations, we can understand those who would make things simpler by a limited definition; however, we cannot join them. The therapist is both responsive to the patient and comes into the clinical situation with responses "set to go," that is, there are unconscious images of the patient independent of the patient. Either kind of responses may be triggered during the course of therapy, separately or in some kind of combination, and it is useful to distinguish what comes initially from the patient (as projection) and what comes from the therapist in response to the patient, what comes as a response from the therapist's own inner, irrational attitudes, and what comes as a response to the patient and the therapist's own inner irrational attitudes combined.

All manner of therapist-response is worthy of exploration and understanding, and all could be classified as countertransference. Not that this means countertransference should be broadly defined and left at that. To the contrary, we are proposing a scheme to be both inclusive of the possible responses, and give them some order.

One way to classify countertransference response is to think of it in terms of it being a "universal" response or a "particular" response. The universal response is simply the response *any* therapist would have to the patient, a response based on what the patient brings to the situation that would call out similar reactions from therapist to therapist.

Here it makes sense to think of such responses as the "homogeneous" aspects of countertransference (Giovacchini, 1989), having something to do with certain psychic mechanisms or operations evoking rather consistent, predictable responses from therapists of diverse personality structure and dynamics. Cohen (1952) would point to the "objective reality" of such circumstances, as would Singer (1980), noting that "countertransference interactions always have . . . 'objective' components" (p. 263), as does Armony's (1975) "syntactic level" (borrowing from Sullivan's syntactic mode of experience concept). Winnicott (1947), in a major break with classical definition of the time, speaks of the "objective countertransference" prompted by the patient, a response called out in anyone.

Here too would seem to fit Racker's (1953) "complementary identifications," those therapist reactions felt as one's own; those internal objects or dimensions of the patient that the patient cannot tolerate and so projects onto the therapist, whose objects or dimensions they then "become." (Sometimes there is a projection and they also originate in the therapist; then there would exist both *universal* and *particular responses*.) Searles' (1971/1979) concept of pathological symbiosis contains projective dimensions.

Grinberg (1979) describes "projective counter-identification," a term also to be classified as a universal response. There, the therapist's reaction is "independent of his own conflicts and corresponds in a predominant or exclusive way to the intensity and quality of the patient's projective identification" (p. 234). The universal response, then, originates with the patient as opposed to the therapist, and in one way or another it is a reflection of or response to the patient's internalized objects and patterns of relating.

On the other side, there is the "particular response," that therapist response that is idiosyncratic. Such a response is peculiar to a particular therapist, with particular personality features and problems called out in response to the patient. They are, in effect, the reactions or features that the therapist (as opposed to the patient) brings to the situation although they may be called out by the patient. Racker's (1953) "concordant identifications," the reliving of the therapist's problems and processes stimulated by the patient, fit in this category. Too, Racker's (1953) "complementary countertransference" reaction would be classified as a particular response in that it is a patient-induced activation of the therapist's preexisting neurotic elements to the point that the patient comes to stand for the therapist's internalized objects. The reaction, in other words, would not be likely to occur without the conflict that the therapist brings to the situation.

Also in the category of particular response would fall the "subjective countertransference" described by Spotnitz (1979) and the "fantasy world" reaction of Cohen (1952), based on the unresolved neurotic problems of the therapist, and Armony's (1975) "parataxic level," a fantasy-tinged kind of reality he describes, again borrowing from Sullivan.

Probably the following, which is one of the best examples of the universal and the particular countertransference responses, is a bit extreme, but it should clarify the distinction. It seems that nothing in particular had happened during a certain therapeutic session to explain the therapist's fantasy, but it occurred to her that she suddenly pictured this particular patient, who was mildly talking to her across the room, as shouting. It was one of those flash impressions, those clear images that sometimes came to her but that she could not link to any conscious observation of the patient or the content or theme at the moment or in the recent past. Nevertheless, the impression was there.

At once the patient proceeded to tell this story. As a child, she was at a friend's house for lunch when with only a moment's warning she threw up on the table, neatly though, right in her own place, next to her friend's mother. Obviously annoyed but appropriately concerned, the mother was solicitous, inquiring as to what was wrong, how she felt, and the like. The patient remembered feeling fine after the event. "It was like a big liquid burp and I had a sense of relief," she said, "not at all sick or anything." In fact, she went on to recall that even at the time, she felt sort of casual about the whole thing. And even back then, it ran through her mind that she hated this child's mother while she coolly watched the mother help clean up the mess, though she made no direct association between the hatred and the vomiting. The therapist responded with what could mildly be termed preoccupation. She worried that the patient was angry at her and would proceed to "show her." She wanted the patient to sit away from her fine rug and maybe even in a wooden desk chair instead of curled up in the big stuffed chair the patient always sat in; and on and on.

It so happens that his therapist was, as a child, a frequent vomiter. Starting out as a sign of what today would be called separation anxiety, the anxiety and vomiting came to be used as an expression of defiance and anger as well as anxiety. The point is that behind the therapist's obsessional focus, this therapist, reminded of herself, was reacting to the patient as a reflection of herself, and did not want further reminders. Surely her response would be a *particular countertransference* response.

The probability is that most therapists would not welcome vomiting in their presence; thus one might expect the unwelcome response to be in the *universal countertransference* category. The distaste would not be an exceptional response, but it would be an expected response. Moreover, the likelihood is strong that the distaste is a reflection of the patient's internalized other's distaste. Such an occurrence is not pleasant, it is a mess, and even the most determined of chronic helpers might feel pushed too far.

Anybody might react with distaste and annoyance. However, had the therapist not come to the situation predisposed to the identification she would not have reacted so automatically and so strongly, and she even may not have been so in touch with the patient in those moments before the patient told the story. Certainly too, the therapist's dynamics would have at least a measure of influence in calling out the patient's content, though obviously the patient comes with it to the therapy situation.

As a final consideration, we want to comment on the views of Reich (1951, 1960), who has no truck with countertransference as a useful guide or tool in the therapeutic process, seeing the "problem" as a failure in identifying with and then detaching from the patient, substituting instead one's own feelings for the patient's. Although she sees countertransference as an inevitable event, she sees it as an interference from which therapists must refrain, an emotional response that does not belong in therapy, an indulgence if you will. She holds a classical position, more classical that Freud's, that countertransference is a pathological, never useful reaction, of which to rid oneself. It is certainly hard to know how a therapist could do that in a vacuum. She seems to imply that if countertransference exists, the therapist will absolutely and unremittingly lose control of his or her impulses, acting them out all over the place, never to stop. Rather, she says, better to stay uninvolved or involved in a severely limited way, as if that were always possible or useful. She would suggest a black or white situation where countertransference either runs amuck or is eliminated, never to be observed, understood, and utilized in the therapeutic process and for the therapeutic good. Obviously, we disagree, and we think seeing countertransference in the context of a human normative process such as fantasy provides a useful rationale for our opinion.

Function of Fantasy

Conceptualizing countertransference as part of the more general fantasy experience broadens its scope. To our mind, countertransference can be seen in a fantasy context because it involves an interaction of affective process states and information processing elements, which certainly is one way of considering fantasy (Singer, 1974). Fantasy starts out in childhood as an attempt to process information, to make sense of experience; and in adulthood it continues to serve that function if in a partially more sophisticated way. In therapy, the therapist's countertransference response may determine the content of the fantasy; it provides the substance for the fantasy. In therapy, the therapist's fantasy can serve to help make sense out of that which the patient cannot articulate, to process incoming and existing interpersonal and intrapersonal information perhaps unconsciously communicated through empathy, or information communicated in an obscure way. On the other hand, because of the therapist's possible distortion of incoming and existing data, especially in the affective sphere, the information processing may go awry so that there is little correlation between what the patient has "communicated" and what the therapist has received. Consequently, the therapist's fantasy would rely more on memory and less on incoming data were that the case. Since long-term memory has a function in fantasy (Singer, 1974), and certain affects are linked with certain percepts, there is always the likelihood of the muddying of the current situation with past reflections. Therefore, one has reason to expect that countertransference is inevitable.

The susceptibility to fantasy varies from therapist to therapist and may depend on the match between patient and therapist (Armony, 1975). Besides, regardless of cognitive styles of storage and retrieval of thought (Broadbent, 1958), or how the fantasy would be classified, therapists have at their disposal their own material to tap. Content of fantasy may be the inner expression of business at hand, or as Singer (1975) puts it, "the unfinished business of our daily lives and, more broadly, the unfinished business of our hierarchies of motives and broader fantasy structures" (p. 219).

Although some countertransference always occurs, its existence does not always make itself known to the therapist, for fantasy in any of its forms may be unconscious. Sometimes, the countertransference is not identified but its fantasy "housing" is conscious; sometimes the counter-transference reaction and its manifestation through fantasy are both consciously recognized; sometimes neither the countertransference nor the fantasy is recognized as occurring, as in the case of the therapist first described in this chapter.

The noteworthy thing is that fantasy and its countertransferential content exist, even if unknown to the therapist. Conscious or unconscious, the reactive content can influence the interaction and ultimately be "known" to the patient, if not the therapist. Although it should seem unlikely, sometimes therapists and patients are totally inattentive to their unconscious processes and their behavioral derivatives, as in the therapist–patient described earlier. Such a situation is worth remedying, for it is through conscious attention to images, to associations, to fantasy, to dreams (which can be seen as extensions of wakeful fantasy) that therapists can better understand their reactions, inordinate or otherwise (Angel, 1979). Furthermore, this activity not only helps the therapist directly, it enables the therapeutic work in the unfolding of new dimensions of the patient's personality heretofore not experienced (Eigen, 1979).

The viewpoint of Singer (1975) on fantasy as behavior certainly holds for therapists: "Fantasy or daydreaming is perhaps best viewed simply as a kind of capacity or skill in us that is part of our overall repertory of behavior" (p. 116). However, although we suggest that the therapist focus attention on his or her fantasy, we are not advocating the use of mental imagery techniques for the therapist in private, or with the patient, regarding the therapist's fantasy.

Unlike those who may use mental imagery techniques to "establish positive affects" or for "role rehearsal" or for "advanced planning" (Singer, 1974), we advocate tuning in to inner process as a method for becoming more aware of the complexity of relating. Since fantasies therapists have may be seen as clues to their countertransferential experiences, our focus is on understanding the countertransference through the fantasy, rather than on using the formal enactment of a fantasy as part of the format of therapy as might be expected in certain kinds of therapy such as transactional analysis (Berne, 1964), or gestalt (Perls, 1972), or psychodrama (Moreno, 1947), or in behavior modification techniques (Wolpe, 1969), or in the European use of imagery techniques originally influenced by Jung (1968).

However, some of the results of using fantasy as a tool for understanding the interpersonal process and the intrapersonal selves of the relating therapist and patient are similar to those occurring when mental imagery techniques are used. Attending to imagery and its context of occurrence can assist therapists in using the imagery as a clue as to what is happening inside the self and the patient. Moreover, it can be a clue as to an emotional response, not for control of the imagery or affective reactions as would be done with mental imagery techniques, but more in the original Freudian sense as a representation of emotional "activity" to understand and work with.

Sullivan (1953a) and Singer (1974), from different vantage points, point out that through development, particularly when school attendance starts, people are called on to filter out or to ignore or inattend "private" or fantasy experience in order to get on with business. In one way, this can be a problem in that at times of less vigilance, awareness of fantasy can be startling and frightening. In therapists, the problem can be far-reaching because of the many external stimuli (from the patient) touching off private, internal processes in the therapist. The private material is touched off whether or not the therapist is aware of the process or the content, and in any event, the therapist's behavior is affected. The more tuned-in to the process and to the content of inner response, the more he or she is in a position to make sense of the current interpersonal experience.

Central to our view that the state of the therapist's fantasy is important in psychotherapeutic work is the following theoretical position on perception and imagery set forth by Singer (1974). He says that, "Perception and imagery both are part of a general process of representation of experience" (p. 200) involving: (1) anticipation of new situations; (2) filtering of external information; (3) coding incoming material or "reports" from long-term memory and assigning it to retrieval programs; (4) attributing various meanings or causes to experiences as they occur. And to these we add (5) discriminating between old and new information, for this is the dimension where we think therapists may particularly get into trouble, for it is this relationship that comes into play in countertransference. It becomes clear that whereas in daily life primary and secondary processes are necessary for effective thought (Neisser, 1967), in doing therapy, the strength of the therapist lies in an ability to harness his or her "internal information," the inner, primitive life for use in combination with secondary process (Rouslin, 1975a). In creative activity, which in many respects psychotherapy is, there must be integrative control of the primary process, a special use of primary process (Suler, 1980). Making sense of interpersonal experience is not the exclusive territory of the psychotherapist, although it is certainly an active responsibility. The task actually begins in childhood, through play (Groos, 1901; Winnicott, 1971). Through play, a child learns tactics and techniques for how to get along in the world. And one cannot talk about play without considering that fantasy helps make sense out of the world, that fantasy provides the roles and experiences to be played. Fantasy, then, can be seen as central to future experience, to future life.

Although the classical psychoanalytic viewpoint holds that the origin of fantasy and play is in the need for a tool for dealing with instinctual drive versus reality demands, another viewpoint (Singer, 1975) suggests that play and fantasy games represent attempted solutions and manifestations of the various developmental orientations or levels of the child. The wish-fulfillment function or catharsis function, stressing a primary process orientation, would seem to us to be only part of the story, as would Singer's view, stressing primarily secondary process orientation. Piaget (1962), however, seems to contain both primary and secondary process orientations. He suggests that fantasy is more than a method of discharging the energy from conflict. It represents an attempt to accommodate to the environment, to understand and to internalize through systematic memory operations the external environment. There are then, implicit (at least by our reading) preexisting internal processes that somehow need reorientation, external events; and the secondary process is developed to deal with and make sense of the external world. In other words, we believe that he implies that fantasy activity is a kind of bridge between primary and secondary processes, representing both states.

According to Singer (1975), "results do not support the notion of a drive-reducing function of fantasy, at least on the basis of projective techniques" (p. 111). He thinks that fantasy has a broader role "as a general response possibility," not simply as a replacement for emotional expressiveness. To us it would seem that projective techniques do not tell the whole story, and too, Singer's viewpoint seems limited, especially when trying to understand countertransference response in terms of fantasy.

From our clinical observation, we would conclude that for the therapist fantasy has multiple, related functions:

1. Drive reduction.
2. A defense against emotional expression while at the same time being a representative of unconscious emotional experience.
3. Both a healthy and pathological way to process or make sense of interpersonal events, particularly the affective dimension of interpersonal events.

It is when fantasy is used primarily for indiscriminate drive reduction, or as a defense against awareness of emotional experience and expression by the therapist, that fantasy becomes a pathological vehicle for dealing with interpersonal events. It is then that problematic countertransference reactions implicit in the fantasy response impede rather than facilitate relatedness and treatment.

Therapists' Shared Fantasy

In the broad perspective, the "rescue fantasy" feature shared by so many therapists does little to foster therapy. Indeed, unchecked, that kind of "assistance" is but an expression of the therapist's needs. Surely there is a place for therapists to progress from seeing patients as extensions of themselves or their internalized parents or the internalized relationship pattern of themselves and their parents. Hardy (1979) assures therapists: "When we advance from our earlier zeal to the cooler stance of the seasoned professional . . . we can let go of our past . . ." (p. 78), at least in terms of unconsciously and compulsively needing to use the rescue fantasy as an expression of our own needs. This kind of countertransference expression can be seen as a lack in the ability to discriminate between old and new experience, what Armony (1975) might call a kind of "parataxic level" fantasy.

As Singer (1975) says:

> Most people in the course of the many daydreams they generate are piecing together complex clusters of fantasy that become in effect their view of what "real" and "ideal" human relationships are and ought to be. These longstanding fantasies become the basis for our hopes and expectations. To the extent that they are grossly distorted because our own childhood experience was necessarily limited in scope to a particular family in a particular cultural milieu, we experience painful disappointments and social confusion. (p. 200)

And if the therapist is like "most people" the trouble goes beyond disappointment and social confusion, impeding the patient's development and so, the therapist is not really being as therapeutic as he or she might like to believe. Neither patient nor therapist can truly fit into a given "model" of helper or helpee, though they try.

Just as there is a "love–hate polarity" in the transference (Arlow & Brenner, 1964), there exists the same polarity in countertransference. Each may stand on its own or be a defense against the other. These features operate in life and in therapy as part of life (Strean, 1979). Therapists who are encumbered by their need to help, by their fantasy as an omnipotent rescuer, actually collude with the patient in his or her wish to have only the good, loving therapist, an all-need-meeting therapist. Such collusion aids and abets the continuance of fantasy-as-reality and reality-as-fantasy in both patient and therapist. Moreover, it interferes with the emergence of hateful fantasies representing dimensions of the therapist and the patient, transferentially and nontransferentially, and countertransferentially. Consequently, there is diminished and distorted perception, offering little chance of integration of the good and the bad dimensions of the object and the relationship, an important developmental and therapeutic phenomenon.

Regarding patients, Corwin (1972) has talked about the "narcissistic alliance," a term he attributes to Mehlman. This phenomenon, he says, is seen as an unconscious alliance whereby the patient seeks to gain an unrealistic position through association with the therapist, a kind of magical way of overcoming limitations; a kind of fantasy as to where the patient will end up through the alliance with the therapist. In our opinion, this kind of alliance is ofttimes sought by therapists as well as patients, to the detriment of both. Its very essence spells the eventual demise of an effective therapist–patient relationship, if it can ever begin, for the "fantastic" qualities inherent in the narcissistic alliance are inimical to the qualities we see comprising the therapist–patient alliance.

However, it is our observation that narcissistic alliances are often seen as desirable by the mental health caretakers. Here is a case in point. A narcissistic alliance was what the junior professional staff on a psychiatric unit seemed to want, and unfortunately, the senior supervising staff never identified the situation as problematic.

It happened that one night, a patient, who heretofore in her week of hospitalization had shown no psychotic symptoms, had a fierce psychotic episode. She just about broke up the unit dayroom and anyone in it. Predictably, patients and staff were terribly upset, in the interest of the patient and themselves. So in the morning, the staff planned a meeting with the patients, ostensibly to offer them an opportunity to talk about their distress at what had happened. Instead, there was a diabolical turn of events, a hidden agenda. Quickly it became clear that the staff apparently had decided beforehand that another patient or patients had somehow gotten hold of some kind of drug which had then been given to the patient they never suspected of being psychotic; and the staff wanted to find the culprits.

The "presentation" by the staff (and it can *only* be called that) bristled with not-quite-spoken accusation in the guise of the helpfulness of explaining, repeatedly, why drugs need to be prescribed. In such an emotional context, the staff expected the patients to feel free to discuss their observations of what had happened and their reactions to the patient. When the patients did not speak, some were called on by staff who seemed to be putting words in their mouths, almost insuring that no other patients would talk. But the staff relentlessly proceeded while the patients sank deeper into silence. The despairing tone of the silent patients was leavened only by the acrid, ironic inquiry of one patient who put into words what others were thinking: "Are you crazy enough to think that we would tell you doctors what we feel or if we know anything when you got your minds made up anyway?"

In essence, the patients had caught on that the staff wanted to trap somebody, but more than that, that the staff wanted to engage them in a narcissistic alliance whereby the staff would be seen in the omnipotent position in which they felt comfortable. That way, the staff could confirm that, indeed, they had not missed the boat with the now clinically psychotic patient, and, moreover, it was not through their treatment that the patient had become psychotic. Rather, it was the fault of the patients, and it was the need of the staff to maintain their fantasy of themselves as all-knowing, omniscient clinicians at the expense of the patients, which the patients sensed. The staff clung to their idealized concept of "professional" at the expense of object reality and the patients. The patients would have nothing of the narcissistic alliance needed to help the staff maintain their fantasy, so the staff had a bit of trouble indiscriminately discharging their anxiety by foisting the fantasy on the patients. But only the one patient could articulate their position in any way.

Like frightened captives, the patients were not very good at expressing their thoughts, or would not take the risk in this mixed message environment even though *their* perception was not faulty. Like frightened captives, their immediate innermost frustrations could not be exposed in front of their accusers. And like some frightened captives, they were being blamed for problems they did not create and asked to join in others that would be created. Yet it did not consciously occur to the staff that the patients may have had no hand in the event, just as it did not unconsciously occur to them that they, the staff, may have had no hand in what happened, nor were they necessarily at fault for not predicting it.

Clearly, this was an example of shared countertransference response where the narcissistic fantasy of ominpotent, omniscient caretaker is used indiscriminately for drive reduction, that is to reduce the anxiety related to a situation being out of control. Further, fantasy was used as a defense against the awareness of the experience and expression of the anxiety, and the attached narcissism of the staff was threatened. What could be seen as the failure of the fantasy was blamed on the patients, the fantasy thereby becoming a highly pathological vehicle for dealing with interpersonal events.

Patients in such situations are realistically helpless figures, victims whom the staff try to use for their own narcissistic purposes. Staff in such situations are ambivalent figures, both helpless victims of their unconscious needs and processes and persons given a chance to create themselves anew. The appropriate use of the fantasy would have involved recognition of the need for it, and the recreation of self-images so threatened as to have to engage in such distortions.

FINAL NOTES

In conclusion, the therapist's fantasy and its countertransferential underpinnings are not something about which to cheer or groan, even after reading our examples. We can only hope they will be attended to and tended to so that the potential of fantasy as a "scientific instrument" (Searles, 1975a) can be realized, not as a tool for narcissistic gratification or a weapon for narcissistic acting out, but as a vehicle for helping patients. Therapy outcome, although certainly determined by patient characteristics, is also a function of how well equipped the therapist is to deal with the patient's characteristics and transference reactions (Strupp, 1980). Even if countertransference were always positive, it is now clear (Strupp, 1980) that empathy, warmth, and unconditional positive regard are not enough. The therapist must contribute more than that.

We have tried in this chapter to demonstrate that the therapist's fantasy operations affect not only the patient but the therapist as well. These operations affect not only direct clinical practice, but certainly have a place in how the therapist sees his or her practice. This becomes abundantly clear when a therapist enters private practice as the major, if not exclusive, income-producing source. Often, the pragmatics of the move take on significance beyond their explicit meaning because there appear to be developmental issues of separation-individuation that come up for review as the therapist enters this new developmental era of professional life.

II

The Therapy Process

*W*hereas the therapist's narcissism designates the route to a helping profession, it also interferes with the therapeutic process once practice is under way. In fact, problems in therapy begin immediately if the therapist holds an "irrational contract" with the patient, whereby the therapist has a privately held conception of how things "should" proceed, namely, which therapist narcissistic needs will be met through the process and the relationship, including the "meta-need" that the patient fit in with the unshared, unconscious conception. Since the therapy experience is a natural replication of the original parent–child relationship where supposedly the parent is there in the service of the child, early narcissistic need is expressed by both therapist and patient no matter what the "rational" contract holds. The therapist must be vigilant in scanning his or her current irrational behavior for its unconscious interpersonal roots.

It is assumed that when a therapist is relatively free of irrational need, he or she is freer to recognize, use, and develop theory. Unfortunately, that is not always the case. Seasoned therapists are often reluctant to admit their deficits in theory and its application. Further, they may use theory in a distorted, stereotypic way, force-fitting clinical data into theory never subject to evaluation or refutation. Or, they may proudly go by the seat of their pants, "sensing" or "experiencing," an internally omniscient form of the narcissistic therapist as opposed to the externally omnipotent, grand-theory–design therapist who fits all data into an established unitary theory to explain all behavior.

Our aim is to conceptualize theory development and its clinical use as free from narcissistic need as possible. Somewhat at odds with the conflict-free use of theory are idiosyncratic responses of therapists. Although they are part of personal style and the art of therapy, idiosyncratic

responses hold high potential for becoming ritualized responses to patients. The automatic, idiosyncratic response then, as an unconscious
expression of the therapist's narcissistic need, may become an unrecognized barrier that crops up when least expected. It is only when the
response leads to obvious trouble that it is recognized as automatic and
stereotypic and in need of reappraisal so as not to limit the range of
therapist behaviors and patient potential. In other words, for the therapist, the characteristic way of being oneself may not always work therapeutically. There is a need to move beyond narcissism to scan and
explore our usual responses, responses so part of our being we do not
know they are there until there is an untoward reaction to them. This
need to attend to behavior is inclusive of therapist changes in the therapy
process as well as patient changes.

   Indeed, the patient and the process certainly change the therapist.
The narcissism of the therapist is surely at stake when the "good therapeutic self" is assaulted with anxiety, boredom, anger, eroticism, and
confusion. Can a therapist remain constant? Can a therapist change and
survive or change and return to the original position if need be? A healthy
narcissistic structure is essential to accommodate the uncertainty, openness, and flexibility required for the gamut of change possibilities, and to
attend to the communication at hand. This includes hearing and observing, as elements of listening.

   The therapist's narcissism not only affects the listening process, it
impinges on the understanding or interpretation of what is heard, thereby
influencing intervention. To better understand "listening with the right
ear," we explore the concept of supervision where trouble spots are often
first brought to the attention of the therapist. It is here we see how the
narcissism of all involved parties facilitates or inhibits the listening process essential for effective supervision and effective therapy.

5

Rational and
Irrational Contracts

In this chapter we consider some unusual and relatively unnoticed, yet very powerful aspects of contracts. However, prior
to introducing these, we want to reaffirm "contracting" as a definite
ingredient of the therapeutic process, regardless of the type of psychotherapy. The concept of the therapist–patient agreement, while varying
in degree and content, has received some mention in all our discussions
thus far, and is a very "alive" topic at the present time.

Montgomery and Montgomery (1975) suggest that contracts can
be efficient in that they may avoid wasted time and game-playing for
client and therapist. They can provide safeguards for the therapist and
insurance for the client. They can define mutual responsibilities and
commitments for the patient to try to change and the therapist to attempt
to help the patient proceed in the direction of the change desired. Of
course the power of a contract in psychotherapy is limited by the difficulties mentioned earlier in this book in regard to defining what can, is, and
will be done, as well as certain limitations on forecasting results. But,
although admitting to these limitations, Strupp (1975) has affirmed that
the client has a right to know what the services are, explicitly, and it is the
therapist who has the obligation to be explicit about these services.

He believes that the nature of the therapeutic process, the aims, and
the probable outcomes, all should be specified so that a specific contractual agreement can be negotiated in all these respects. Unfortunately we
doubt at the present time that it is possible to deal with such complex

This chapter was originally published in *Issues in Psychotherapy*, 1982, New York: Brady-
Prentice Hall. Copyright 1982 by William G. Herron and Sheila Rouslin Welt.

issues so clearly. The idea has more difficulties and hidden traps than most people notice. The results have often tended toward polarities. Either we are offered an overwhelming vagueness about what psychotherapy is and does, or we get some attempts to be very concrete, and somehow the whole process appears diluted into "common sense." Neither can be the answer in terms of establishing a useful, working, client–therapist contract.

DEVELOPING THERAPEUTIC CONTRACTS

Initially, the therapeutic process appears straightforward with respect to procedure and goals. A person is paying for services being received and so is entitled to knowledge about these services. An agreement is reached between the purchaser and the service provider as to the nature of the service, the goals that can be set and reached, the procedures followed, and the delivery date. The expertise of the provider and the characteristics of the purchaser govern the substance of the agreement. The two parties now have a contract, which in therapy is usually verbal, but sometimes written.

Interest in contracts has accelerated in the last 15 years. Motivating forces include increased consumer participation in determining the type and process of their health care services and the increased call for the accountability of health care professionals by people in and outside of the professions. More than ever before, patients' rights are inherent in the substance of the treatment contract concept. Yet the contract in psychotherapy is certainly not a new concept. Freud (1937/1964) used the term "analytic pact" in regard to the psychoanalytic procedure. We describe that pact in more detail later in the chapter. It is of course true that at the time of the analytic pact the setting of treatment conditions and objectives was more private, and less specific. Now it is more collaboratively conceived, and is hopefully aimed at greater clarification and facilitation of psychotherapy.

To do this, and therefore to be considered appropriate, therapy contracts should do the following (Hare-Mustin, Marecek, Kaplan, and Liss-Levenson, 1979): specify the methods and goals of the therapy, the duration and frequency of the sessions and of the total treatment, cost and payment procedures, cancellation and renegotiation provisions, the extent of each party's responsibility, and the degree of confidentiality. The exact issues covered will vary somewhat according to the orientations and inclinations of individual therapists and clients.

Specifying procedures, goals, indirect effects, qualifications, policies, and practices are all complicated activities for therapists, yet it seems to us that the difficulties involved are beginning to be underplayed in an admirable desire to protect the consumer. We have repeatedly urged that the profession aim for more accurate, prescriptive therapies, but making an overt contract with a client is only part of that effort. And that part—contracting—is no easier than the other parts.

Some present the making of a contract as though it were the major answer to many of psychotherapy's woes. Morrison (1979a) has been particularly vocal in advocating a consumer-oriented approach to psychotherapy. This has as integral parts the clients' evaluations of services they receive and therapist–client agreements open to modification based on evaluation by both therapist and client. He suggests strong client involvement in problem definition and a clearly understood therapist–client contract. Although we agree with the principles suggested, we believe that there are severe limitations as to what the therapist and client can be certain about in any contract they make.

Morrison (1979b) wants therapists to specify the effectiveness of a particular type of therapy with particular clients under particular circumstances. As we, and others, have said before, we would like that too, but in most instances it is possible only to approximate what will happen. We are painfully aware of the limitations on our own certitude, and we experience these limitations as being shared by most people in the field. What Morrison and other consumer advocates want we do not contest, but we cannot produce it, and we doubt those who claim they can. Beyond that, we feel that such rather exact promises as are desired may currently contain a hidden danger for the consumer. The specific contract may offer a new variation on convoluted therapist narcissism. These therapists may have unconsciously found a way to offer rationally what their irrational desires and needs demand they seek.

Hare-Mustin et al. (1979) appear aware of a number of the problems that cannot neatly be resolved through the use of a contract. In particular, making a contract is no guarantee that certain clients will be able to keep it, or in some cases, depending on their ego functioning, even be able to try. Nonetheless, we see the potential value of clear contracts. Yet, we insist on a balanced presentation that includes the realities of the current state of psychotherapeutic practice. We do not think the contract ought to take on a significance and life of its own, thereby becoming an end in itself instead of being a possible means to an end. We will continue to support the idea of making contracts for the good of all concerned, but it is erroneous to consider that this is a simple undertaking, particularly if we now look at an aspect of contracting thus far avoided.

It is our contention that a contract as most therapists and patients conceive of it goes beyond its rational intention. Actually, Hare-Mustin et al. (1979), in describing and illustrating a patient's right to challenge the competence of the therapist, to disagree, or to criticize the therapist, are implying that there is more to a contract than meets the eye, but they do not say there may be two levels of contract operating simultaneously. We believe this to be the case, and we call these the "rational contract" and the "irrational contract."

From our own clinical work and that of our colleagues and supervisees, we have found that it is something more than the details of a given contract *per se* that become really problematic in the process of therapy. What becomes clear is that there is a level of contract that is irrational, a level often interfering with carrying out the rational contract. Thus we see in operation two levels of contracts, one rational and one irrational. The levels indeed may have conflicting intentions, thereby sending out mixed messages and placing therapist and patient in a most confusing position.

Conflicting levels make for the kind of therapeutic impasses where neither therapist nor patient knows exactly what went wrong or how it happened, but each feels intense and uncomfortable about the experience. Interestingly, this description can also be applied to the pathological dimensions of the parent–child relationship. The subsequent development of defenses to explain, inattend to, or obscure one's inner perception of noxious experience provides the substance for neurosis and psychosis. This is not the aim of the therapeutic experience, at least from the therapist's vantage point, yet it becomes a possibility.

It is with the desire in mind to assure that therapy be a therapeutic experience that we address ourselves in this chapter to the genesis of irrational contracts, suggesting ways in which irrational contracts impede or impinge on rational contracts, rendering rational contracts impotent. To this end we define rational and irrational contracts and discuss related concepts of "therapeutic alliances" and "working alliances." We focus our attention on the irrational contract as the more problematic contract because of its insidious negative consequences and its customary low visibility in contrast to the problems of rational contracts.

Through question, commentary, and presentation of clinical data we will now explore how an intricate combination of therapist need and misconception makes way for the use of irrational contracts. Our aim, as when we discussed the therapist's narcissism, is not to indict the therapist. Rather it is to examine and clarify a process occurring naturally in human experience and inevitably in the therapy experience. By doing so, our desire is to help the therapist increase awareness of the complexity of the patient–therapist experience. With increased perception, it is hoped that the therapist's clinical use of self can be understood and refined in such a way as to be truly therapeutic.

Definitions and Related Concepts

Our definition of "rational contract" presumes a conscious intent and plan. It is a verbal or written agreement between therapist and patient that has four components:

1. What the patient wants from the treatment process, for example, changes regarding personality and behavior, intrapsychic and interpersonal problems.
2. What the therapist is willing and able to agree to or offer to the treatment process, for example, expected changes regarding personality and behavior, intrapsychic and interpersonal problems.
3. Time arrangements, including frequency and length of sessions and duration of treatment.
4. Financial arrangements.

Our definition of "irrational contract" is more complicated. For the most part, it is presumed to take place on an unconscious level. Even if the contract terms are consciously recognized by the user, the idea that the contract has an irrational base is rarely recognized without assistance. There are two related types. Type A has to do with the agreement a patient or therapist has with the other that the other has no knowledge of, and therefore has not agreed to. Further, not only is the establisher of the contract unaware of it or its irrationality at the outset, but the he or she becomes aware of the contract only after the other person breaks it. The contract is held "privately" by either patient or therapist.

The following illustrates what we mean. It is a prototype in kind and complexity, and so it is presented in some detail. A supervisee-patient was reporting to his supervisor that a problem he had not experienced in some time was reemerging. It seems he felt unusually angry with several patients because they were not "appreciating" him. Although they "allowed" him to help, he nevertheless felt superfluous. He said he thought the problem had become worse because of his dissertation, with which he was having a terrible time. On the face of it, the reaction he had to his patients did not make sense, but when he amplified on what he had been going through, the situation became clear:

> I got the proposal done for the last time and sent it out. At first I felt relieved, but then when I went to a party with people from another program they were so disparaging of "my" university I felt horrible. I started to think I looked like hell and about what was wrong with my proposal and how everyone else's was better. I thought they

would be happy for me or at least not criticize my program. Then I
heard a friend had twins and that was the last straw; I felt even more
defeated.

The explanation for what was going on was part and parcel of his
narcissistic tie to his mother, which at this point, he was seeing in every
relationship, including those with his patients. Although this therapist
desperately wanted his doctoral degree, the fact that the desire was his
alone was not enough. First, "who was he anyway," since he could not
receive standing or respect from his family, even with a degree. So
entering into a situation with shaky regard, as he said, "How can what a
nobody does count, anyway?" To have it count for himself obviously
was not enough, for who was *he?*

In addition to everything else, the supervisee–patient had been
having unexplainable anxiety. In fact, on his way to the session he kept
looking over his shoulder, thinking someone was following him. Indeed,
figuratively, it was the mother he was leaving behind but obviously not
quite, for he had a menacing feeling that some piece of bad luck would
befall him on the way. In other words, separating from the symbiotic tie
with his mother, particularly from the struggle to get from her the
confirmation he needed, was occurring, loosening a lifelong grip. But in
the transition to autonomy, he thought he would surely be punished for
breaking their bond. Here he was, relating this to not feeling appreciated
by his patients, when he was "the diligent therapist, working hard and
doing what he should despite the terrible pressure of a dissertation." It
seems that the terms of the irrational contract in operation were: If he did
all he should for the patients, despite personal suffering, the patients were
expected, at the very least, to appreciate him, certainly to let him know
that somehow he was having an impact on them. Obviously, they neither
knew about nor agreed to the terms of such a contract, and therefore, did
not know they were breaking the rules. (It is useful to note that they
could have been unconsciously compliant, which will be discussed in
regard to type B; or they could have negativistically resisted the therapist's demand, neither of which seemed to be taking place. Rather, the
therapist's problem was short-lived enough so that the patients weath-
ered it without too much trouble.)

The irrational contract established by this therapist had a parataxic
basis, as all irrational contracts do. The original contract ran something
like this: If he produced well, surely he would be loved and respected by
his parents. The hitch, really a double bind, was that if he produced *for*
his parents he felt diminished, and so, unappreciated, which was how he
continually felt too in his early years of working with patients. If, on the
other hand, he produced for himself, and so, without parental approba-

tion and appreciation, he was on his own, which was how he now felt with his patients. His patients then, were being asked to appreciate him for far more than their therapy. And as he perceived it, they could not or would not, which at least could prevent them from buying into that irrational contract.

Another example of a type A irrational contract comes to mind: This one was held by the patient and imposed on the therapist. The gist of it was that if the patient deigned to let the therapist in on her life, the therapist was to be thoroughly consistent. Not knowing of the contract and not having agreed to its terms, the therapist made a "mistake" during a group therapy session. She interpreted another patient's behavior in a way different from the way she had interpreted similar behavior of the patient with the contract. Indeed, the behavior was similar, but the two patients' dynamics, needs, and levels in therapy were quite different.

When the event occurred, the contract patient was unexplainably enraged, saying only that she felt betrayed and wanted to leave, *had* to leave treatment. During the weeks following her initial response, she was able to figure out that she had been furious because there existed what amounted to several levels of irrational contracts: If she were to be involved with the therapist, such involvement should not come to her (the patient's) attention. If the therapist happened to have caught on, the therapist should keep the knowledge secret. The therapist, in demonstrating involvement with someone else, was not seen so much as deserting the patient, but as reminding the patient of their involvement, so she could no longer ignore it. Too, since it was so difficult for the patient to let the therapist know her, the therapist was not to become close to any other patient with a tailor-made, "special" interpretation. In addition, for the patient to feel relatively comfortable in putting herself in a position where the therapist would finally be admitted to the patient's inner sanctum, the therapist was to be totally predictable, which obviously she was not.

This very bright patient kept repeating, "How could the same behavior mean two different things?" On an intellectual level she understood the difference a context could make, but on an emotional level, an admonition imbedded in her by her mother of not to let anyone in on her business caused her not to trust any outsider. As a child, when approached by other children as to what she was doing or where she was going, she had told them, "business is business, so please mind your own." Only her mother was to be confided in and trusted. Now, the therapist at once was seen as the transferential mother in whom the patient put her trust and the outsider who proved not to be trustworthy.

During this time, the patient was also very anxious. She dreamed often of her mother locking her in her mother's room. This content pointed to the patient's fear of punishment lest she let anyone in but her mother. Here, yet another irrational contract dimension emerged, which came down to the patient wanting the therapist exclusively, the way her mother had wanted her.

The therapist neither knew of nor had agreed to any of these levels of contracts, nor should she have. The contracts arose spontaneously and proved to be a most useful indicant of the patient's dynamics and progress. Interestingly, the expression of these particular irrational contracts could never have been predicated, although in retrospect their existence seemed logical in an irrational system. For several years, this well-functioning patient had carefully avoided looking at the therapist directly or even calling her by name. She had even said there was no relationship between them. During those years, there had been what now could clearly be identified as a reaction-formation against allowing the recreation of the original symbiotic bond on one level, whereas on another level, there existed a defense against allowing "the outsider" to intrude on the original bond. The protection had now worn thin.

Type B irrational contract is that agreement, quite unspoken, into which therapist and patient have entered in partnership without awareness or acknowledgment on either of their parts. The contract can be initiated by either patient or therapist. To illustrate: A therapist had several sessions with a young man in his first year of college. The fellow could not bring himself to go to classes, even at the urging of parents and friends. He came to treatment reluctantly, quite depressed to the point of having made at least one suicide attempt prior to coming for help. He thought there was no hope for his very disturbed parents to change, there was no hope for his lot in life, or for his feelings to change. He had come to therapy because his parents wanted him to, and although he held no hope for it helping him, he came anyway.

The therapist had been in the business and in her own treatment for a long time, and had very little hope left that she would get gratification from either her patients or her parents. Too, she was aware of the suicidal risk and felt appropriately anxious about it. What she did not realize was that from the first moment of the first session until the middle of the sixth session, with all her emotional growth and smartness, she had been in partnership with the patient, joined in an irrational contract initiated by the patient. It went something like this: "I am depressed, suicidal, maybe even homicidal. If in any way you reach me, I may explode, so stay away. Ask me questions maybe, but don't 'disturb' me. I propose to sit here and control everything that happens here by saying nothing and you are to say nothing, at least nothing of significance." And the therapist agreed. But the therapist's "agreement" was not rational. It went beyond the reasonable, theoretically and clinically based caution one would ordinarily have with such a patient to not intrude, to not push, to not struggle for power. It was an irrationally based agreement. Obviously, it was wise neither to say anything inflammatory nor to force a reaction from this "time bomb" nor to have him set goals for treatment that he volunteered was probably useless anyway.

During the sessions, the therapist began to realize that she felt intimidated by the patient, feeling both anxious when she made even a benign comment and ever vigilant to his response. The anxiety went beyond worry about suicide, homicide, being sued, and all the regular worries. Interestingly, it never occurred to the therapist she could be a homicidal victim of her patient's rage. She apparently was so concerned about the immediate situation that concrete realities took a back seat. Although indeed she felt intimidated by the patient and was not sure why, in the sixth session she forced herself to ask him a question about what qualities in his parents he thought he was reacting to. The patient had just finished saying he was angry at them for certain concrete things they did or did not do and for their doing nothing about fixing their relationship and "cleaning up the house." The therapist's question did not seem inappropriate in level, time, or placement. Yet he claimed he did not understand. A look of disdain appeared on his face that the therapist should ask such an obscure question.

The therapist was to become aware that indeed this sensitive, schizoid young man did understand the question. He understood, too, that his depressive stance had enormous power to control this therapist and make her quake by turning her into a powerless child subjected to the power of her depressed mother. It was not until this moment that the therapist realized the full extent of her participation in the irrational contract and what its dimensions were.

Although intuitively she realized he had understood the question she asked, she rephrased it, not out of need to penetrate or ingratiate, but to give him another chance, lest he change his mind. When he still did not understand, for one second it ran through her mind, "Is a thought disorder interfering? Is his preoccupation with his problems and depression stopping him? Am I really being obtuse?" Simultaneous with these thoughts, she found herself saying, without anger or force but with conviction, "I find that awfully hard to believe. You're really a smart guy." His look of surprise and glare of hatred were unmistakable. The therapist had received the message of the patient and of the irrational contract; and receiving messages was not the wont of this young man's parents. Thus the surprise, and the transferential hatred. In addition, however, the therapist would not be intimidated further into joining in partnership in the irrational contract, adding to the surprise and hatred.

It is only natural that because of the existence of irrational contracts in everyday life such contracts will be replicated in the therapist–

patient relationship. It becomes academic, therefore, and a bit naive, to think that if goals in a rational contract are set, goals will automatically or easily be adhered to. Acknowledging the existence of irrational contracts helps facilitate the treatment process once it has started and may hold lessons for therapists as they debate a wide variety of schemes for contractual agreement with their patients. In essence, we are asking therapists to recognize that irrational contracts are made all the time, throughout the course of treatment, not just initially, so they must look out for them. We are asking therapists to go beyond the rational contract, to notice a deeper dimension of relatedness and communication, not because that is "the analytic way," but because it seems the only way to assure that any rational contract can be carried out. More important, such scrutiny assures that the process is not therapy in name only. In essence, such examination is part of the therapist's accountability.

The Alliance

In one form or another, contracts have been written about for some time. As early as 1893–95, Breuer and Freud (1964) were writing about the patient as a collaborator in treatment, although the collaboration itself as a process was rather taken for granted. There were hints in Freud's later papers that, through his emerging theories of transference and his enlarging on the process of analysis, he was moving in the direction of what might be seen as an early conceptualization of what today might be called a contract. Indeed, Freud (1937/1964, 1940/1964) coined the term "analytic pact."

The major terms of the pact were simple and referred mostly to the conduct of the session. During the session, to the extent it was possible, the patient was to say everything that came to mind. On the analyst's side, there was one essential rule (aside from the abstinence rule, which both therapist and patient were to follow with each other), namely, to utilize the patient's distortion (transference) of him for therapeutic purposes, for "after-education" as Freud put it. Actually, this was more of a cooperative than collaborative effort in that the thrust seemed to be that the patient defer to the therapist–parent by doing, in at least the session, what the therapist indicated, albeit for the patient's benefit. The therapist indicated what to do to help him provide a corrective emotional and intellectual experience. The context for such an experience was respectful, permissive, and growth-facilitating and not really as authoritarian as it would appear. There was, however, certainly an element of "parental" control over the patient's personal life at times.

Although Freud (1916–17/1964) introduced the idea that the therapist in an alliance with the patient became a "new [parental] object" in the process of being seen as the original object, it was Anna Freud (1965) who extended and elaborated on the new object concept as a facilitator of growth beyond the original after-educator and transference-interpreter roles of the therapist. Thus it seems to us, the way was paved for development of the concepts "therapeutic alliance" (Sterba, 1975; Zetzel, 1956, 1966) and "working alliance" (Greenson, 1965; Greenson and Wexler, 1969).

According to Sterba (1975), he coined the term "therapeutic alliance" in 1932, in a paper presented at the International Psychoanalytic Congress in Wiesbaden, although the literature often attributes the term to Zetzel. Whereas at first Zetzel (1956) used the term interchangeably with what Greenson (1965) called the "working alliance," later she distinguished between the two (Zetzel, 1966). Greenson (1965) also initially drew no distinction between the two, but he focused on the nonneurotic relationship with the therapist. Frequently the two concepts are used interchangeably even today, which made our task of finding clear definitions difficult. To make matters worse, variations in the definition of therapeutic alliance and working alliance are anything but consistent and are often couched in jargon.

As we understand it, the concepts are seen by many as the operations involved in the patient's alliance with the therapist. Each concept presents a difference in emphasis for understanding the therapist-patient relationship, but each seems to focus on the patient end. Zetzel (1966) emphasizes that the alliance is based on positive transference. The current relationship is meaningful and potentially helpful mostly in light of the patient's earliest experiences. On the other hand, Greenson (1965) stresses that the alliance is based on the current, nondistorted relationship and the nonneurotic dimensions of the patient's personality that make this "real" relationship possible. Therefore, both authors attest to the positive value of the relationship with the therapist for the progress of therapy, one from a transferential view and one from a nontransferential view. But interestingly, both exclude negative transference as part of the alliance; rather they see negative transference as separate from the alliance; any irrational aspects of the relationship are seen as the so-called "transference neurosis." To us this separation seems artificial in light of the replication of both good and bad parent images in the one therapist-patient bond.

As Arlow (1975) sees it, "Both Greenson and Zetzel establish an artificial dichotomy between external reality and internal fantasy life. Each one sees the need to breach this dichotomy with a bridge of reassurance and interpretation of the so-called 'real relationship.' Both deemphasize thereby the dynamic interplay of the mutual influence of perception and fantasy, memory and reality, past and present" (p. 72). We agree and would add some.

A compromise approach to the problem of defining the nature of the alliance between therapist and patient has been suggested by Dickes (1975), although he too does not see the negative transference as in any way part of the alliance. He does, however, use both the therapeutic alliance and working alliance concepts to explain the therapist–patient alliance. He sees the therapeutic alliance as the full-scale therapeutic rapport including all elements facilitating progress in therapy; "factors as the patient's motivation for treatment based on ego-alien symptoms, positive transference, and the rational relationship between therapist and patient" (p. 1). He sees the working alliance as also operating in the relationship but as more limited in scope than the therapeutic alliance. He thinks the working alliance refers to the healthier interpersonal exchange between therapist and patient and is a reflection of the mature state of many of the ego's functions. Dickes's package is a bit neat and a bit incomplete for us, but we do agree with his idea that the two dimensions of alliance coexist.

The point is, there exists "an alliance" in the therapist–patient relationship promoting emotional development through some kind of interpersonal, emotional process. It is neither Zetzel's therapeutic alliance nor Greenson's working alliance. It is both. These alliances cross and blend and separate from one another, and when seen as coexisting in therapeutic work, each is an integral part of the therapeutic process. In addition, we add that the disturbed dimension of the patient is also part of the alliance. For example, the healthier dimension of an alliance or the positive transferential dimension of an alliance allows the sicker dimension to manifest itself as an integrated part of that alliance—for many patients the forerunner to integration of the good and the bad dimensions of the parent. In operation, it is as if the rational, reasonable, or positive portion says to the irrational portion, "Right, I feel comfortable here with this person, this therapist, to react any way I feel, so here goes, you son of a bitch!"

Our consideration of the illustrations and the definitions of therapeutic and working alliances leads us to conclude the existence of what we will simply call the "therapist–patient alliance" in psychotherapy. This alliance contains dimensions of both Zetzel's and Greenson's alliances but goes beyond them in a few major ways. The therapist–patient alliance as we see it is an unconscious, unspoken commitment on the part of both therapist and patient to allow the emotional relationship between these partners to develop in whatever direction the patient points it. This does not mean the patient or therapist has permission to act out against one another or with one another for destructive ends. Nor does it mean the therapist is free (with clear conscience) to burden the patient with his or her emotional needs. It does mean that at some level, undiscussed and even privately unarticulated or unformulated, the therapist provides a "holding environment" (Winnicott, 1960/1974; 1963/1974) for the patient in which the patient "agrees" to "be him or herself" to the degree possible, and in so doing, uses the therapist in a way suitable at any given point in time to the patient's needs and emotional life. The "uses" include various distortion experiences and nondistortion experiences. The uses are bound only by the patient's capacity and the therapist's emotional and social limitations and those uses could be seen as destructive to the patient or as a patient response to the therapist's own need.

Further, the therapist "agrees" not to retaliate against the patient and if it happens, then to examine the precipitant as a force evoked by or arising not simply from the patient but from the therapist's internal life. In short, the therapist and patient unconsciously agree to stick together while the very forces against a positive alliance are operating. The patient vents rage and empathically communicates anxiety to the therapist. At the same time that it could logically be assumed that such goings on would herald the end of an alliance, there is an unconscious agreement the therapist makes and the patient "learns" about. This dimension of the agreement is that the therapist will not be frightened away by the threat and not be demolished by the mutually shared anxiety. To the extent that the therapist can tolerate this incredible disequilibrium, the patient will benefit with a beginning awareness and acceptance of psychic imbalance and interpersonal imbalance.

We know only too well from our own experience and that of our colleagues and supervisees that what we describe as the therapist–patient alliance is an ideal to be aimed for and one that must be worked on constantly. It does not just happen. Sometimes it does not happen at all. And sometimes it does not happen completely enough to salvage a relationship. Of course, then we lose patients, but we like to think it is possible to learn from these experiences. This is what a contract is about. This is what patients' rights and a therapist's responsibilities are about. This is what being an "expert" and "participant observer" (Sullivan, 1954) and being accountable are about. No terms drawn up by patient and therapist can promise the sort of therapist–patient alliance we have described, for each relationship is different and sets off different features of our dynamics and the patient's dynamics. But the definition can serve as a guide for the growth of the therapist. And if the therapist benefits from the guidance, the patient will benefit, and to that contract we can agree.

Questions and Misconceptions

The use of contracts altogether and what features (aside from time and financial arrangements) comprise them provoke spirited debate among therapists over questions such as this: What if the patient or the therapist breaks the terms of the contract? For example, a patient and therapist contracted for 12 sessions to direct their efforts at understanding why the patient chose the man with whom she had recently broken off after a peculiarly satisfying, yet stormy affair. After the third session, the patient was no longer focusing on the relationship or its meaning, at least on a discernible level. In such an instance, should the contract be renegotiated? If so, with every apparent shift in focus on the part of the patient, should the contract be renegotiated? Could such contract rigidity interfere with the unfolding of the meaning the patient seeks and the development of relatedness between patient and therapist? Is it possible that a therapist's need to negotiate or renegotiate is based on a need, in a most acceptable and benevolent way, to control the process, the patient, and the therapist, thereby establishing boundaries for who is where, who is who, and who is in charge, all in the guise of clarifying direction in the patient's interest?

This brings us to another point. The therapist in the example cited earlier was found to be nodding off at times during some of the sessions. If a therapist breaks his or her end of the bargain, in this case, to at least stay awake in order to raise questions and make comments leading to understanding of the patient's choice of partner, should the patient break the contract? If the patient decides to explore the situation by bringing out in the open the therapist's failure, should the therapist simply attribute it to a response to the patient's drifting off the subject? Or should the therapist sever the contract on the grounds that the therapist has been an obvious failure at performing the task? Perhaps by this time you can see how the questions proliferate and how difficult it is to respond with certitude, which is a major burden for rational contracts.

Perhaps too by this time it has become abundantly clear there is more to this contract business than the written or verbalized word. Adding to the confusion, we have noticed in patients and therapists a certain belief in the magic of words. Here, we are not necessarily talking about psychotics in whom we might expect such thinking. We are referring to a kind of approach to words whereby words are taken as the sole communication dimension, whereby what is put into words is taken as the only reflection of one's motivation, or whereby words are used as a basic outline, the details to be filled in differently by patient and therapist.

In writing about the "uses" of interpretation by narcissistic patients, Rosenfeld (1964) says about interpretation what could easily be said about mutually agreed upon rational contracts. Whereas the patient uses intellectual insight to agree with the therapist, the patient puts the insight into his or her own words in such a way as to deprive the interpretations of life, leaving words bereft of all meaning except that they belong to the patient. So too can a patient or a therapist "use" a rational contract. Each can put the terms of the contract into his or her own system, thereby adding a private dimension to the contract that in Sullivan's terms is not consensually validated.

Akin to the private use of the contract is the capitalizing on ambiguity that is bound to occur no matter how tightly drawn the contract terms. Bion (1963) coined the term "reversed perspective" in writing about distortion or misuse of interpretations. In such instances, the patient and therapist appear to agree on an interpretation but the patient capitalizes on an ambiguity in the therapist's presentation to give the interpretation a slightly different meaning than intended.

In establishing a rational contract, patient and therapist might appear to agree on terms, but one or the other may capitalize on an ambiguity, frequently something not said rather than something that has been said, in order to turn the treatment into what one or the other wants it to be. Often this distortion does not occur until the therapy process is well under way, when the need for maintaining distance may become paramount. It occurs as a defensive operation to hold the other person at bay. It keeps the person from intruding on one's emotional territory, except in a way one deems acceptable, and fits the other person into one's own system so as not to experience the other as separate from the self, and to experience the other as being in the service of the self. In the extreme, the feared dynamic would be that the therapist or patient would be so undifferentiated as to be unable to distinguish between the "outside" and "inside" in Searles' (1963/1965) terms, or the "me" from the "not me" in Winnicott's (1960/1974) terms; or to see that there was not a proper fit between the self and the other (Balint, 1968), that the other could not yield to be there in the service of the self of the partner. So, "fixing" the contract to fit one's system has a primitive narcissistic basis dynamically, a symbiosis to which every patient and every therapist is susceptible.

Then there are those to whom the words of the rational contract make it irrevocable. The goals and procedures are absolute. To such therapists and patients, there is no such thing as unconscious motivation. The stated intention is the only intention. No levels of intention are thought to exist, no conflicting motivations operating. The implication here too is that words have a kind of magic, a kind of structural magic. The existence of the contract assures both therapist and patient that neither person is there for any reasons other than those stated. Such thinking implies that as unconscious motivation emerges, a person cannot have a change of mind without renegotiating the contract. For example, it would seem conceivable that with every shift of intention and surfacing of resistance, more intellectual and emotional effort would be spent on renegotiating to "get the process on a clear track" than would be spent on allowing the process to proceed unimpeded by the therapist's need to keep things straight, to have an exact match between the contract terms and the process experienced. Furthermore, inattention to the therapist's levels of intention and motivation as they emerge promotes proliferation of irrational contracts and is just plain denial.

We come now directly to discussion of possible misconceptions on the part of the therapist, misconceptions that render rational contracts impotent, misconceptions that are at the heart of irrational contracts in that they combine with irrational need, producing irrational contracts. For much of what we think along these lines we are grateful to Sullivan (1954), who, although not talking about irrational contracts *per se*, recognized there were assumptions therapists held, assumptions that served to make for difficulties in the psychiatric interview.

Our understanding of assumptions implicit in Sullivan's work and of his ideas on what he thought the psychiatric interview should be has helped us conceptualize misconceptions we think many therapists bring to the therapeutic situation. For the most part, these misconceptions appear to arise from a narcissistic need. They provide a general context in which various irrational reactions find themselves a rationalized base, albeit a misconceived theoretical base.

A frequently noted misconception is that *the verbal character of communication in psychotherapy is emphasized.* Thus, whereas open communication is often praised as an effective therapeutic tool, in practice, it may be ineffective because it is limited to what is spoken. Yet there is a nonverbal dimension to communication. The nonverbal level may be consonant with the verbal, or, unfortunately, it may communicate a totally different message from the verbal one. Thus, "open communication" as it is generally used, which tends to be in the verbal sense, is not necessarily as open as it would appear or as we might like it to be.

Sullivan (1954) long recognized that nonverbal levels of communication operated in conjunction with the verbal. If there is incongruence between the verbal and nonverbal levels, the discordance will eventually be perceived, and even before it is consciously perceived, it will interfere with the sending and receiving of verbal messages. Communication then, has two levels, as do contracts. The nonverbal level has great significance in determining the quality of and influencing the therapist–patient relationship, just as the irrational level of contract does. The double dose here is that obviously, an irrational contract itself is replete with nonverbal communication. In fact, from a communication standpoint, an irrational contract is a nonverbal pact.

A focus on verbal behavior alone implies that statements have unquestionable meaning. Thus, although "communication is the channel of interchange between patient and therapist" (Wolberg, 1977, p. 44) words mean different things to different people. How often clinicians have noticed that patients of all kinds, from schizophrenics with blatantly psychotic, private usage of public words, to obsessionals with skillful use of words intended to obscure communication, are not saying what we think they are saying. One cannot, therefore, assume that communication is so exclusively verbal or that there is an exact fit in meaning between sender and receiver. In other words, communication must be scrutinized. Although we agree with Wolberg (1977) who writes that the therapist "must be able to subject the patient's communication to selective scrutiny" (p. 44), we would extend that scrutiny to the therapist's communication. The implication of this misconception for contracts is that although words are exchanged in the formation and process of a rational contract, that is all they are. This is not to say that rational contracts are hogwash; it is to note their limitations, limitations that may not manifest themselves until the relationship is well under way.

Would not it be a pleasure if a patient's motivation for treatment was not mixed? Too, would it not be less complicated if a therapist's motivation for being a helping professional was not mixed? As Enright (1975) says, "Motivation is a complex variable [only one] facet [of which] is the expressed willingness to be there" (p. 344). The assumption that patients and therapists do not have mixed motivation is another misconception bringing trouble to the therapist–patient relationship. Certainly, as Wolberg (1977) indicates, without a patient's motivation to relieve personal suffering, it is difficult to treat him or her. Then, says Wolberg, there are "defective motivations" (p. 424), simply "irrational needs" in our language, needs such as projecting hated dimensions of the self onto the therapist, needs beautifully described by Searles (1971/1979) in writing about pathological symbiosis in the therapist–patient relationship, needs such as idealizing the therapist, therapist and patient needs for perfection, power, and so on, which Wolberg seems to imply will interfere with the outcome of treatment. Although irrational needs make treatment difficult, such difficulties are essential aspects of treatment. We see such motivations as part and parcel of characteristic patterns of living and think of the therapy experience as an uncommon opportunity for patient and therapist to gain understanding of these patterns in themselves.

No matter how tightly drawn a rational contract is, therapist and patient needs will be revealed through irrational contracts operating. In

our view, the goal is not to stamp out the needs, these irrational motivations for treatment, so that a rational contract may be designed and the
therapy may "begin." Instead, these motivations become part of the
therapy process itself. Certainly there are virtues in paying attention to
stated motives, virtues to setting a structure, establishing limits or long-
range planning or however one might express the structure and establishment of the rational contract. The issue is whether adherence to the
patient's stated motive, to the contract derived on the basis of that
motive, takes precedence over the patient's initial irrational motive, or an
emerging irrational (or unaccounted for) need to experiment with, to
resist, to act out, to manipulate and control the therapy and the therapist.
Maybe the issue comes down to how much latitude a therapist is able to
give a patient, how much respect a therapist has for the patient's need to
proceed at the patient's own pace and way, no matter what rational
"terms" for goals and process the patient has agreed to. It is, after all, the
patient's nickel.

Speaking of it being the patient's life brings us to an allied misconception—that *a patient must be "properly motivated" to derive benefit from
therapy.* Blanck and Blanck (1974) point out that many therapists are
prejudiced against "unmotivated" patients, yet these patients make up a
large segment of the patients in psychotherapy. Dynamically, such patients show enough of a desire for help to talk to a therapist. But, using
projection and displacement, they display a conscious reluctance to
commit themselves to therapy. In fact, our experience indicates that
therapists feel terribly uncomfortable with patients who may come because they have to, or with patients who really cannot articulate why they
are coming. In either case, the patients would be unable to establish
major elements of a rational contract. Obviously, it is easier for the
therapist when the patient is clearly "motivated" or has an idea of why he
or she is there and can say what is desired from the treatment.

We think therapists react poorly to these patients who can but
"present" themselves for treatment. First the therapist feels anxious and
perhaps angry about being unwanted, not being "allowed" to help by the
patient whose major contribution to the rational contract is to show up.
Second, although there may be good, rational reasons for providing a
patient with information and obtaining agreement through the rational
contract (Hare-Mustin et al., 1979), the therapist's need to define the
therapeutic relationship as a mutual, equal endeavor is not so entirely
rational as many would choose to believe, nor is it done solely out of
patient concern.

The therapist's need for a "motivated" patient is often based on the
therapist's need to assure at least some measure of gratification from
being a therapist to this patient. In addition, the therapist may have a

need for structure in relationships, a discomfort in allowing relationships to proceed in an undefined and unpredetermined way. Too, the therapist may need to control the parameters of the process lest the therapist lose control (which to those therapists worried about such matters would mean the patient would be in control of them).

After practicing for a while, most therapists learn that there may be little gratification derived from patients—any patients—even those eager and grateful for their effort and expertise. Ultimately, a therapist learns not to count on the gratification; if it comes one's way, that's a fortunate experience. They also learn that no rational contract can really clarify the therapeutic relationship. Neither can a rational contract prevent all false expectations and disappointment inherent in relationships, any relationships. Certainly the rational contract cannot prevent all those events with "motivated" or "unmotivated" patients.

In short, we think the therapist's motivation for needing a rational contract with clear-cut goals relating to specific problems may be based on both irrational need and rationality. The former too often has gone unrecognized, helping to perpetuate some unfortunate contracts. This becomes startlingly clear when a therapist works with overtly schizophrenic patients who may not really be speaking our language. In the therapy of potentially mature, adult "neurotics," arriving at a mutually agreeable rational contract would seem a reasonable possibility. It seems unreasonable to assume, however, that schizophrenic or severely regressed patients, or compensated psychotic patients with a high potential for ego disorganization would have sufficient ego functions of self-observation and reality testing to negotiate a substantive rational contract. For such patients, patients who live in a world of pathological symbiosis (Searles, 1971/1979) or defend against pathological symbiosis by living in an autistic world (Searles, 1970/1979; 1971/1979), the fact that they come to therapy can be seen as motivation enough for treatment to proceed, if the therapist can tolerate the ambiguity, vagueness, and lack of order. It is a distinct possibility that this "unmotivated" psychotic is not terribly different under the skin from the "motivated" patient who comes with a million irrational contracts covered over by a beautifully articulated rational contract. The psychotic may be just clearer about the motivation issue!

We are not advocating discontinuing the use of rational contracts. Nor are we saying there should never be exploration of why a patient veers from the contract, although we do think that much of that exploration could be unconsciously designed by the therapist merely to bring the patient in line or to gain control over the patient in a "benevolent" way. We are suggesting that when a therapist starts with the assumption that a patient's motives are or should be "pure," it is not simply a reflection of the therapist's naiveté or trusting nature. Rather, it would seem to be some manifestation of the therapist's need to help at all costs (Searles, 1967/1979), in short, the general irrational contract that "if a patient comes to see me, that patient will let me help." Or, put another way, "if a patient comes to see me, he or she will help me out, be a mother-therapist to me by meeting my need to be helpful."

This brings us to another misconception—that *the needs of the therapist, such as those for personal satisfaction, prestige, and companionship in the relationship with the patient, can be eliminated through the contracting process.* As indicated in previous chapters, therapists have been trying to fool themselves for years in regard to lacking needs. Here we are concerned with the recognition of the effect of those existing needs on the contract. The danger is not so much that the therapist has needs. It is if the therapist does not sufficiently recognize certain needs, needs that may impinge on the patient, burdening the patient to meet them through the therapist's irrational contract that the therapist does not know about, but the patient senses. In that respect, the irrational contract is reminiscent of Winnicott's (1947) description of the parents who cannot accept those self-images reflecting negative attitudes toward their child. The parents try to alter the situation by implicitly or explicitly demanding that the child facilitate a loving parental image instead, but not without cost to the child. The child gets the message that if the child were to be better, then the parents could be better parents, and thereby see themselves as better people. Or as Saretsky (1980) suggests, "Just as in the case of the pathological mother–child situation, the [therapist's] activity often succeeds in interrupting the patient's presentation of self so as to quiet the [therapist's] own internal objects" (p. 86).

An important misconception (held by therapists and patients alike) about the therapist is that, *as an "expert" the therapist is "a purveyor of exact information"* (Sullivan, 1954, p. 12). Whereas it is understandable that this attitude about the therapist is a generalization applied to all so-called experts in our society, it becomes a significant problem if the therapist needs to believe it, if the therapist needs to assert authority, needs to force-fit clinical data into existing theory, needs to impress upon the patient the true–truth. The irrational contract would then be developed on the assumption that the therapist had all the answers, knew the true-truth, and that indeed there existed absolute answers. In that event, the patient had better listen or at least act in a fashion allowing the therapist to impart wisdom.

Although human behavior shows certain phenomena and patterns, and concepts have been identified and developed to explain the phenomena and patterns, in some ways the study of people remains an inexact science. In our estimation that's not so bad. The study of human beings is inexact because there exist multiple variables in infinite variation expressed on many levels. In one sense, the therapist can be a true scientist: When "answers" are found that explain experience, the door can remain open to elaboration and revision of the explanations with further receipt and search for data. Not only does such an approach pave the way for therapist and patient to understand further experiences in living, it aids in the constant growth of theory derived from clinical practice.

Just as it is important to have theory-based clinical practice as opposed to a do-one's-own-thing practice attitude, it is important for the therapist to remain open enough to allow that theory will be revised under the influence of the living situation. Furthermore, at the very least, such an attitude communicates to patients that indeed, when they can be unafraid or undefended against doing and knowing and feeling, they can be "experts" on their own lives, certainly better able to live and to cope with the problems in living.

Many therapists, including psychoanalytic therapists, pay lipservice to taking note of and working on their countertransference reactions. Although we will discussed countertransference at length, here we want to point up a major misconception based on what too often seems a fear of really understanding what countertransference and transference are all about. This highly unconscious misconception seems to be that *parataxic distortion can be ignored without consequence to the therapist–patient relationship in general and to a rational contract in particular.* In actuality, every relationship and therapy process is affected by it, even if the type of therapy does not focus on understanding the distortions.

Sullivan (1954) puts it well when he says,

> Parataxic distortion is one way the personality displays before another some of its gravest problems. In other words, parataxic distortion may actually be an obscure attempt to communicate something that really needs to be grasped by the therapist and perhaps finally grasped by the patient. Needless to say, if such distortions go unnoted, if they are not expected, if the possibility of their existence is ignored, some of the most important things about the psychiatric interview may go by default. (p. 27)

Although Sullivan seems to be talking about the patient's parataxic distortion, what he says applies as well to the therapist. In short, we are affected by what the patient brings to the therapeutic situation and by what we bring. It may be entirely possible for the therapist not to notice those influences, but it is absurd to think the process remains untouched, unaffected.

That distortion occurs then, is only natural on both sides. It tells us something about the interaction, about what makes each person tick, about areas of response and living that are peaceful and troublesome. Consequently it is not the fact that parataxis occurs that is the issue. It is whether the therapist recognizes it, how he or she uses it or does not use it, that is of primary importance. The hope is, in psychoanalytic psychotherapy in any event, that the distortion will be harnessed in a way to promote understanding of patterns of experience and to facilitate the growth of the therapist–patient relationship as an emotional model for other relationships.

Just as parataxis goes on, so too will irrational contracts, for this kind of distortion of experience is central to the needs expressed through irrational contracts. The distortions may be a projection of dimensions of the self or of parents. The occurrence of distortion is as great, if not always of the same quality, in therapists as in patients. And why would it be different?

Transference and countertransference phenomena are "set to go" even prior to the first visit to the therapist (Adatto, 1977). Adatto calls them "preformed transference expectations . . . more often out of awareness [that] surfaces throughout [therapy], beginning with the initial interview" (p. 12) Therapists have a professional obligation to remember that when they establish a rational contract and when they and the patients hit snags in fulfilling the contract. It is safe to say that these preformed transference expectations, these distortions of present experience in light of past experience, this interpersonal expression of intrapsychic experience being relived and expressed interpersonally as it was in the past, constitute the substance of therapy, but they are also the fuel for irrational contracts. Unless irrational contracts are acknowledged and examined by the therapist on his or her own, and by the patient in the treatment situation, we have little hope that either therapist or patient will be able to come to terms with the image of a relationship as each wants or needs it. Unless this can happen, one is ruled by one's parataxic distortions, by one's original symbiotic bond. True individuation and emotional separation become impossible.

Sullivan's work with schizophrenics and Searles' work with and writings about the quality of the therapist–patient bond in the therapy of schizophrenics has forced the field to go beyond old definitions of such concepts as therapeutic alliance and working alliance, with their narrow range of application. We see that as good and have been influenced by this kind of flexibility and receptivity to experiencing and rethinking clinical experience. When existing concepts do not jibe with clinical observation, the object is to study the situation in a way as to make sense out of what is going on, to try to conceptualize in order to help.

Anna Freud (1976), in discussing changes in psychoanalytic practice and experience, writes of how the widening scope of psychoanalysis in treating many conditions for which the original techniques were designed (and certain concepts formulated) caused a terrible strain. Therapists had to confront "significant changes in the therapeutic atmosphere governing the analyst–patient relationship and, thus, unfamiliar problems for which they had not bargained" (p. 258).

In treating patients there are always problems for which therapists do not bargain in the rational contract, so they manifest themselves through the terms of irrational contracts. Just as clinicians such as Sullivan and Searles have abandoned that classical theory and technique that was not useful and have instead formulated new conceptions and techniques, so too let us not hold on to new conceptions such as the (rational) contract as today's therapeutic model, a shibolleth not to be revised or discarded or reconsidered in light of other formulations such as the irrational contract. Conceptions must fit clinical data, or they haven't much meaning for our clinical work.

6

Theory Development and Clinical Applications

This chapter is prompted by our impression that a major source of therapeutic ineffectiveness is a lack of knowledge by therapists. Although therapists will concede that mistakes may be made because of the human failings of therapists, these are generally ascribed to emotional, countertransferential sources. For example, a therapist may be seen as overly responsive to a patient's dependency because of his or her own rescue fantasies, or a therapist may be seduced by a patient's manipulations because of fear of retaliation. These are considered understandable errors that, although not admired, are quite admissible and traceable so that a remedy can accompany their discovery.

In contrast, ignorance is a far greater narcissistic injury than a countertransference, so it is less readily recognized. Experienced therapists are very reluctant to consider what they have not learned or do not know about theory and its application. Neophytes can admit to relative ignorance, and continuing education is acceptable from time to time. However, many experienced therapists like to believe they know what they are doing after (or because) they have been doing it for some time. Length of time in practice or professional status become equated with a more complete knowledge base than is warranted.

Granted, most psychotherapists will attempt to inform themselves about treatment procedures when confronted with an issue that they see as clearly out of their current range of knowledge. However, there can be reluctance to have such vision about competency. More common is the establishment of a chronic comfortable relationship with certain psychopathologies. This comfort is thought of as part of knowledge and competency. The therapist's theory becomes whatever he or she does, with limited reevaluation. The articulation of theory and congruent technique become thought of as unnecessary. A large number of therapists are on-the-line workers, not prone to listening to other therapists or to explaining themselves. They simply act with the apparent validation of their competence based on the continued existence of their practice. The current emphasis on marketing services within a competitive environment increases the focus on action without a corresponding concern for the learning and relearning that really support effectiveness. Theoretical orientation is self-designated with a personally negotiated meaning that may come to have only a remote connection to current developments in the nominated orientation. Also, the technical maneuvers, such as the use of free association, position of the patient, and session frequency, may pass for theory in the minds of its users.

As theoretical updatedness gets neglected, so the therapist slips into ignorance and increases the possibility of doing ineffective work. Considering the extent to which most therapists become caught up in what they do, the neglect will usually be insidious. After all, therapists do have baseline training that, although varying in length by difference in speciality, tends to be at least appropriate to initial designated areas of competence. Continuing education and specialization are further possibilities, but new learning often tends to be practice-oriented, coming about when problems appear. Although practice and theory are designed to be partners, doing what appears to work frequently takes precedence over understanding thoroughly the reasons for techniques or their possible ramifications. Theory construction, development, and revision are left to a minority of psychotherapists. In addition, a number of therapists disdain theory as an obsessive intellectual exercise divorced from clinical reality.

The neglect of theory is understandable in terms of short-term expediency, yet such neglect can become lifetime ignorance. Whereas therapists may often be unaware of what they do not know, and certainly do not intend to harm their patients, the current state of affairs is unacceptable. Limitations in theoretical knowledge are overlooked contributors to psychotherapeutic ineffectiveness that can and should be remedied.

Lawrence Friedman, in a substantial and compelling treatise on the structure of psychotherapy, states: "Theory is needed. It is all that distinguishes the therapist from the rest of humanity" (1988, p. 533).

The context of Friedman's comments is the uses of theory in psychotherapy. These include: the mechanics of change in psychotherapy, such as the use of insight; assurances for the therapist that there are definite perceptions, that some objectivity can exist in the process; and, the most common usage, to give order to what happens.

Theory is both an explanation and a demand. It has assumptions, termed metapsychology, and then these wait for validation. Failing validation, theory should be modified or retired. A number of things seem to happen in this regard. One is that theory is applied as once learned and not considered subject to revision. Another is that theory is apparently revised in terms of technical changes but the therapist remains unaware, or unacknowledging, of any theoretical alterations. A variation on these possibilities is that techniques masquerade as theory, so that the therapist comes to believe that by doing the same things over and over again theory is both viable and clearly understood. Actually the reasons for the techniques may have long since been forgotten or become invalid.

All of these abuses of therapy appear to be represented by what Peterfreund (1983) has termed "stereotyped approaches." Such approaches are characterized by rapid and far-reaching initial formulations that do not seem to be subject to revision. In turn, patients are "shaped" into the formulations, with patient data selectively attuned to so that a fit has to take place. All patient objections are viewed as resistance to the correct conceptions of the analyst, and the resistances are also interpreted according to the original formulations. Thus, "an oedipal problem is an oedipal problem is an oedipal problem, etc."

Although practitioners of stereotyped approaches are not so dogmatic as to avoid saying that their theories are more than hypotheses, they seem quick to believe in and insist on the accuracy of their hypotheses. Their patients are scarcely partners in the development of the hypotheses, but merely suppliers of confirming material. Some refinements undoubtedly take place, but ambiguity, uncertainty, and ongoing revision are rare. The result is circular, self-confirming work that particularly ignores the uniqueness of patients and the role of patients as true working partners in the therapeutic endeavor. Such therapists have a theory, but they misuse it, particularly distorting its purpose and limiting its growth, and in turn doing the same thing to themselves and to their patients.

The narcissistic appeal in such approaches is their certainty, their protection from confusion and error on the therapist's part. There is an appealing dogmatism about such theorizing. Once past the possible uncertainty of initiating the formulation, which is less of a problem as one gains knowledge through experience, a formula is put into place, and if it does not work, the patient is at fault. That such certainty exists in the therapeutic situation ought to be seen by now as nonsense, but often it is not, and in fact may get deified as "classical" or "original" theory, equivalent to "truth." In this regard Peterfreund comments about the actual practice of an established classicist: "His clinical hypotheses can never be subject to refutation" (p. 42).

At the other extreme lie the eliminators, and as Friedman (1988) has indicated, there is no shortage of theory bashers. These range from revisionists, "clinical" theorists, and minimalists to nontheorists. As an example of how far this approach can be carried, one of us, when a candidate in a psychoanalytic institute, asked an instructor who seemed particularly "free-floating," what his theory was. He replied, "I have no theory."

However, what he did have was patients, some of them analysands, and students. Several then asked, how did he do it? He replied, "Experience, a sense of things." No one pursued the issue further, but we were less than impressed. A new form of narcissism, the therapist as internally omniscient, was offered in place of dogmatic formula. Of course other revisionists have been less radical, recognizing and building on the body of existing theory as well as challenging it. They are responding to the ills of stereotyping and embracing the idea that theory is meant to be tested. Sometimes this has resulted in a new area of focus, such as preoedipal relative to oedipal, or stages of the development of object relations that in a fashion parallel stages of psychosexual development.

The relatively slow pace of change often disturbs therapists, and many times that leads to such a narrowing in the revisionist's emphasis that history is neglected in an attempt to give birth to a new and better psychoanalysis. The typical progression is described by Gedo (1986) as follows. A neglected part of clinical theory is apparently discovered and turned into a new type of pathology, which then has a rippling effect so that all pathology appears to be embraced within the classification that in turn becomes the linchpin of a new psychoanalytic theory. That theory moves in the direction of becoming the generic psychoanalysis, until critics raise questions about such generalization, and discovery and revision start once again. As Gedo points out, such a pattern repeatedly results in a lack of consensus, and so therapists remain heterogeneous in the revisions.

Add the amount of clinical information presented to the complexity of theoretical development, and it is easy to see why there is a tendency among therapists to establish some type of theoretical beachhead, even if it still leaves the therapist really tossing in the waves. Theory offers identity and fraternity, certainly more than passable narcissistic supplies, even though all theories have their critics.

Theory criticism is far easier than theory construction, but that does not reduce the necessity or validity of appraisal. We know of no psychoanalytic theory that is free from limitations. Drive theory is probably both the most abused and used, particularly as a point of origination for theory development. Ego psychology has the taint of mustiness and disuse relative to object relations theory, which in turn appears to have its own areas of neglect. Self theory, the current controversial contender, is experiencing its own personal round of continued evaluation (Rubovits-Seitz, 1988).

Given the admitted state of diversity and probable accompanying confusion, numerous solutions have appeared to try to satisfy the need for theory. In addition to the "classicist" and "no-theory theory" approaches already described, it is possible to choose a theory that appears to have the fewest limitations and/or the greatest probability of ultimately being *"the* theory." Also, many people select the theory that affords them the greatest degree of personal comfort. This may mean they experience it as translating well into clinical practice, or they like the sound and status of being called, for example, an "interpersonalist." Security in a theoretical position can also be enhanced by avoiding and ignoring what other theorists are promulgating. Another possibility is to use a smorgasbord approach, although that contains the dangers of unexpected contradictions. Greenberg and Mitchell (1983) suggest that attempts to mix models and somehow develop a consensus have not been successful. There are also "theorizers" who offer pathways to clarity regarding all theories without necessarily providing the details of a complete theory. For example, we have the description by Peterfreund (1983) of psychoanalysis as heuristic process, or the descriptions by Gedo (1988) of the problems of deficit and repetition, or the work of Schafer (1983), to name only some of the more influential writers in this vein.

As a psychoanalyst or psychoanalytic psychotherapist, one is trained within certain theoretical boundaries, and an impression is usually given by the trainers that the theorists outside of what is being taught are less than accurate. This is an understandable approach to training, but if the spirit of inquiry is indeed to be fostered, then an openness to other possibilities certainly can and ought to remain alive. The renewal of interest in people such as Otto Rank (Menaker, 1982) and Melanie Klein (Caper, 1988) are examples of how this occurs, as well as the writings of a more contemporary theorist such as George Klein (1976).

Our concerns are that although psychoanalytic training, to be practical, will have specialization, exposure to a great variety of psychoanalytic thinkers needs to accompany the focused learning. In addition, practitioners need to carry out a process of theoretical reappraisal throughout their careers. However, our most basic concern is that whatever one claims to be, theory is indeed understood and practiced in accord with that understanding. We believe such is too often not the case. Instead, theoretical atrophy occurs, many times unwittingly and without recognition. The result is the inefficient, less adequate, and less effective practice of what is being called psychoanalytic psychotherapy.

The preceding comments are of course not limited to psychoanalytic therapy and theory, but all psychotherapies and their theories. Our conclusion that therapist ignorance is more of a problem than is generally acknowledged is, we admit, an impression developed over considerable time and lacks "hard-data support." There is no *psychotherapist test* for experienced therapists, but we know many therapists, and we have had experience with patients of other therapists, so that we have developed an awareness of a knowledge gap that appears to us to be restricting the effectiveness of psychotherapy.

Lest this appear as an indictment of others in contrast to our own attitude, we emphasize that it is an understandable problem, for the many reasons already cited, but one that still needs to be recognized. Then, too, we recognize the problem well because we have seen it in ourselves. At times we have been complacent with our supposed knowledge only to have our heads turned by the word of a colleague, a patient's reaction, what we read in a new, or old, book.

At this point, we are ready to consider specific developments in theory. The focus is psychoanalytic theory, with the aim of proposing a blueprint continually open to specific modifications. The map we currently draw we believe must continue to be redrawn, yet at the moment it provides an estimate of current knowledge and possibilities that can translate into effective practice. First, we will consider theoretical development and then focus on clinical application.

THEORY DEVELOPMENT

In discussing the development of theory, we are selecting what we consider areas of major concern, recognizing that others might well construct a different list. For example, Issacs (1988), in a brief article on affect theory, also includes as issues for exploration REM, frequency of sessions, the anxiety process, and differentiation of narcissism. The point is not his list, or ours, or yet another person's, but that questions exist, hypotheses are formed, and theory is put to various tests in terms of logic, supporting data, and applicability.

Psychoanalysis is historically and currently a developmental psychology stressing the effect of the past on the present but also seeing development as reciprocal interaction with the weight of relative influence subject to variability. It is a theory of *ongoing* development, although the past may seem disproportionately dominant in the psychoanalytic model. Of course the past has the lure of causality, of explaining an apparently unexplainable present, and it is hard to discover, yet it is discovered in the context of the present analytic setting. The patient's memories of his or her mother as depicted in the words of an analytic session are *now* words, and the portraits of remembered scenes and figures change again and again, so that there will be new versions of the truth as already found yet only to be rediscovered. Any analysis is just a developmental fragment, even if it is lengthy. Discoveries have relative stability, although the process of gaining and using intellectual and emotional understanding certainly has the potential for permanence.

As a psychology of an unfolding developmental process, psychoanalytic thought is open to many directions and emphases, with understandable contention as to what really matters. The work of Pine (1985, 1988) is particularly helpful in gaining perspective on the leading challenges for the psychoanalytic title. He suggests four major psychoanalytic psychologies of drive, ego, object relations, and self. They are embedded within theoretical systems of the same names, and it is there that they vie with each other for dominance, particularly in regard to motivational concerns and corresponding areas to be addressed in treatment. However, Pine emphasizes the conceptual separateness of these psychologies and the applicability of all their emphases to clinical work. Furthermore, he makes the point that they are all psychoanalytic, and in so doing illustrates a psychoanalytic core.

Thus, a distinguishing feature of theoretical identity, and in turn knowledge, has to be certain defining characteristics. For psychoanalysis, Pine suggests psychic determinism, unconscious mental functioning, primary process thinking, the significant influence of interconnected early, bodily based, object-related experiences, and the importance of conflict, repetition, and development. He also mentions the technical aspects of listening; working with resistance and transference; and neutrality, anonymity, and abstinence. Although not claiming to produce an exhaustive universal group of criteria, Pine is making the point that there are many perspectives to psychoanalytic work, that these viewpoints all have utility, and that one is not inherently superior to another by virtue of being "more psychoanalytic."

In our view the psychoanalytic identity does not rest on adherence to drive theory, or any of the other possibilities mentioned, but in a belief in a psychoanalytic view of how people function. This emphasizes the existence and influence of the unconscious as well as the importance of developmental influences in creating and shaping personality. It is understood that there is an interaction between constitutional and environmental forces in this process. Principal motivators appear as drives, needs, and wishes operating within a context of affects and object relations. Developmental difficulties are the source of mental disorders, and overcoming them leads to mental health. The psychoanalytic therapeutic process requires the creation of an environment in which there is opportunity to discover and learn about the operation of previously unconscious factors. This requires the use of an associative process on the part of the patient and an interpretive one by the therapist. The concepts of transference, countertransference, and resistance are integral to the therapeutic work. There is a metapsychology with a variety of concepts used to provide contextual understanding. The ultimate goal is the translation of intellectual and emotional insight into constructive action.

This is a general outline of the psychoanalytic view, and it may well be subject to criticism as either being too inclusive or exclusive, but our impression is that most psychoanalytically oriented people would be comfortable with it. The specifics are another matter, and they are definitely of interest. First, the degree and manner of unconscious influence remains subject to study. What we do know is that such influence exists and appears powerful but is certainly subject to individual variation. That point is unflagging and restricts generalization. In any given instance, an analyst may be aware that the patient is unaware, and therapists have learned a number of things about how the unconscious operates, particularly the presence of primary process thinking, but the unique aspect of a person's unconscious content and operations remains in each case to be discovered.

The same can be said regarding the developmental process. Again there are normative data such as when people usually start doing important things that are observable, as walking and talking, as well as more inferential information, for example, the formation of concepts. Certainly a wealth of information has been provided by developmental research as well as clinical work so that the complexity of developmental influence is now more apparent, with a particular emphasis on early development. Although the nature–nurture controversy is by no means solved, an interaction is evident.

Constitutional factors that tend to be assumed are capacities for pleasure–unpleasure, manifest in the broad based categories of sexuality and aggression embracing drive–affect–object triads, and capacities for psychic structuralization, manifest in the self, ego functions, and the superego, as well as those for physical structure and genetic endowment. Environmental factors include external happenings and society's rules and institutions, but the major focus is on significant others, particularly family and the interpersonal world that is subsequently created. Although it is understood that there is an interaction of heredity and environment, in practice we tend to focus on the environment since it is accessible for the therapeutic process. It is a mistake, however, to lose sight of the interaction concept and become exclusive in theorizing or in practice.

In the same vein, at the moment we see no evidence to support the dominance of one or the other psychoanalytic ways of theorizing about psychic experience. As Pine has stated: "There *is* hierarchichal organization in every individual, but this is a matter of personal history and not general theory" (1985, p. 16). This means a therapist's preference for a particular theory's importance is based on personal taste, experience, and conviction rather than on an unequivocal body of evidence or consensus.

Where does that leave us, or anyone for that matter? The possibilities remain of choosing a particular theory, such as drive theory, and operating within its boundaries, or using the different theories as perspectives of emphasis to be varied depending on the patient in analysis at a particular time. In the first approach the other perspectives are not ignored, but they are considered secondary. Thus, in drive theory, the objects serve the drives, whereas in object-relations theory, the drives serve the objects. The focus of the analyst is seen as the same as that of the patient from the outset because the analyst assumes a position of correctness before the patient is even seen. It must be emphasized that such a position is not whimsical but assumed out of conviction based on an interpretation of the evidence for the theory.

For example, Klein (1983) maintains that ego psychology has failed to be consistent with key propositions of Freudian theory, that there appear to be inconsistent ego psychologies rather than a consensual psychology, and that libido and aggression are redefined and transformed radically in the process, but not for the better. Klein depicts ego psychology as "a smorgasbord of Freudian concepts where one can take what one likes and leave or change what one doesn't" (p. 508).

Sternbach (1983) has a similar criticism of object-relations theory, and actually he and Klein appear to disdain both object relations and ego psychology. As already noted, self theory has numerous detractors, so it is certainly possible to conclude that drive theory is really the answer. However, the same probability exists in regard to the other theories as well, since in varying degrees, they oppose drive theory and each other. To complicate the matter still further, some theorists, such as Blanck and Blanck (1986), tie the theories together in such a way that they appear to present a logical elaboration of what Freud really would have said if he had time. Such an approach has an even greater appeal than adhering to one theory because it does not require disproving or even disparaging other theories. However, it does involve considerable reinterpretation that is not extremely convincing. It appears that the logically consistent position is to protect the boundaries of one theory by limiting elaborations and keeping revolutionaries off of one's coattails. However, such an approach may have little to do with the validity of the theory and offer little or no chance to test hypotheses because there is an overwhelming need to act as if one already has such validation.

It is pertinent to add here that it is difficult to categorize accurately when it comes to psychoanalytic theorists and theories. Classification is of a rough order based on enough similarity with tendencies toward overlooking or reinterpreting apparent differences. For example, it is possible to say that Sullivan and Winnicott have more in common than they have apart, or that they are more akin to each other than to Freud, and so based on their interpersonal emphasis, they are object-relations theorists. There is truth in that, but it does not at the same time provide a coherent picture of an object-relations theory because of the differences that exist between Sullivan and Winnicott and other object-relations theorists.

Also, ego psychology as originally formulated by Hartmann as well as by Anna Freud appears very similar to drive theory and, thus, really not that much of a separate theory. Ego psychology as formulated by Blanck and Blanck seems to be something else entirely, as already noted, moving in the direction of an object-seeking motivational theory. Object-relations theory appears to aim at changing the basic drive theory formulations of libido as pleasure seeking and aggression as destructive into libido as object seeking and aggression as constructive. This approach is not in accord with Freudian metapsychology, so the connections to it that are customarily attempted are strained. Also, the comprehensiveness of object-relations theory, particularly as it is represented by the British School, who should get credit for the name, is limited in comparison to drive theory. The latter also has numerous detractors, since object-relations theory, self theory, and ego psychology to some degree arose as expressions of dissatisfaction with drive theory. Some of its more problematic concepts are the death instinct and psychic energy. Self theory is even more of a one-horse approach than the other three possibilities and, in turn, is limited.

None of the above comments mean that a particular theory is true or false, but there is a clear indication of disagreement among psychoanalytic theorists. Since it is with some caution that analysts say or imply that Freud was wrong, most theorists try to keep connected to what he said. Often when they want to disagree, they ignore or reinterpret a Freudian explanation, and thus stated loyalists remain. Implicit, however, in the current development of psychoanalysis is that Freud made mistakes. It is also possible that had he lived longer he would have changed his mind about a number of issues, just as he did while he was alive. Examples of this include the switch from the importance of actual trauma to fantasy and the changed role of anxiety.

Since the spirit of theory development requires hypotheses testing and reevaluation, permanent oracles are doubtful and certainly not necessary. The problem with the theories mentioned is their insistence on exclusivity in regard to being the essence of psychoanalysis. It is an understandable urge, for theory development is indeed difficult, and since it is in search of truth, it is painful to remain tentative. Yet tentative therapists will have to be, the whole truth still being quite elusive. Our theoretical connections are based on what each of us believes is the best answer at the moment, but certainly not the final or exclusive answer.

Of course we will always be in awe of Freud and notably impressed with theorists since then, such as Sullivan, as well as more contemporary theorists such as Kernberg. However, we are not ready to accept any one of them or any one school of psychoanalysis exclusively and without the reservation that our spirit of inquiry remains free and very much alive. Does that then mean we are after all promoting definite eclecticism? Not really. What we are suggesting is the knowledgeable yet questioning use of a theoretical position that appears most accurate right now. Specifically, one of us is inclined to favor drive theory, with the belief that an appropriate theory of ego development, object-relations, and self-development is contained therein. The other takes a similar approach, but interpersonal relations are the main theoretical construct. This means we will look at the same clinical material from different vantage points and have a different slant to our interpretations, but we still tend to be more alike than different. Our approach to the particular theory is broad based, open to the complexity of personality, and moving toward some type of integration.

Two strands of thought are prominent for each of us. One idea is that there usually are dominant motivators, but whatever one calls them, they are broad and open to dilution. For example, the libidinal interest in objects can be seen as part of the libidinal drive from a drive-theory point of view, but libidinal interests can be construed as positive cathexes allowing for a large variety of object relationships that are valued by the person. This libidinal drive, however, is the focus rather than the interest in objects or the objects themselves. Conversely, a relational point of view emphasizes the relationship and the objects but is also open enough to consider the drive aspect of the interest. Thus, similar ground is covered but with a different view about the origins of the motivations.

The second conception is based on people varying their interests and capabilities to explore different types of psychic material. As a result, rather than attempt to force a fit to us, we try to work at a level that accommodates the patient. The material then does not always conform to our presumed emphasis in terms of both content and interpretation. We see this as the patient developing one way of understanding that is helpful, although we may think there is yet another way that is still a more satisfactory explanation, but the patient seems to "catch on" only in the one mode, not necessarily our preferred one. In essence, some patients seem more relational, others more drive-oriented. This kind of clinical finding raises a question for us. Although, for example, a thera pist may be able to conceptualize a patient's primarily relational approach in primarily drive terms, if the patient cannot do so, is such an exercise on the therapist's part of value? It ensures a type of theoretical consistency, but perhaps it is the therapist who "doesn't get it," not the patient.

Thus, an ambivalence on our part exists in regard to theoretical conviction. We would certainly like to be consistent, comfortable, even secure in our specific theoretical position, but we are only relatively so, and we expect to remain in some discomfort. Reformulation of motivational concepts continues to be an ongoing process (Freedman, 1984; Parens, 1984) and belies definitive, and particularly reductionistic, formulations. As a result, we find ourselves moving more in a direction suggested by these comments from Pine:

> There are indeed four psychologies *of psychoanalysis* . . . they do not simply fit into the traditional confines of psychoanalysis. Rather, they require us to see psychoanalysis not only as a psychology of *conflict*, but also of *repetition* and of *development* . . . The use of the four psychologies . . . provides a fuller approximation to the phenomena of human development and clinical psychoanalysis than any one or two alone. (1988, pp. 594–595)

A similar idea has been expressed by Silverman (1986) though with the three models of drive-defense, object-relations and self, apparently including ego psychology in the first model. She believes that although one may favor a particular model as a description of the most basic motivation, mixed models are required to work with patients. Further, she believes that empirical research and clinical evidence support a multimodel approach. Although she appears to favor the primacy of relational needs, she describes case material that was approached using the three models. The emphasis is on utilizing all the perspectives in considering the meaning of material rather than blending techniques particular to specific models. She made interpretations from three vantage points, rather than one, with interpretation being a constant technique.

It is easier to work within one model, since expansion means a thorough knowledge of all models to be employed. There is a related question of whether one also then employs the particular techniques attached to the model when the particular perspective of the model is being used, but we will get to the application issue later. A more logical question exists in regard to the issue of primary motivation. If we assume that drive needs are the most basic for everybody, yet relational issues appear more important in a particular patient or group of patients, then ultimately will not the therapist have to frame the material in a drive context? Greenberg and Mitchell (1983) highlight this as a problem with mixed models. Silverman (1986) disagrees, taking the view that the needs that are the source of the psychopathology get the focus in treatment. These needs would be learned from the patient rather than preconceived by the therapist in accord with one model only.

This is appealing as logic for a mixed-model strategy, but it side-steps the issue. In a practical sense, psychotherapy or even a lengthy analysis may conclude with a resolution of psychopathology that does not require a focus on the basic need as stressed by only one model. However, in terms of *really understanding*, the patient would be incomplete, albeit satisfied with the results of the therapeutic work. This may be a better alternative than rigidly adhering to an exclusive model, considering the hypothetical essence of all models. Nonetheless, it is a compromise solution, and would have to be used and understood in that manner.

Also, there is a question as to how well psychoanalytic therapists would master all the models available, particularly if, as seems to be the tendency, they favor one. How satisfying will it be to the therapist if the patient insists on emphasizing what ought to be less important from the therapist's point of view? How can the therapist refrain from trying to at least slant the therapy? Can therapists even approach therapy with an objective openmindedness in regard to need emphasis by patients?

Pure theoretical orthodoxy has the potential liability of being completely wrong, whereas mixed models could deteriorate into truth fragments that fail to coalesce, the ultimate nontheory theory of infinite possibilities. What will probably happen then? Our best guess is that there will be an increased movement toward the mixed-model approach, but with apparent parsimony. Thus, Pine suggests four models, Silverman three, and Greenberg and Mitchell two. We incline toward two ourselves, drive and relational, and manage to embrace the others within those two, granting that we, as well as others, slight some psychoanalytic models in favor of others. Also there is the possible paradox that reducing the number of general categories multiplies their specifics, so complexity appears inevitable.

At the same time, the search for the ultimate model will continue. Some of this now takes place in terms of clarification of an existing model so that limitations and objections are addressed and mitigated. Two examples of this approach are the elaboration of psychosexual stages by Juni (1984) and the 1982 American Psychoanalytic Association Symposium (Compton et al., 1982) on the concept "object." Both are thought-ful preservations of drive theory but are probably more convincing to drive theorists than to anybody else.

Although the roots of other prominent psychoanalytic models can usually be found in the works of Freud, those models are not designed to be drive-theory models, even when they customarily give credit to Freud's conceptions. This is particularly marked in the area of early childhood development, where the original model was psychosexual stages but with an oedipal emphasis. Revisionists such as Melanie Klein (Segal, 1974), Mahler (Mahler, Pine, & Bergman, 1975), Kernberg (1976), Kohut (1971, 1977), Fairbairn (1952), Sullivan (1953b), and Winnicott (1965b) emphasize preoedipal development. Also, they represent a shift from drive motivation to relational motivation, and the description of stages of object-relations development (Mahler et al., 1975) has become a popular and useful conception to accompany psychosexual stages.

Thus, a central unifying element in major revisionist theories tends to be the developmental thrust and the increased importance of early object-relations. This is also true in ego psychology, although the tie to drive theory is more apparent. At the same time, most of the theorists mentioned based their theorizing on clinical material rather than having derived it from research or a combination of the two. Also, developmental hypotheses have been advanced by some theorists not working directly with children or not with the age group under consideration. Granting exceptions, there was and is considerable reason to search for validation, which brings us to the area of research on early development.

A major work in this area is the overview presented by Lichtenberg (1983). This work, as well as others in this area, is subject to a number of interpretations, but there does appear to be an agreement that such research supports the conception of an active, alert, responsive infant. This view contrasts with the idea of a normal autistic stage as well as a symbiotic stage. The work of Stern (1985) is particularly challenging as he describes the first 2 months of life as a time when a sense of an emergent self is actively being formed by the infant. Differentiation precedes fusion, in his view, and in turn makes joining with another possible. In Gedo's evaluation of Lichtenberg's work, he states, "The Mahlerian schema of development during the first year of life is utterly refuted" (1986, p. 170).

Silverman (1986) believes that infant research supports the basic primacy of relational needs, particularly attachment to the mother. Although Gedo admits that such findings support some type of object-relations approach, he agrees with Freedman (1984) about the inadequacies of object-relations theories to explain early behavior regulation, particularly sensorimotor phase development. Whereas Silverman

(1987) believes the research supports Melanie Klein's view of the infant's early awareness and maternal connection, Gedo dismisses Klein's view on the grounds that it requires too early an age to form mental representations of self and object.

Gedo makes the point that infant studies ". . . challenge the adequacy of *every* prominent psychoanalytic schema about early development . . ." (1986, p. 161). Gedo understandably concludes that research results provide more support for his views than those of most other theorists. Our narcissism has to travel a different path because we do not have the conviction of such strong opposition, or even an attachment such as Silverman to Klein and her ideas on female bonding. At the same time, we are struck by the fact that numerous viewpoints are possible and probable, again being drawn to the multitheoretical or integrative stance of Silverman (1986), Eagle (1984), and Pine (1985). We also remain aware of the difficulties, many already noted, in developing workable integrative models. The broad-based model of Blanck and Blanck (1974) that attempts an integration of developmental stages for psychosexual maturation, drive taming, object relations, adaptation, anxiety level, defenses, identity formation, and internalization unfortunately has too many "forced-fit" characteristics. Brown (1985) tries a similar approach with developmental stages for concreteness, but it also left us more impressed with the inconsistencies than the feasibility of mixing these models.

Fortunately, Pine has a softer touch in pointing to integrative possibilities, beginning with the idea of a number of motivational systems without necessarily giving universal primacy to one, an idea also advanced by Stern. Whereas Pine sees research on infant competencies (Stone, Smith, & Murphy, 1973) as requiring a revision in developmental conceptions, he does not argue for abandonment of the prevalent psychosexual and object-relations stages. These stages are depicted as "moments" of experience based on critical events in development that are affectively intense but at other times are quiet moments. The concept of experiential periods offers the possibility of accomodating the needs of drive, ego, object relations, and self-motivations, since primacy varies with the "moment." Multiple function in turn allows for integration.

Pine also makes the point that the use of terms to describe certain developmental stages emphasizes key moments, not exclusive behavior. Thus, normal autism stresses the fact that the infant sleeps a lot, while deemphasizing awareness and responsiveness. The use of the word "autism" then has to be qualified and may well be replaced with a better term to give a more balanced picture. A similar view can be taken about all the described stages, with both descriptions and names subject to change as more data are provided for both developmental and clinical theories.

Of course the question of the major motivator, *the* universal explanation, still hangs there. Pine is cautious about this, although he certainly seems to be inclining away from such an idea. Rapaport (1960) had proposed the five metapsychological viewpoints of structural, economic, dynamic, adaptive, and genetic, really within a framework of drive–ego psychology. Such an expansion of motivations then presented integrative and validation problems. Metapsychology, construed as the minimum number of explanatory assumptions, was increasing in complexity and unwieldiness. When Pine approaches these concerns in a different manner, designating functional descriptions of behavior as focused on drive satisfaction, reality adaptation, conscience, repetition of past relationships, and self consensus, he is furthering the expansion. This contrasts with the relative simplicity of having one theory, one major viewpoint to apply that explains all. It is very difficult for the practicing clinician to synthesize theoretical viewpoints and approach each patient with a thorough knowledge of all significant viewpoints, along with an openness to revision in any or all of the perspectives.

Nonetheless, we sense that Pine's work is prognostic. A new and complex metapsychology will have to come into being with an emphasis on explaining a developing theoretical integration that can also be translated into treatment. In a review of the Pine book, Frank (1987) points out the lack of a "modern-day Fenichel" and makes it clear that although his effort is laudable, Pine has not filled the gap. Actually, we find the work of Pine to be clear and specific but appropriately cautious. The literature on early development has raised many questions, some of which Pine answers, whereas others, many others, remain open. He does provide a framework for integration of knowledge as well as its application. In this regard the works of Doris Silverman and Daniel Stern, both already cited, are also particularly valuable.

We would like, at this point, to provide a more complete answer, a better integration, the hoped-for definitive theory with a full-blown accompanying clinical technique, but we cannot. At the same time, we are interested in and applaud efforts to try to do it as well as efforts that do even a little bit. One contribution of the moment will be to stress that this is a pressing task that all clinicians need to address. The rehashing of old material without looking at the new, or the presentation of new material while ignoring the old will not advance the field. A defensive stance about any particular point is also of little value unless it is truly open to an understanding of all the possibilities. The struggle to produce an effective integrated psychoanalytic theory is in its inception, and we all need to be part of it.

Although there are many other areas of theory development open to inquiry, we mention only one more as an example of new conceptions being needed. This is the area of identity development, especially sexual identity. Identity can be thought of as the sense of "who am I," with sexual identity, boy–man, girl–woman, as a major component of this. The original psychosexual stage development emphasized the appearance of male–female differentiation and sexual identity in the phallic–oedipal stages. The material previously discussed on infantile development indicates an earlier differentiation. As Flugel (1982) points out, there were early dissenters, including Horney, Jones, and Melanie Klein, but their views had a limited impact. The recent work of Stoller (1968, 1976) has been more influential with its concept that core gender identity is established in the preoedipal phases. Thus, the sense of being masculine or feminine appears to be in place earlier than originally thought.

    As a result, there has been considerable reevaluation, particularly of the development of female sexuality (Galenson & Riophe, 1977; Kestenberg, 1980; Moore, 1976). Although these authors have found points of dissent with previous theory, they tend to reinterpret in such a way as to keep drive theory relatively intact. Formanek (1982) approaches it differently, focusing on gender identity as an aspect of self-development that is initially concrete and based on stereotypes. The genital differences are noted by each sex, viewed narcissistically, and associated with gender identity as another attribute of being a boy or girl. Her view attempts some integration of theory, which can also be seen in the work of Fast (1984). She proposes a gender differentiation model for both sexes that follows a developmental pattern from narcissism to recognition of limits and then recategorization of experience. Thus, one differentiation aspect is integrated, the other seen as independent of the self, but both are conceptualized in relationship to each other. Although she emphasizes ideas such as narcissism being a mode of understanding one's experience rather than a bodily focus, the integrative possibilities of both perspectives are there. Most of the revisionist approaches we have mentioned thus far have emphasized female development, so we would add the work of Tyson (1986) in regard to male gender identity.

    The thrust of the literature on the development of sexual identity is that Freud came to erroneous conclusions, particularly in regard to women. This is usually followed by the now familiar attempt to recast Freud's meanings or in some fashion to salvage the psychosexual stages and their attendant features such as sublimation and superego formation. As Flugel said: "The impact of all of Freud's ideas, both within psychoanalysis and in the culture at large is such that they cannot be ignored and for that reason they cannot simply be discarded; they must be addressed" (1982, p. 8).

    The following is an example of the difficulties involved: If sexual identity is based on object choice, then boys and girls start with mother as their first object, and girls have to make a switch, which requires an explanation. In contrast, if identification is primary, then boys have to make the change, and that requires an explanation. Drive theory offers an explanation for the first alternative, although it has certainly been well criticized. Object-relations theory works better with the second alternative, although sexual development is not well articulated in object-relations theories. Also, whereas a sexual drive can easily be formulated as a given, a sexual preference is more complicated. Identification would certainly appear to come into play, but the individual differences of parents in their sexual expressions and attitudes have to be legion. Does the child then merely identify with the concept of an opposite-sex target? Homosexuality poses an obvious problem in that line of reasoning. Unfortunately, psychoanalytic theories usually have offered little except pathology to explain anything that does not appear to constitute "normal sexual development" (Friedman, 1986).

Sexual development theory is beginning to sound more convoluted than that of infantile development, with specific motivations more of a problem than general areas of causality. The problems are really very similar, however, because there are more exceptions, more factors involved than first thought, more developmental lives with greater significance than previously imagined. An awareness of this complexity has increased, and so more complex explanations tend to be involved in the service of accuracy. Again, both of us attempt to cope with this theoretical confusion by attempting relative integrations, admittedly incomplete.

Male and female homosexuality are good examples of the need for creative theory development. Instead of seeing homosexuality as pathological, such theory permits this type of sexual preference to be viewed as one avenue of sexual development. The option of homosexuality is then akin to heterosexuality albeit one not as frequent as the dominant sexual preference, or as deliberately fostered by either parents or society. Furthermore, neither homosexuality or heterosexuality are viewed as homogeneous, but rather as representing a range of intensities and frequencies. There is some mixture of heterosexual and homosexual preferences in varying degrees in most people over their life span, despite heterosexuality being more common. This is supportive of innate bisexuality, an original conception of Freud's, although he saw the repression of homosexuality as the usual, and healthier, developmental path. Rado (1940) closed out the bisexuality hypothesis, leaving psychoanalysis with the view of homosexuality as reparative and thus pathological. This view has persisted, with an ongoing search for the psychodynamics of homosexuality in a model of presumed psychological etiology. Although the search has been less than successful in distinguishing specific, differentiating homosexual dynamics to support an exclusive psychological etiology, such a view is supported by the available evidence on biological factors. For example, in concluding his review, Money states ". . . available evidence supports a nongenetic hypothesis for the origin not only of homosexuality, but of psychosexual differences and variations of all types" (1980, p. 70).

Even an analyst as sympathetic to the positive possibilities of a lesbian relationship as Eisenbud (1982) rules out a genetic explanation. She postulates an etiology in precocious sexual arousal used by the ego to cope with difficulties in the mother–child interaction, particularly too much exclusion or merging. The problem with this approach, however, is that while one can certainly find psychodynamic constellations that provide explanatory power for a lesbian choice, very similar constellations appear in women who do not make such a choice. In fact, considering sexual orientation, much of a choice is questionable if the pleasure component is to be included. To many, if not most people, sexual orientation appears natural, something that instinctively happened. A change in orientation, although possible, would not be conceptualized as "feeling good." Sexual arousal and sexual pleasure tend to be experienced as part of what feels like a predetermined preference. Whereas people can act in a bisexual manner, or even be celibate, there is a preference for sexual pleasure. Some of the details of that preference appear to be learned, but the orientation, same-sex or opposite-sex primarily, appears more instinctive. Thus, even when one sexual orientation is encouraged by society and significant others, a given person may still prefer a different orientation. The assumption tends to be that heterosexuality is the natural way and homosexuality an unnatural choice, but it is from homosexuals that therapists are more likely to hear, "I don't feel I had any choice."

In essence, clinical data are not convincing in regard to the learned nature of homosexual orientation, unless the therapist begins by assuming such an orientation is pathological. Of course it could be learned, and there are numerous instances where such a conception does seem accurate, but that is in accord with the heterogeneity of sexual orientations. Also, regardless of etiology, there is value in exploring the development of a person's sexuality through the psychoanalytic method. The problem lies in the frequent assumption of psychopathology as well as the insistence on attempting to change homosexuals into heterosexuals. Different assumptions can be made, starting with the etiology of homosexuality being unknown, but considering a variety of possibilities correlates with the varieties of homosexuality. This is not the usual psychoanalytic viewpoint, but it is in accord with a recent publication by the Federation of Parents and Friends of Lesbians and Gays as reported by Landers (1989). This brochure, based on the responses of researchers active in regard to sexual orientation, suggests a combination of genetic, hormonal, and environmental causes. It also indicates that although therapy may affect sexual behavior, the basic sexual orientation stays the same. One can learn to act like a heterosexual, but the desire for homosexuality will remain, and as an erotic pleasure, still be preferred.

The viewpoint then is that sexual orientation has a number of developmental pathways, that homosexuality can be a viable one, and that the purposes of therapy with a person regardless of sexual orientation is the understanding of personal development and the effective use of that understanding. Considering the heterogeneity of homosexuality, an adaptive solution to the life of a person self-designated as homosexual may or may not involve a change in sexual behavior and orientation. In this regard, most of the gay and lesbian people we have worked with in psychoanalytic therapy have opted for an effective life as a homosexual.

We have described our views on homosexuality to provide a specific example of the development of theory by individual therapists in an area where the existing theory did not seem to us to be adequate to support the range of clinical data. Although a minority, we are not alone among psychoanalytic writers in thinking this way (Friedman, 1986; Isay, 1986; Leary, 1985). Reformulation in this area does appear to strike an even more dissonant chord than reevaluation of the theory of female development, although the bulk of psychoanalytic theorizing about homosexuality is certainly an example of gender ideology. Implicit is the expression of theory as a narcissistic exercise that can be cloaked in the striving for objectivity. Theory is needed for self-expression as well as for the acquisition and application of knowledge, so that subjectivity and objectivity are indeed delicately related in science, and certainly in therapy, despite an emphasis on correctness and truth above all. Not a great deal of attention is paid to this relationship, despite an awareness that theorists are discovering others within the context of trying to know themselves. The work of Keller (1985) is of interest in this regard as an attempt to explore the relationship between the knower and the known using the metaphor of gender. Our emphasis is more on an awareness of the personal, subjective side in theory development as an expression of narcissistic needs. This leads into the exploration of theory as translated into practice where the "you factor" and its possible consequences are particularly striking.

CLINICAL APPLICATIONS

Although our specific concerns are with psychoanalytic formulations and applications, the areas to be discussed here are certainly applicable to other theories and therapeutic procedures as well. The first subject is the psychodynamic formulation, followed by specific techniques for con-ducting psychoanalytic therapy. The basic idea is that the therapist's theory provides a necessary and practical rationale for the use of specific procedures, with this rationale first appearing in the psychodynamic description inherent in a developmental approach. Personal vagaries, the narcissistic loading, are certainly interwoven in psychodynamics and related techniques, and we take note of their possible influence.

Psychodynamic Formulation

This is essentially a diagnostic plan, sometimes called a genetic-dynamic explanation to emphasize the attempt to ascertain the causes of the patient's problems as well as the subsequent development and current expression of personal history. The plan is formulated early in the treatment, is open to continual revision, and includes what is adaptive as well as what is maladaptive. The plan's advantage lies in the therapist potentially being more able to understand what is happening to the patient, why it is happening, and what to do about it. The danger of psychodynamic formulation is that initial conceptions may be rigidly adhered to by the therapist regardless of unfolding evidence that is not confirming. The flexibility and hypothetical nature of the plan are essen-tial to protect against possible narcissistic blindness unconsciously tail-ored to ensure the therapist's security.

An experienced therapist recognizes symptoms and characteristic behavioral patterns as preliminary indicators for tentative psychodynam-ics. For example, depression is generally related to loss, whether real, imagined, or symbolic, and it usually takes the form of damaged self-esteem. However, that is a very broad categorization, so that it is neces-sary to explore the origins and continuing development of the self in respect to esteem. Such exploration brings into play numerous descrip-tive as well as enhancing possibilities. Because similar developmental patterns appear to give rise to different major problem constellations, such as damaged self-esteem appearing in anxious people, schizoid peo-ple, narcissistic people, etc., more specific explanations attached to each individual will be required. Thus, both therapist's and patient's psycho-dynamic knowledge ought to be greater at the end of a course of therapy than at the beginning. However, the psychodynamic formulation offers a way to begin, and it is easy for both parties to flounder when the therapist has not been diligent in this respect.

A basic feature of psychodynamics is a tentative sketch of a per-son's development providing possible sources of current difficulties, including conflict, repetition, and deficit. Although such a formulation is familiar in psychoanalytic theory, a formal statement is often lacking in practice. Case presentations generally contain such material, but frequently in a relatively unorganized form so that the theory–treatment connection is unclear. The relative dearth of comprehensive psychodynamic formulations has been noted by Perry, Cooper, and Michels (1987), who suggest a number of contributing causes. These include misconceptions that psychodynamic formulations are only for patients in expressive long-term therapy, are primarily for training and so must be lengthy and elaborate, do not need to be written, and that therapists become too invested in them. As we have noted, the last issue often may not be a misconception, but the psychodynamic formulation is actually designed to be tentative and exploratory.

Perry et al. (1987) see the formulation as relatively brief, with four parts. The first is an introductory outline of the clinical situation, including the patient's current problems, precipitating events, type of interpersonal relationships, major predisposing factors, and the behaviors that the psychodynamics will try to explain. This summary description of the case essentials is followed by listing possible nondynamic contributors to the patient's problems, such as drugs, physical illness, and socioeconomic factors. The point is also made that even if nondynamic factors appear as the major cause, psychodynamics should also be considered, since both sets of factors are related.

The third part of the formulation is the identification of central conflicts and themes followed by their psychodynamic formulations, using primarily one of three models, ego, self, and object-relations. The final section is a prognostic estimate of how the patient is likely to use the treatment. Perry et al. (1987) present examples of psychodynamic formulations using each of the models with the same depressed patient. It is clear that the formulations arise from the central concept of psychoanalysis as a developmental approach emphasizing the influence of the unconscious and personal history. It is also clear that the models serve as predictive guides for the therapist and are open to modification.

Specifically, the ego model emphasizes drive derivatives, oedipal resolution, and intrapsychic conflicts and defenses. Thus one patient's central conflict was seen as between an aggressive wish and the fear of retaliation. Intellectual defenses and passive–aggressive behavior were used to contain the anxiety engendered by the conflict. His depressive episodes were triggered by competitive factors, and his tendency to view life as a continual competition was traced to unresolved oral and oedipal situations. He had a depressed, demanding mother who had stifled his assertiveness as well as a controlling father with chronic heart disease who died when the patient was an adolescent, further increasing his guilt and need to control his anger. In therapy, we can expect that he will feel competitive with the therapist, devalue therapy with passive–aggressive maneuvers, and in response to guilt, have difficulty allowing himself to improve.

The self model stresses the patient's low self-esteem, his need for approval, and his inability to accept limitations in others or himself. These problems were traced to narcissistic parents who were unable to respond empathically to his needs and invested him with their grandiose ambitions to compensate for their own failures. The patient's failures damaged his self-esteem and in turn resulted in depression. In therapy, we may expect him to show a great need for admiration and to have grandiose expectations. He will be discouraged as the therapist demonstrates realistic limitations, and he will display anger passively.

The object-relations model views the central problem as a failure to integrate good and bad self and object representations. Both parents fostered the repression of the patient's bad self to the point of splitting. The depression was related to guilt for projected hostile wishes as well as failure to meet perfectionistic ideals. In therapy he may begin with apparent compliance, but, subsequently, the projection of his angry self will reactivate the impression of controlling parents and result in denigration of the therapist.

Given the psychodynamic formulations, the guides for the therapist fall into place. In the ego focus, the therapist will work on the relationship between current difficulties and earlier struggles with the parents. Resistances will include guilt about improvement, passive-aggressive defenses, and the possibility of competitive struggles with the therapist.

In the self model, understanding of the patient's delicate grandiosity will be prominent with an uncovering of the relationship between perceived therapist empathic failures and the lack of empathy in the patient's childhood. Resistances will involve discouragement and devaluation of the therapist.

With the object-relations model, we may expect interpretations to be made regarding parental control of the patient, and the therapist will encourage the expression of repressed feelings illustrating the capacity for tolerance of such affect. Resistances will include increased depression in reaction to the emergence of the angry self and projection of the bad self onto the therapist.

Another example of psychodynamic conceptions has been presented in the treatment of bulimia, using the three models of drive, relations, and masochism (Herron et al., 1988). Blanck and Blanck (1974, 1979, 1986) describe a developmental diagnosis that aims to be integrative, although it is more detailed than what is suggested by Perry et al. (1987).

Sources that are particularly useful for formulating develo
stages are Mahler et al. (1975) and Kernberg (1976). The work of Bellak,
Hurvich, and Gediman (1973) is useful in operationalizing psychic structures and their functions. In an earlier part of this chapter we indicated
the limitations in such a schema, but these can be kept in mind without
eliminating the utility of the works suggested.

Psychodynamics becomes more valuable when used with caution,
discretion, and flexibility, since narcissism is certainly operable. One
tempting direction is to be as elaborate as possible, to leave listeners and
readers in wonderment. Yet because of the apparent labor and erudition
involved, this may actually reduce the attraction for many therapists to
make such a formulation. Such conceptions also become hard to consider as hypotheses, so that a relatively inflexible investment in them may
take hold. In addition, sometimes the elaboration may turn out to be
confusing rather than clarifying. Of course, none of these problems has
to occur, but they are pitfalls to consider when one attempts such
detailed explanations.

The second temptation is not to bother with details or written
formulations. Instead the position taken is one of implicit dynamics more
or less intuited by the therapist and not requiring a formal statement. The
role of intuition is quite probable, but the explicit formulation is a very
useful clarifier. Neglecting it goes in the direction of "my theory is
whatever I do." This seems to be a more dangerous alternative than the
first possibility of overkill.

We prefer a third possibility that is practical, brief, and integrative.
This psychodynamic formulation is conceptualized in terms of three
main overlapping emphases—drives, structures, and relationships. A
therapist more wedded to one model than another will naturally give it
the central position. Also, the specific patient with his or her problems
may stimulate a focus. Regardless, attention can be usefully directed to
the three categories.

The drives include libido and aggression. The structures are id, ego,
superego, and self, as well as their functions. Relationships embrace the
concepts of self-representations and object representations as well as
object relations. Furthermore, a patient's difficulties are seen as resulting
from conflict and/or deficit, both accompanied by the tendency for
repetition in a variety of forms. The patient's problems are discussed in a
therapeutic situation involving transference, resistance, and countertransference.

This type of psychodynamic formulation can be illustrated by a
middle-aged man who came to therapy after a series of failed relationships, including several marriages. He was attempting a new relationship,
which had deteriorated to the point where the woman involved insisted

that he get therapy or she would end the relationship. He admitted that he needed some help, but it was a reluctant admission, so that he immediately assumed an antagonistic stance with the therapist. This patient presented major problems in the three areas of drives, structural development, and object relations. The initial psychodynamic formulation did not attempt to pinpoint the locus of the patient's difficulties within his personal history. The patient's subsequent verbalizations were used to become more precise, but there were early hints.

First, the patient had arrived with a stated relational issue. From his aggressive behavior and attitude in the early sessions, it was clear that drive expression was also quite a problem. Then, he moved quickly from acknowledgment of his own apparent unreasonableness and paranoid sensitivity to an emphasis on how badly others treated him. Thus, his hostility was now turned into a superego issue where he was really right and so merely reactive to others being wrong. Cognitive and affective deficits appeared, as well as intense conflicts around drive expression and object attachment. Limited self-esteem and the recurrent need for approval were striking.

His demandingness had an oral quality, his object-attachment issues raised questions about symbiosis, and his damaged self-esteem highlighted narcissistic difficulties. Thus, the therapist was given focal possibilities in recapitulating psychosexual stages, object-relations phases, and self-development. As the patient's personal history unfolded, the psychodynamic formulation became less tentative. For example, the patient's relationship with both his parents had been very frustrating, and repetitive attempts to gain the missing gratification had been unsuccessful, although it was difficult for the patient to see that he had a role in the outcome of interpersonal events.

With ensuing sessions, it became more apparent how his conflicts and deficits came about, how they were being played out in the transference, and what interventions tended to be effective. A promising line of inquiry was his relationship with his mother. She was enticing but rarely forthcoming, and now he pictured most women in that way. In turn, he demanded whatever he could, expected to get only a little, yet resented the power of women and remained angry. His omnipresent anger offered another area of exploration. Expressions of anger in his household had been allowed only when the anger could be justified. He remained attached to that model, with limited spontaneity as a protection against making a mistake, but with weak impulse control under the guise of justification. His superego development had involved a punitive, righteous father who distorted events to suit his wish to be angry. The patient followed suit only to be rejected by people who mainly found him too annoying over time and became tired of wrangling about right and wrong.

These reactions left him hurt and perplexed, feeling victimized and out of touch with his own maneuvers.

In addition to indicating some of the lines of inquiry suggested by the psychodynamic formulation and subsequently pursued, it was also possible to predict how the patient would operate in the therapy. The patient demanded from the therapist, yet criticized whatever the therapist did. Trust was a major concern, and it was very difficult to form an enduring therapeutic alliance. Transference was intense, but erratic, with splitting and acting out as prominent features. Resistance was very frequent, and despite the patient's obvious emotional pain, there was considerable denial. Thus, therapy often seemed to be starting all over again.

This patient stimulated intense countertransference. Two major trends appeared. At times, the therapist had a strong desire to get rid of the patient, which was easy to justify based on the strong resistance. At other periods, the therapist found himself caught in masochistic efforts somehow to make the therapy work even though the patient was really avoiding dealing with his own issues.

Although interpretation was a therapeutic goal, the patient needed the therapist to structure yet be flexible because the patient had fluid boundaries and was beset by a harsh superego. Before, in, and around interpretation, the therapist needed to work with structure building and deficit repair to create an appropriate therapeutic holding environment. The psychodynamic formulation offered the tentative lines of engagement, starting with the idea that the patient would have to learn to trust the therapist enough to allow sufficient self-appraisal. Furthermore, the therapist had to learn to withstand the onslaught of hostility generated by the patient's projections. In an intriguing moment of insight, this patient said to the therapist, "You know, at times I can't stand myself, but the real question in this therapy is, can you stand me?"

Familial patterns of distrust certainly seemed to underlie the patient's struggle with himself and others. These pointed to a broad area of psychogenesis. The elaboration over time offered interpretive possibilities, and these ultimately had positive effects. This was a difficult case, and the changes made were hard to come by as well as relatively limited. The patient did not end up living happily, or at all, with the woman who helped him enter therapy. However, his relationships did improve along with his manner of affective expression, self-esteem, and ego strength, and the psychodynamic formulation played a significant role in facilitating the therapeutic effects.

Let us consider one more example. The patient was an attractive, thin, verbal, young married woman whose presenting problem was anxiety over rejection by a lover. In the early sessions, it was discovered that the woman had some form of eating disorder, poor body image, limited sexual desire, and difficulty identifying herself as a woman. Shifting to psychogenesis, possible lines of inquiry were difficulties in the oral stage, problems in identifying with her mother and still being sexual, and repression of sexual desire to please her mother. Probable transference manifestations were a struggle with respect to dependency, separation-individuation problems, the degree of acceptable togetherness, and the need for reinforcement of an insatiable self that could not feed itself.

Whereas this case was easier to work with than the first, and the outcome more positive, the value of psychodynamic formulation was again evident. It provided a place to begin, an initial mode of understanding to be enriched as therapy continued. In the examples cited, we have the benefit of hindsight, but the initial questions and lines of inquiry were our original formulations. Even when their accuracy was in question, they were at least helpful. They gave us a tentative plan, the confidence to begin, and the flexibility to shift when necessary. The theory provided a framework for understanding. Of course, successful clinical application is also a matter of technique, which we now consider.

Clinical Procedures

Our discussion is about psychotherapy that is conducted from a psychoanalytic point of view, and therefore we refer to it as psychoanalytic therapy. This is not intended to distinguish it from psychoanalysis, although such a distinction can be made. Paolino (1981) presents a detailed consideration of the distinction, in which he suggests an essential similarity between "intensive investigative" psychoanalytically oriented psychotherapy and psychoanalysis. Supportive psychoanalytic therapy is differentiated from the other two based on its emphasis on symptom relief. Luborsky (1984) distinguishes supportive–expressive psychoanalytic psychotherapy from psychoanalysis. Lines are also drawn between time-limited short-term psychoanalytic therapy and psychoanalysis. Our description of techniques in turn will refer to a variety of techniques to be used in psychoanalytic therapies. The use of the technique will depend on the goal desired.

Freud provided six papers on technique but not a thorough or definitive exposition. As a result, technique has developed slowly, and the essentials of technique have been open to question. Greenson (1967) indicates that increasing insight is the main goal and requires analytic techniques. However, there are a variety of other techniques, and he cites abreaction as one example that strengthens functions to be used to eventually gain insight. The analytic or insight techniques themselves he describes as confrontation, clarification, interpretation, and working through. Nichols and Paolino (1986) recently suggested six major techniques: suggestion, catharsis, manipulation, confrontation, clarification, and interpretation. Luborsky (1984) provides in manual form specific techniques for being supportive, as well as how to listen, understand and respond from a psychoanalytic frame of reference. Peterfreund (1983) describes strategies to be used by the therapist, first general possibilities, then the three specifics of being a participant observer, including the patient as participant, and establishment of meanings, as well as strategies to be used by the patient.

The authors cited are only a sample of the possibilities, but what they have in common begins with Freud (1914) and is an emphasis on patient understanding. For our purposes, we will use the four techniques suggested by Greenson (1967) as our basic outline. Prior to this, it is important to note that there is agreement that other techniques will have to be used in order to make the patient able to benefit from the principal technique of interpretation. Luborsky (1984) refers to these as supportive techniques and indicates that the therapeutic relationship itself is really the first of these. Thus the structure of the analytic situation is designed to establish an atmosphere of mutual respect and trust.

An issue arises when this is not sufficient, in which case other techniques must be used. Luborsky divides these into a grouping in which the therapist is experienced as giving help, the patient as receiving it, and a grouping in which the patient experiences working together with the therapist. The first group includes conveying support for the patient to achieve the goals of therapy (goal setting having begun in the initial session) through words and manner, conveying a sense of understanding and acceptance, developing a liking for the patient, helping the maintenance of defenses and competencies that support the patient's level of functioning, communicating a realistically hopeful attitude and giving recognition to the progress being made, and encouraging selective expression. The second grouping involves encouraging a mutual bond and a joint search for understanding, including references to a backlog of familiar therapy experiences, conveying respect for the patient and giving the patient recognition for developing parallel therapeutic abilities.

These are all useful therapeutic activities displayed in other therapies as well, and we have discussed in other chapters issues in regard to their use, such as working with a patient the therapist does not like. The point of mentioning them here is to indicate that they are derived from the therapist's theory. For psychoanalytic therapies, they are used to develop or maintain situations in which both therapist and patient are able to use procedures directly aimed at insight, such as interpretation.

Peterfreund's (1983) description of the components of a working model for psychoanalysts is useful here. Psychoanalytic therapies are concerned with the patient's inner world, subjective emotional states, personal meanings and motives, unconscious processes. The therapist starts and fosters a process of analyzing these concerns in each patient, using the basic rule of having the patient associate as freely as possible. If the process is effectively in place, then insight and change can take place. Varying degrees of support are required to initiate and maintain the process, and this is the purpose of supportive techniques in psychoanalytic therapies. In other therapies, such approaches may actually be the ultimate goals of the therapies, or they may be used as intermediate steps in developing a process, akin to the way they are employed in psychoanalytic work even if the process is different.

The risks connected to the use of supportive measures are overutilization and underutilization. A therapist who needs the narcissistic gratifications that can come from being actively supportive will be likely to overuse the approach and in turn limit the patient's ability to use the analytic process. Such a therapist will too often believe the patient is inadequate for the task at hand and in turn "help," not realizing the extent to which the patient is being restricted from making progress. Patients in which deficits are more apparent than conflicts certainly set the stage for the need for support. Yet the therapist must keep in mind that the patient has his or her work to do in the therapy. If the therapist takes over the patient's work, the process is curtailed. Thus, the therapist using supportive measures must remain aware of his or her intermediate purpose.

The contrasting problem may also occur where the therapist is so invested in keeping a distance and having the patient struggle with the task that needed support is not forthcoming. The therapist's narcissistic protection from responsibility will result in irresponsibility as the patient's inadequacies for participating in the process go unrecognized. Patients whose conflicts appear more obvious than their deficits are most likely to be treated this way. Any apparent difficulties with the process are interpreted as resistance without an accompanying consideration of a willingness by the therapist to be supportive in overcoming the resistance. The extremes of this are to dismiss a patient as unmotivated or unsuitable for analytic work when, really, the therapist does not want to do the work needed to help the patient carry out the process. In this instance, it is the therapist who lacks the motivation and self-sufficiency. Thus, the therapist not using supportive measures must recognize the necessity of intermediate steps in analytic therapies.

Supportive measures actually appear when the therapist sets the structure of the therapy, as in schedule, fees, the patient's work of free association, and describes the goals, essentially developing a process leading to insight and change. A contract is then formed, a helping alliance, and analytic techniques will become more prominent.

We now turn to a discussion of the specific procedures of confrontation, clarification, interpretation, and working through that are prescribed by psychoanalytic theory as ways to produce insight. Although these techniques can be demarcated, they are not so differentiated in practice. Also, often, but not always, they occur in the analytic process in the order given. Finally, they are not the creators of insight, but ways to facilitate an introspective process that can lead to change.

Confrontation

Confrontation means that the therapist directs the patient's attention to something that the patient seems not to notice. This "something" that the patient appears to be avoiding could be intrapsychic or external. The emphasis is on the avoidance, not the reason for the avoidance. As such, confrontation prepares the patient for clarification and interpretation and may not appear to be directly aimed at insight. However, since it is designed to get the patient to understand something that was not apparently acknowledged, it produces one level of insight. The patient now has information previously lacking. It could be that what is being confronted was out of consciousness, or if it was conscious, now the patient is aware that the therapist also knows, so that, at the very least, a communication of understanding has taken place.

Karpf (1986) sees confrontation as having two main functions: as a preparation for an interpretation and, by itself, as a challenge to defenses, thus improving judgments. These tend to overlap because the therapist is essentially telling a patient that something needs to be looked at that is currently being avoided. The confrontation is successful if the patient agrees and is willing to explore the issue. This depends a great deal on the manner in which a confrontation is delivered, since this technique provides many unfortunate opportunities for error.

The patient is frustrating the therapist by being resistant, and the therapist in turn moves to confront, ostensibly for therapeutic reasons. The questions arising are: Is the patient ready to hear this, and how can the therapist say this? The possibilities for mistakes lie in misjudgment of the patient's preparedness for the confrontation, and in expressing the information in a way that either has no apparent effect, or a harmful effect. The judgment of patient readiness is a clinical assessment, but it may be clouded by the therapist's feelings. If the therapist is impatient, then there will be a tendency to move quickly and be rather insistent. If the therapist is intimidated by the patient, there will be an inclination to avoid confrontations and make them tentative when they do occur. Reaction formations or counterphobic moves are also possible by the therapist in response to personal feelings of impatience or reticence.

Thus, in confrontation, therapists have to be particularly attuned to timing and their motives and then present the material in such a way that the patient does not feel injured and can use the observation offered. There is considerable intuition involved in both timing and manner of confronting. Although psychoanalytic theory postulates the use of confrontation in service of the process, that is not a license to psychologically assault the patient in service of the therapist's feelings.

With the patients described in the previous section on psychodynamic formulation, the difficult man required more confrontations than the woman. He also presented more of a temptation for the therapist to be sadistic, as well as avoidant, because of the tedious aspects of dealing with his continual resistances. Confrontations tended to be gentle, in deference to the fragility of his self-esteem, but firm because of his need for structure and his loose boundaries. Also, because of the strong negative countertransference potential, the interventions were generally thought out very carefully in advance. With the woman patient, confrontations were less frequent because she was more cooperative about the process, and they were more spontaneous because she was less defensive. Most of the time they were presented in a calm, neutral manner, though with a definite indication of their importance. There were times, however, when in both cases there was considerable affective interchange in confrontations, representative of the therapist attempting to be attuned to the patients' moods. The therapist wanted to make a sufficient impact on the patient to cause effective processing of the material, and the attunement was integral to the success of such an effort.

There have been some comments that confrontation is really not an analytic technique, but a parameter or deviation, since it is not directly interpretive, but preparatory to insight. In our view, it does aim at a type of insight, and Karpf (1986) considers it primarily an analytic technique because of its role in the development of insight, as does Greenson (1967). In essence, it is more of a direct path to insight than other measures we have termed supportive, and since we see it as also producing some insight, we classify it as analytic. We acknowledge, however, that there are analysts who disagree, insisting on interpretation exclusively as *the* analytic technique.

Clarification

Clarification is similar to confrontation and interpretation. Attention is drawn to material in order to increase the patient's awareness and understanding of it. In confrontation, the emphasis is more on getting the patient's attention. Clarification would then customarily follow, increasing the focus with the patient prepared for the therapist's observations.

Brown (1986) describes three functions of clarification: conscious re-statement of the patient's material, conscious–conscious linkage, and conscious–preconscious linkage.

The first function emphasizes surface material in order to refine consciousness, and as such, it is the least directly aimed at insight. In the second function, a connection is made that was previously missing, whereas in the conscious–preconscious model there is both a new connection and new material. Although the latter two are more directly concerned with insight, in all three possibilities new understanding is imparted. Clarifications are differentiated from interpretations primarily in terms of the level of access, with interpretations being explanations of material that is deeper, that is, unconscious rather than preconscious. We can use a clarification here by pointing out that depth is a metaphor for the degree to which material is distant in time from the patient's present and the degree to which it is repressed or otherwise defended.

Clarifications are explanations that prepare the patient for interpretations. They imply a sense of working together by therapist and patient that is based on a foundation of successful confrontation. As such, the countertransference probabilities are less likely, but they can occur if the therapist is either too persistent about what is really the picture, or if the therapist is too cautious. In the first instance, the patient may be forced to submit to error, whereas in the second, error is perpetuated because of a lack of clarity. The narcissistic contributors are here on the therapist's part as they were in regard to confrontation, but they tend to be less of an issue because clarification usually occurs within a firmer patient–therapist alliance.

However, there are some additional considerations. If there is an insufficient working alliance, the therapist may be continually clarifying because the patient is resisting through an apparent lack of understanding, even at relatively obvious levels of experience. This in turn means a return to confrontation and that the therapist had misjudged the degree of alliance, probably out of a need to increase the progression of the therapy. In the same vein, therapists may assume the patient knows more than is the case and do little clarification. The patient is then poorly prepared for interpretations.

Both confrontation and clarification are in the service of interpretation. For example, a patient avoids talking about a woman with whom he is involved. His behavior is pictured as reactive to hers rather than as having motivation initiated by the patient. He externalizes as resistance, and the therapist uses confrontation to deal with this. Once this is accepted by the patient, the therapist uses clarification to begin an understanding of the resistance, pointing out the anxiety and anger engendered in the patient in regard to discussing his relationship with this woman. The reasons for the feelings that necessitated the resistance are what is being traced, with the interpretation next in line as an explanation of unconscious causes. The progression is appropriate to all models of psychoanalytic theory, but the model of preference for the therapist will usually dictate the emphasis of the interpretation. In the case of this patient, the focus could be on drive expression, with the relationship secondary; or it could be reversed. We will elaborate in the next section on interpretation.

Interpretation

Interpretation is a statement to the patient of hidden meaning. It is an explanation in which the unconscious is made conscious. Generally considered the premier and particularly distinguishing technique of all psychoanalytic therapies, its purpose is increased self-understanding for the patient, understanding that will lead to change. To be effective, interpretations need to be accurate, delivered in a way that is congruent for the patient, and emotional as well as intellectual.

The accuracy of an interpretation is based on the therapist's understanding of the patient's life. There are a number of possible accurate interpretations of a patient's material, with the therapist presenting what he or she believes is the answer, which in turn is a function of the therapist's particular model. The more integrative the model, the easier it is to be flexible in emphasis and content. However, the therapist tries to be correct within the boundaries of whatever model or models are being used. Of course, there is the possibility of error. The therapist may misunderstand the patient or misunderstand theory. In addition, the therapist may have an intense narcissistic investment in being correct that will be symbolized in the interpretation. Then, even though interpretations are hypotheses, the therapist will start to treat them as facts. Validation rests on the patient's acceptance and use of the interpretation, but it can be difficult to know whether the acceptance is based on understanding or a desire to please. In addition, an interpretation can be correct but be rejected by the patient. Nonetheless, the therapist's first task is to think of an interpretation as a hypothesis that hopefully is correct, but is to be reformulated until a correct explanation is discovered.

The congruence for the patient is based on the therapist's attunement to him or her. If this is good, the therapist interprets when the patient is receptive and can make use of the interpretation. If there is an alliance, if confrontation and clarification have been well received, then interpretation should be appropriate. Boris said "The therapist's patience is the patient's best friend" (1986, p. 294). The message here is: Give the patient time for self-understanding as well as give the therapist time to understand the patient.

In many instances, patients will learn to make their own interpretations. Patients are capable of knowing a great deal about themselves provided they feel safe and capable of exploring, and the therapeutic situation tries to provide the facilitating conditions. The intervention of the therapist as an interpreter is needed when the patient cannot seem to comprehend but may be close to understanding and is therefore open to the interpretation. Thus, "Recognizing the 'truth' of an interpretation is only partially mutative. . . . Only when the 'truth' takes on an air of inevitability does an interpretation do its work" (Boris, 1986, p. 295).

Since interpretations are ways for therapists to exhibit themselves, there is a temptation to "look smart often." This results in frequent and rapid interpretations, with the therapist implanting insight that is probably artificial at best. The other side of this approach is the insecure therapist who lets the patient reside with only what the patient already understands.

Natterson (1986) has suggested the following categories of interpretation: past–present, intellectualized, empathic, transference, resistance, and affective. Although we have indicated the necessity of both intellectual and emotional components for the effectiveness of interpretation, the categorization makes the point of understanding the circumstances of the interpretive situation. Thus, an anxious patient may become better organized because of the structuring effects of a relatively intellectual explanation since it is emotionally distant. The reverse may be true with a patient who is excessively intellectualized. However, these are way stations, serving a purpose for the moment and, it is to be hoped, allowing later interpretations that are understood cognitively and affectively. This means the patient will understand meaning and experience meaning, new information being both known and felt so that the patient can understand what was not previously understood, look at life differently, and act accordingly. A major criticism of interpretation has been that it is primarily an intellectual exercise in which both therapist and patient get to look smart, but when it concludes, they do not act intelligently because neither has really learned anything. Thus, the therapist has to be concerned with more than giving insight and the patient with more than receiving insight. Both have to be concerned with the patient's use of insight, which brings us to the next topic, working through.

Working Through

This is the most mysterious of all the analytic techniques because it is the mechanism of translating insight into action. If a therapist successfully interprets to a patient the early origins of the patient's fear of women, can it be reasonably expected that the patient will now feel differently about women and act differently with women? The answer is, it depends, and what it depends on is whether or not the issue was worked through.

Greenson (1967) sees working through as a separate analytic technique that follows insight via interpretation. It is a repetitive analysis of resistances to change as well as repeated reconstructions. Nichols and Paolino (1986) consider it a form of interpretation, although they describe it in a manner similar to Greenson as involving the repetition of interpretations. The upshot of this is the recognition that analysis takes a long time, meaning that the actual changes in the patient are slow in coming about, and the exact mechanism of changing is unclear.

Brenner (1987) reviewed the literature on working through, concluding that there had been a variety of explanations offered, that none were satisfactory, including his own, and that the question of why analysis takes so long is at the moment unanswerable. What happens is that the patient continues to resist progress, and if therapy ends or goes on, more still needs to be accomplished. The mystery in this is why some patients do change when others do not despite what appears to be in each case some definite signs of progress. Also, the mechanism of change when it occurs is relatively individualized, so that insight leads to change sometimes. Our impression is that some combinations of patients and therapists work better than others, but the ingredients of success are at times hard to discern and hard to generalize. We believe that if most people stay in therapy long enough with a competent therapist, change will occur. However, we recognize that "long enough" is an individual variable, and there is no definitive time line. Patients and therapists become impatient and often act on this via arbitrary time limits that produce failures that could have been successes, as well as designated successes that do not remain that way. It is incorrect to assume that a person who has been in therapy a long time is either very disturbed or has an incompetent therapist. People vary in their abilities to change, probably because of a variety of predisposing developmental events and factors that can be difficult to identify. There is an anxiety about change and dealing with the unfamiliar that is often more compelling than a current distressing situation or than repetitive ineffective patterns from the past. Working through has to deal with that anxiety, and there is no accurate way to specify how long that will take. People make judgments and set limits because they want and think therapy ought to work that way, but it does not. Therapists need to learn to be patient, and to help others understand the need for time as well as the need not to be threatened by all the "hurry-up" clamor of our society. Our position has been, and remains, that we will try to work with people for as long as it takes them to achieve their therapeutic goals

Although we cannot solve some of the mysteries of working through, an example will cast some light on the process. A young unmarried woman seemed unable to become involved with any appropriate man despite a stated desire to do so and no obvious impediments. The major interpretation placed the psychogenesis on an inability to separate from her parents. Despite the patient's acceptance of this relational interpretation, she seemed to ignore the insight into her behavior. Then at some point, after seducing and then abandoning a much older man, she started to go with a man who appeared as a plausible marital choice. She had made such switches before, only to destroy or have destroyed the new possibility. However, this time she seemed willing to have something positive happen. She viewed it as an opportunity to free herself from her father in particular, and she worked at this new relationship. She became engaged and then married, and the relationship with her father, previously very stormy, greatly improved. She attributed her ability to do all this to finally "really understanding" the separation issue. She felt more independent yet also closer to her parents than before. She married a man who was very interested in her and focused on pleasing her, a role her mother played with her father. The patient had always imagined she would be like her mother and marry a strong, demanding man like her father, but she tended to reverse the process and in turn learned to enjoy her strength.

Why did she "catch on" at the point she did and become able to lead her own life? We do not know. The therapist just kept at it, and conviction on the therapist's part was undoubtedly helpful. The transference had always contained the patient's projection that the therapist wanted to control her, either by preventing her from being with people she wanted, a trait she ascribed to her father, or placing her with someone the therapist endorsed, a trait she gave to her mother. When she allowed herself to become engaged, she no longer saw the therapist as trying to control her. Perhaps it is as Brenner remarked, "there is nothing special about a patient's failure to improve that requires anything other than good, solid, analytic work, usually—perhaps invariably—centered on the transference" (1987, p. 106).

CONCLUDING REMARKS

Holt (1985), in a sympathetically devastating paper, made explicit how tentative psychoanalytic theory appears to be. Although we found no evidence of many theorists paying attention to Holt, part of learning any theory is to pay attention to critics, particularly in terms of criteria for theory validation. Holt's approach is that of a psychoanalytic scientist, whereas most therapists are concerned about the practice of therapy. However, that does not remove them from an obligatory interest in theory and its development. We believe there is a "knowledge neglect" about theory that in turn has been reflected in practice.

Using psychoanalysis as our example, we have stressed the value of theory, given examples of theory development, discussed the trend toward an integrative approach, and showed the application of theory in practice. We have also pointed out how the therapist's narcissism can resist new knowledge and contribute to the misapplication of theory. For a time in psychoanalytic therapies, the emphasis was on the method, but as understanding of the therapy relationship increased, the focus shifted to the personality of the therapist. Certainly we consider the therapist a major factor, with much of this book reflecting that emphasis. But here, we wanted to adjust the balance to give knowledge more weight. Therapists have learned that knowing a method is not effective without having the personal qualities necessary to apply it. At the same time, empathy is not a substitute for knowledge or knowing what to do.

7

Idiosyncratic Responses

Idiosyncratic responses are characteristic ways a particular therapist behaves in the therapy session. These are not conceptualized by the therapist as especially patient-specific but, rather, as special to that therapist. They are thought of as facilitating the therapy or neutral in the sense of not being essential. They are just the way the therapist habitually operates as a therapist regardless of such designations as theoretical orientation or professional affiliations. A basic example is the way a therapist usually greets patients, whereas a more complex example would be the manner in which a therapist usually makes interpretations.

Idiosyncratic responses can be categorized conceptually as secondarily autonomous ego functions, indicating their probable derived origins and providing a reminder that they are not guaranteed to remain conflict-free. Unfortunately, in that regard, the narcissism of the therapist facilitates repression. The idiosyncratic responses do not include errors. Instead they represent a therapeutic style that is believed to be only good in the exclusionary sense of never being really harmful. The model for this may be in the self-protection of early differentiation where the good precedes the bad, and the bad is still seen as part of the good. The therapist has integrated and automatized a personal style that no longer receives reflection, and the therapist has an investment in keeping it that way.

A reinforcement for this unscrutinized safe harbor of therapists' behavior is the fact that psychotherapists have spent decades trying to standardize their clinical techniques. This work continues with much of the effort in the service of developing coherent theory so that technical procedures and theoretical propositions can be integrated to produce change in patients. Such a match could indeed contribute a greater sense of probability and respect to the field of psychotherapy. At the very least, the hope has been that two therapists of the same theoretical persuasion would practice psychotherapy in approximately the same way. On this basis, the results of therapeutic endeavors would become more predictable rather than rest with the degree of uncertainty that now surrounds them.

The goal is admirable in many respects, but the degree of success may always be limited because so much of it depends on the psychotherapist. As a major player in the psychotherapeutic process, the therapist presents a situation in which no aspect of his or her individuality can be treated as mere white noise. Increased elaboration and understanding of both theory and technique does not equivalently reduce the tendency of therapists to remain quite idiosyncratic. As a result, a fundamental neglected issue is the effects of the idiosyncratic ways in which therapists use clinical techniques.

There are definite barriers to even the realization of the issue. Acknowledging a significant presence of individual variability that is markedly resilient in its destiny does emphasize the artistic component of therapy in contrast to the scientific. This can have some appeal but probably a limited one. Such a view makes techniques hard to duplicate, results difficult to replicate, and undoubtedly illustrates a discrepancy between what therapists do and what they often say they do. All of this is indeed problematic, but it cannot be solved by neglect or by what Gedo refers to as "an unfortunate tendency toward ritualizing our therapeutic techniques" (1979, p. 15).

In one sense idiosyncratic responses represent the personal artistry of the therapist, giving the same message unique flavor depending on who is sending it. Yet, in another sense, they are insidious dangers because their potential impact goes unrecognized by the therapist. They can include, or indeed, be the countertransferences that nobody knows about, or even cares to know. They are the ways in which the therapist characteristically deals with patients and to which there has been little or no negative feedback. For the therapist, they are representations of who he or she is as a person in the role of therapist, and because they are so incorporated, they are considered safe. In addition, they are really little things, distinctive but scarcely discernible in their effortless facilitation of therapeutic possibilities. They may not explicitly be thought of as therapeutic techniques but, rather as habitual ways the therapist operates in the therapeutic setting. Although for therapists life is usually filled with relatively complex meanings, these responses are not. If they are thought of as having meaning at all, then it can only be positive. They are simply not to be considered issues.

Some of the time they may not be, but following the principle of overdetermination, they deserve more evaluation, as tiresome and troublesome as it may seem to extend the range of possible countertransferential behavior. The need for such an extension is reinforced by the fact that, at times, therapists are forced by patient reactions to examine some behavior that becomes unexpectedly troublesome. Then the therapist is compelled to reevaluate what was not even thought about as ever becoming a problem. The need for painful reevaluation and the accompanying insecurity about one's self-image could be reduced by the adoption of a more preventitive approach about the possible effects of idiosyncratic responses.

Of course it remains understandable, if not really acceptable, that therapists may be reluctant to adopt the strategy we are suggesting. Naturally therapists are not keen on appearing different from what they claim to be, and certainly that could happen more often with the process of reappraisals under consideration here. Also, within any given theoretical orientation, there is very little official room for the individual differences that surely do exist. As a result, therapists who may seem often, and in detail, to be examining their behavior in therapy sessions may be subject to unwelcome criticism from the apparently more orthodox who have no such need. All this limits the range of therapist behaviors subject to continuing scrutiny, thus facilitating the unexplored character of idiosyncratic responses. Psychoanalysis is a major example of how the field struggles with the broad issue of therapists' personal reactions, including idiosyncracies, classed under the rubric of countertransference.

We will return to a consideration of the countertransference concept later in the chapter, but first we want to explore in more detail the hidden effects of idiosyncratic responses. We are interested in a greater recognition of the pragmatic artistry of all therapists, which in turn means that all therapists could have greater necessity as well as opportunity to be accountable for all their idiosyncracies. These can be intriguing facets of the human condition, and our aim in highlighting their effects is not so much to consider their possible elimination, but to delve into ways to mold them into effective tools of the trade.

All therapists develop characteristic ways of being themselves in the therapeutic interaction, even if they are trying not to be themselves. Schafer (1983) has described an analyst as having a "second self," distinct from the self of usual social and interpersonal interaction. Yet this self retains elements of the total personality, including at least some of its uniqueness. Although in psychotherapy the very purpose of the endeavor provides a recognized and somewhat standardized framework for expression, the boundaries of that structure have a fluidity when it comes to the manner of expression. Eventually we may develop distinct methods of personal interaction as psychotherapists that are different in significant ways from how we react and present ourselves in many other situations.

The development of a personal therapeutic style is of course intended to be effective and, as such, congruent with the therapist's theoretical orientation. Many times such styles are expertly honed with experience to present a very special productive context for each patient. Even when therapists are not outstanding, they can create quite a facilitating environment. Numerous stylistic errors have their own punishments through the negative responses of patients. As a result, the *known* good and bad aspects of style can be accounted for in the process of therapy. At issue, however, are the frequently unnoticed and therefore unknown stylistic features that also affect the therapy.

The conscious and unconscious formal establishment of a therapeutic style begins in training under supervision. This involves learning how to be helpful as well as how not to get in the way. The result is a particularized way of working with patients that therapists come to believe in as their unique style. It is validated by the manner in which patients respond and by the "fit" of the style with the therapists' personalities. All concerned become happy enough with it so that the style becomes a comfortable background for therapeutic interaction.

Missing from this pleasant sketch are the elements of style that have gone unnoticed in the training process, and those that remain so despite further training, as well as new features added almost imperceptibly. Also, the maintenance of a style is subject to limited scrutiny and probably limited revision. There is a lulling familiarity to being one's usual therapeutic self. Although the results of a therapist's current efforts may be personally satisfying, more can be discovered by casting a discerning eye on what the therapist customarily does and by examining all the probable effects of this behavior that has become so natural. We now provide some examples of such scrutiny, starting with how therapists begin and end sessions, make interpretations, and finally how therapists relate to patients outside sessions.

BEGINNINGS AND ENDINGS

In the following example, a therapist greets a new patient. The patient is sitting in the therapist's waiting room. The door to the therapist's office is closed. Then it opens, the therapist steps out and walks toward the patient. The patient stands up. The therapist extends his hand and says, "Hello, I'm Morton Gordon."

The patient shakes the therapist's hand and replies, "Hello, I'm Dennis White."

This therapist routinely introduced himself without his title. His original reason for doing this was to decrease the patient's probable anxiety at being there for the first time. He believed the relative informality furthered this and established the relationship as more of an equal one in the collaborative sense as opposed to a superior–doctor and inferior-patient relationship. Such an approach became routine, and the therapist felt no continuing need to reexamine his rationale. He had also received reinforcement over time from two types of patient responses. One was directly positive, commending him for his very human and understanding way of presenting himself, which made these patients feel accepted. The other was from patients who reported difficulty in knowing what to call him because they had trouble with authority figures. His approach led them right into a problem area, and they ultimately liked that. He really had no negative responses to his manner of introducing himself, so he stopped evaluating it.

This particular patient appeared to fall into the second category. He did feel uncomfortable with the initial greeting by the therapist, but he did not indicate his discomfort immediately. Instead he called his therapist Dr. Gordon until at one point the therapist asked Dennis about what the therapist perceived as unnecessary formality. This led to interpretations about the patient's relationships to authority figures, in particular, a need to keep them in a place above the patient. This was indeed true, and in fact the patient was unable to call his in-laws by their first names. He did not call them Mom or Dad, or any variation on that theme, because he did not like them that much. They did not want to be called Mr. and Mrs., so he avoided calling them by any name. In the light of his insight he was now reluctant to use any of his old patterns with his therapist, so he uncomfortably called him Morton. In time his reluctance seemed to fade, and his new skill even generalized to his in-laws so that progress was apparent.

However, his problem was not solved because there was an additional reason for the patient's discomfort. The therapist's first name, Morton, was a name in a "dirty joke" the patient had been told by another boy when he was a child. Unwittingly he had regaled his parents with the joke one night at the dinner table, and to his astonishment, he had been punished. The joke with all its implications was never forgotten, but he never told his therapist about that part of the discomfort. The association was revealed when he began therapy with another therapist. His reasoning to support the previous concealment was that his therapist had acted as though the name issue had been resolved. Since the patient wanted it to be that way, he concurred. It was discovered only when in his new therapy he was asked what he had called his first therapist. His reply was hesitant, and when the hesitancy was discussed, he told the story of his difficulty with authority figures. It might have rested there, except that over the course of the therapy, the patient seemed to have little trouble calling his new therapist by her first name even though she had been introduced to him as "Doctor." At the same time, whenever the previous therapist came up in the associative process, the patient hesitated in saying his name. The new therapist investigated this hestiancy, and the patient spontaneously called the previous therapist a "dirty man." The patient then went on to relate the associations between the first therapist's name and the joke.

There was considerable significance to this revelation. The patient had terminated his first therapy because of his continuing discomfort with using the therapist's name, although he had trouble admitting that even to himself. He did not mention it when terminating, or when beginning a second course of treatment. Instead, he used different, and what he saw as more psychologically palatable, reasons that were accepted by both therapists at the time they were offered. Furthermore, the "dirty man" and the problem with authority figures turned out to be related in ways that had not been explored before. They well might have been except that the name issue was negatively idiosyncratic for the first therapist. However, he closed that avenue of investigation because he believed he already knew the answer to "what's in a name." Either patients called him by his first name, as he did to them, or they had a problem with authority, as indeed this patient had, but that was only the more accessible concern. The possibility that his name might have certain other meanings to a patient was not part of his therapeutic rationale. As a result, he missed a significant issue and lost a patient.

The categories for introduction can be grouped generally into formal and informal. In the example cited, the informal ultimately posed a problem that the formal did not. However, our emphasis is not on a preference for one category over another, since either can be comforting or threatening depending on the patient's expectations. If introduction by title is used and the patient is indeed expecting a "doctor," then the title is reassuring. In contrast, if the patient associates words such as "doctor," "patient," and "therapy" with "crazy," which in turn the patient has a deep fear of being, then the title and all the structures that can go with it loom cold and hard in the patient's path. Also, even with a category, there will be variations with possible differential impacts.

Formality in the therapy field does not automatically mean "doctor," since many therapists are not doctors by title, and again this could be disturbing or reassuring relative to the patient's preconceptions. The consequences of the form of introduction, which has to be, at least in part, idiosyncratic can be rather apparent on the level we are now describing. However, our concern is with the therapist's willingness or unwillingness to look beyond usual expectations.

Another example of the hidden possibilities in idiosyncratic responses can be seen in the ending of a session. A patient had been talking about her sexual difficulties with her husband. That morning they had sexual relations and she had found the event particularly unsatisfying. She also felt that her husband had not really enjoyed it either. However, he acted as though nothing disturbing had occurred, and on leaving for work, kissed her and said, "have a nice day." Although his tone was not sarcastic, she questioned the remark to herself and doubted his sincerity and felt attacked by him in a passive–aggressive way. She contrasted this with her relations with another man with whom she was having an affair. The experience with her husband had preceded the therapy session. She was to see the other man following the session. She was talking about her positive anticipation of that meeting when the session ended. At that point the therapist said to her "well, that's it. I hope you enjoy yourself."

She turned to him and said with considerable anger, "screw you," and stormed out.

The therapist was taken back. He had expected either a positive response or a noncommittal one, but not anger. He had felt that he was being empathic, connecting with the final material of the session and in that way with her in providing a bridge from the session to the outer world. It was a routine idiosyncratic pattern he followed in ending sessions that he believed was an appropriate and therapeutic effort. His view of the results of doing this was that patients reacted positively to it, experiencing it as a statement of understanding on his part. This was validated either by immediate patient response, or if not immediate, by subsequent reports even if the first response of the patient was to feel uncomfortable. The latter type of patient admitted to having trouble taking, and at first had felt something was being demanded personally, but then realized he or she did not have to do anything and, as a result, appreciated the therapist's concern. The therapist did not consider the possibility that both his technique and his attitude might be working to keep out any patient responses except the two categories he was getting.

When this patient responded angrily, he did question what he had said to her, thinking he should not have said that, or perhaps he should not have said anything other than indicating the session was finished. He realized his adding a comment was relatively frequent for him, in fact a habit with certain patients with whom he felt it was needed. He had a narcissistic investment in the therapeutic power of his words that was not accompanied by an awareness of the range of possible negative patient reactions.

We are not arguing here for the value of one technique over another, as silence rather than a comment conceived to be empathic. Our concern is the limited scope of his rationale and understanding. His idiosyncratic response allowed no room for reactions he had not experienced before. He had acted in a certain way many times in concluding sessions, and he thought he knew all the effects of what he was doing. This patient fortunately shook his conviction and opened his perceptual field.

When he saw her in her next session, he explored her angry responses. She confirmed her anger stating that he had acted like her husband, that he was being sarcastic, and had even used her husband's very words, "Have a nice day." Of course, his words had not been identical, but he understood the similarity and how she could have thought he was being hostile to her. What now struck him was something that he had missed before. Her concern had been with the difficulty between herself and her husband. The material about her affair may have been at the end of the session, but it was not her major issue. Perhaps she was attempting a reparative or displaced defense for herself, but the rage at her husband was ready to be transferred to the therapist. She suggested that perhaps that was what the therapist had intended by making his remark, but he knew that had not been the case. He had missed what her feelings were at the end of the session and was trying to empathize with what he wanted them to be. In this case the therapist had the opportunity to reexamine an idiosyncratic response and to realize the variety of meanings that could be attached to it as well as the error of assuming that what was relatively habitual on the therapist's part would be greeted with "the usual" by the patient.

As with introductions, our point about endings is that they also lend themselves to idiosyncratic approaches by therapists. In turn, they carry the potential for overlooking possible patient reactions as well as creating concealment on the part of patients in reaction to their perceptions of having "a good fit" with their therapists. Thus, although we are not suggesting that there is a universal best way of beginning or ending sessions, we do suggest a review of how idiosyncratic such responses have become and what this may mean for both therapist and patient. Over time, even the more obvious probabilities may be ignored in deference to a favored one that appears to guarantee some perfunctory time for the therapist. In this profession, nothing can ever be really perfunctory; everything has meaning; and things keep changing. Perhaps the best index of therapist reliability is the remembrance of all that along with the ability to flex accordingly.

INTERPRETATIONS

The essence of analytic therapy is certainly interpretations, and therapists often pride themselves on both the content and manner, including timing, of their interpretive statements. Theoretical adherence is definitely a determinant here, as for example, the use of instinctual interpretations by drive theorists as compared with the use of relational interpretations by interpersonal theorists. However, there is nonetheless a considerable range of idiosyncratic interpretive styles within the boundaries of theory. Therapists develop familiar interpretations that are believed to be appropriate both in content and style. Habituation to these fosters the development of blind spots in regard to the breadth of the context. Something is being missed in terms of the interaction between therapist and patient, but that is not so apparent based on the verbal material presented by the patient. The interpretations may well be accurate, but they are not received as such by the patient. The result is frustration and a stalemate in the therapy.

A good example of this is the use of projective identification, a defensive maneuver by the patient that involves attempts to maneuver the therapist to be in some significant ways identical to the patient. The maneuver is attempted to make certain aspects of the patient more tolerable to the self. For example, if successful, a painful feeling may unconsciously be shifted from the proprietorship of the patient to joint ownership with the therapist. Boundaries are blurred, and responsibility is reduced for the patient whereas it is increased for the therapist. Such a maneuver is threatening to the narcissism of the therapist and often reacted to by repression and denial accompanied by reinforcing activity, such as the usual interpretations.

Ogden (1982) describes projective identification as having three main interdependent components. The first of these is the desire of the projector to put a part of the self in the therapist in such a way that the part indeed becomes a real aspect of the therapist. This is fantasized because the projected aspect, a feeling, an internal representation, is a source of discomfort to the patient. The wish is essentially to inhabit, at least partially, another person and internally control that person. It is that desire for control that is so difficult for the therapist to respond to in a truly understanding way. Instead, the idiosyncratic interpretive process offers an apparently understanding approach that is soothing to the therapist's narcissism while it shifts the burden back to the patient.

Such a maneuver by the therapist runs counter to the second step by the patient, which is to get the therapist both to experience the projection and to behave in a manner that shows this. The boundaries between self- and object representations are to be obliterated in reference to the projection, with a symbiotic union created in their place. The interaction between the patient and therapist will show whether or not the projection has been successfully transplanted, and the patient will struggle with the therapist to bring about such validation. If the therapist is unaware of what is happening, the results will be markedly chaotic. The patient's attempts to control the therapist will be met with the therapist's interpretations of the patient's maneuvers, which in turn will be rejected by the patient who is seeking a verification of the projection. This in turn could result in the therapist becoming more insistent and appearing angry. If this were the sought-after feeling, then the patient could feel relief, although not resolution. If the therapist's response did not fulfill the projection, the struggle could continue or deadlock. In either case, the therapist's unawareness is a major obstacle to any real progression and is really increased by the idiosyncratic belief that the patient is merely resisting true but painful interpretations. Although this may be true, the projective identification has to be considered first and processed by the therapist.

Processing is central to the third phase of projective identification, which begins with the therapist being able to experience the projected feelings. These feelings are not, however, from the therapist's point of view the same as the patient's feelings. Whereas they tend to be similar to what the patient feels, the therapist creates a personal approximation of the original projection that can be dealt with in ways that differ from the patient's methods. The result can be a processed version of the feelings that constitutes a new package of the projection, which the therapist then can make available to the patient for reinternalization. By having the projection processed by the therapist, the patient is able to consider new ways of again owning a feeling that previously needed to be "lent out" to protect the patient from the discomfort of owning the feeling. To make this work, the therapist must be able to show the patient that the projected feeling has been received and can be integrated by the therapist, thus modeling the idea that the therapist's version of the patient's projection is not the problem the patient had found it to be. The therapist's receipt and integration also serve as a model for grappling with unpleasant internal feelings at this source without displaying the need to project them and identify with them as emanating from an external source.

How does the therapist do this? There is considerable disagreement about the answer, and even about the utility of the concept of projective identification as a separate construct. In our discussions, we have been using the framework suggested by Ogden (1982), but since the introduction of the term by Melanie Klein (1975) in 1946, it has often been reshaped and used with a variety of meanings (Finell, 1986). Grotstein (1981), for example, does not distinguish it from projection, as does Ogden, nor does Grotstein see the therapist as the processor in the manner described by Ogden. However, all authors who recognize this concept as a clinical reality agree that the patient is trying to do something to the therapist and that the therapist can feel this and react either defensively or constructively. We consider it quite useful both theoretically and clinically, as well as particularly apt for the illustration of the idiosyncratic interpretive response. Finell, although recognizing the problematic aspects of the concept, stresses the frequency and ease with which patients' projective identifications result in therapists' misuse of interpretations. Also, Ogden makes the point that projective identification does not have to be thought of as a metapsychological concept to be recognized. Its clinical phenomena of the patient's unconscious fantasies projected to the therapist that result in congruent or defensive feelings in the therapist are well documented. The value we see in using the particular term and describing it in terms of the patient's specific type of projections as well as the feelings engendered in the therapist is that this distinguishes relatively unique patient projections and therapist responses. As such, particular therapist responses of containment and subsequent interpretations are called for and are subject to specific countertransferential responses that differ from what is usually seen in defending against patient manipulations that would not be categorized as projective identifications. It is quite probable that within the broad range of patients' projections, projective identifications are the most likely to trigger idiosyncratic interpretive errors.

Two major possibilities appear. The first is that there will be a relatively complete lack of awareness of what the patient is trying to do, so the interpretation is made almost glibly, and any resistance is considered a sign of the patient's unpleasant affective reaction to the veracity of the interpretation. Such an approach is the idiosyncratic style of "now it is time to interpret," and the patient's associative content calls for a particular type of interpretation that is routinely given. Either there will be resistance, which can in turn be interpreted as such, or the interpretation will be accepted and thus validated. This method completely misses the projective identification and basically ignores the patient.

The second approach is somewhat better in that the projection is felt unconsciously, but the feelings make the therapist uncomfortable and so are defended against by use of interpretation. The content of these interpretations will be similar to the content in the first possibility, but the motivation is different. The therapist is being made uncomfortable and is trying to dissolve this unease through interpretations. There is a recognition that something is being done to the therapist, but there is no interest displayed in really dealing with the provocation. The patient gets recognition that is followed by rejection through the therapist's use of interpretation. The ensuing struggle that may follow between the patient who wants the therapist to keep and share the feelings and the therapist who wants to be rid of them can result in the therapist expressing anger and resentment toward the patient. If angry feelings were being projected, then the identification can be validated without the therapist's awareness. This can be followed by a relaxation in the contentious interaction, which the therapist may experience as validation of the interpretation and dissolution of the resistance. However, as the therapist then relaxes, the patient's projected feelings no longer seem to be present in the therapist so that the whole process needs to be started again by the patient. In both of our possibilities, the idiosyncratic responses of the therapist mean the lack of a therapeutic resolution for the projective identification.

For the therapist to be effective, it is necessary that he or she understand and address all the components of the projective identification. Ogden (1982) has identified these as a defense, a communication, a form of relating, and a way to experience psychological changes. All these components have their origins in early attempts to organize experience within the mother–child interaction. Splitting is used to keep good and bad experiences apart, and projection and interpretation provide methods to insert aspects of the self into others as well as to assimilate aspects of others into the self. Dangerous aspects of the self can, by this devise, be made distinct from the self and be "put into" the mother for security and still be retained at a psychically comfortable distance. By inducing these feelings in the mother, the child can feel understood and have a transitional type of object relatedness. If the mother cannot contain these feelings, her distorted responses will perpetuate the child's negative perceptions of the feelings and the need to be rid of them and will offer the probable internalization of the mother's methods for mishandling the feelings. In contrast, if the mother contains and masters them, then by her psychological integration, she provides a model for the child's reacceptance of the feelings and a sense of a way to integrate them.

Providing standardized habitual interpretation as part of an idiosyncratic response pattern misses what is required of the therapist as the object of a projective identification. Two examples will illustrate the therapist's unawareness, its damaging effect, and how this was corrected, thus answering our previous question of how the therapist can successfully work with projective identification.

The first case is described by Finell (1986) and involved a woman who had been rejected by a rather sadistic lover whose relationship with her was very similar to her relationship with her parents. The love relationship had been a difficult one, but nonetheless she remained preoccupied with the loss. The therapist felt frustrated in her attempts to ease the patient's suffering. The therapist interpreted the patient's masochism and the repeating of early losses, but the patient considered the therapist to be lacking in empathy and actually to be causing the patient to feel more alone. She saw no value in the genetic interpretation, although it appeared appropriate to the content. The patient felt misunderstood because she wanted a container rather than an interpreter who was rejecting her. Fortunately, the therapist examined what was happening and began to realize that a personal desire to save the patient and therefore not to feel helpless and angry toward the patient was motivating the interpretations. The therapist was able to stop interpreting and instead to begin containing the projected feelings. Empathic statements by the therapist and the provision of a holding environment opened the way to subsequent interpretation. The lover had been a projective identification of the patient's dependency and hostility, and she began to see this and to separate from such an ambivalently experienced object. The key was the therapist's recognition and containment of personal feelings of sadism and helplessness, and the use of such recognition by the therapist to now be empathic rather than intellectually interpretive. In this regard, Finell suggests offering questions that give the patients an opportunity to understand their feelings as opposed to statements that inform patients what they are feeling. The message is, listen and contain first, be clearly empathic; interpret later, and the chances for making effective use of projective interpretations are markedly increased.

In our second example, a patient was telling her therapist about responding to a plea by a former male lover that she meet with him. The relationship with this man had been discussed at length in therapy. Akin to the first example by Finell, there was a sadomasochistic interaction wherein the man was angry and destructive. However, in this case, the patient had rejected him but was again drawn to him when he called her. They met, he was drinking, and they had an automobile accident while he was driving. No one was injured, but the car, which belonged to the patient, was badly damaged. The patient felt frustrated and angry with the man, and the therapist in turn felt frustrated and angry with the patient. The patient was projecting her anger and helplessness, and the therapist felt uncomfortable but did not recognize the projection. Instead she interpreted, focusing on the patient's self-destructiveness in reinvolving herself with the man who destroyed the patient's car and could have destroyed the patient as well. The patient reacted angrily to the self-destructiveness designation, denying it and indicating that the therapist did not understand her. The therapist now felt threatened and compelled to prove her point, so she marshaled evidence about the patient. A prominent piece of this, according to the therapist, was the fact that the patient had been careless about birth control at one time, which had resulted in pregnancy and an abortion that had greatly disturbed the patient. The patient also disputed this, pointing out that although there had been times in her life when she had not been careful to use birth control, none of these had resulted in an abortion. She indeed had had an abortion but at a time when despite her best efforts, birth control had been ineffective. The therapist realized the patient was indeed correct and that the therapist had mixed up the facts.

All this took place over a number of sessions during which the therapist felt uncomfortable as she waited for interpretations to take hold and the resistance to dissipate. When the patient pointed out the therapist's error regarding the self-destructive character of the patient's abortion, the therapist reevaluated what was happening. Although the patient may have acted in a masochistic fashion in the relationship with the man, the interpretation was being given for the sake of the therapist who did not want the patient's projective rage. The therapist automatically made an obvious interpretation that was unsuccessful in all endeavors. The patient felt misunderstood, more frustrated, and was more angry at the therapist. The therapist apologized for her error and for misunderstanding the patient. She stated she had been confused but now could understand, and this allowed the patient to refocus on her anger at the man. The patient did this quickly, dropping the overt anger at the therapist but continuing the projection now sensed by the therapist who was experiencing her own anger and self-destructiveness. As the therapist contained the patient's feelings, the patient moved to the genetic antecedents of her rage, and eventually to a consideration of why she had reentered a relationship that she should have known could harm her.

In this case, the therapist was at first unaware of the patient's defense, experienced the communication as immediate material for interpretation of self-destructive tendencies, engaged in an aggressive interaction, and essentially did not process the projection. Her idiosyncratic response was to interpret and to continue doing so in the face of the patient's apparent resistance and as a way to defend against her own anxiety about aggressive and self-destructive feelings. In this process, she appeared to engage in some self-destructive forgetting herself, and the subsequent awareness of that started a chain of reparation working into resolution. The therapist's idiosyncratic mode of standardized interpretation was in the service of protecting her from possible narcissistic injury, but it was unsuccessful. Had she not made the memory error and had the patient not reacted to it, the interpretive approach might have continued to no avail because the idiosyncratic response was so habituated that the therapist did not consider it to be in need of reexamination.

CONTACT OUTSIDE OF THERAPY

Two types of patient–therapist contact are considered here. The first is fantasy, the therapist's imaginings about what it would be like to be with the patient in a variety of situations outside the therapy. Some of this will occur during a therapy session and be prompted by patient comments. For example, a depressed patient stating, "It must be horrible to live with someone like me who can't even stand herself," could lead the therapist to identify with the possibility of both living with the patient and being the patient. This is idiosyncratic to the extent that any therapist would bring personal elements to the identifications, but these are tempered by the array of information the therapist has about the patient. These fantasies are usually conscious or preconscious and serve as a means of being able to understand the patient. They would become a problem if their purpose was more to meet the therapist's needs and, particularly, if the therapist's boundaries became blurred and the fantasies began to have a potential reality. The essential feature needed to keep identification fantasies valuable is the consistent recognition that the patient–therapist roles are not actually going to change. The therapist's projective identifications then serve the therapy, mainly to increase empathy.

However, in the second type of contact the roles do change, at least to some degree. The rules around patient–therapist interactions are designed to protect the therapeutic process from any more intrusions than those that are already inevitable. This means that there will be some possible contacts that have an intrusion potential and that therapists need to be able to deal with these in a therapeutic manner. For example, a therapist may meet a patient on the street, in a store, or at a restaurant. Therapists write books and papers in professional journals. Patients can and do read at least some of them. Therapists make presentations at public meetings and some patients attend. There is a public side to all therapists, and even when it is deliberately restricted, patients have access to it.

The question then is what to do with these interactions, keeping in mind that the patient–therapist roles are the predominant ones and that anything else may impact those roles. That is where an idiosyncratic stance tends to develop, namely a usual way of dealing with such encounters that includes both what the therapist is likely to do in such situations as well as what the therapist will do in the therapy when such contact has occurred. An example would be that the therapist will be polite, but limit the extent of the interaction, and in therapy the therapist will wait to see if the patient brings up anything about the interaction. If the patient does not mention it, the therapist will not. A number of variations on this formula are possible, particularly the therapist's always bringing up the meeting regardless of whether the patient mentions it or not. The theme in whatever approach the therapist adopts is that these extratherapeutic situations have a potential for adding something to the therapy that could be a problem. As a result it would be easier not to have them, so therapists seek to deal with the situations in ways most facilitative for the therapy. The result over time, however, can become an idiosyncratic

formula that the therapist believes is best for all concerned but that tends
to narrow the therapist's vision as to what all this means to the patient.
How one deals with these situations cannot be habitual without a sacrifice of some therapeutic possibilities for the patient in favor of alleviation
of the therapist's anxiety.

These outside-of-session encounters can actually be productive,
depending on how the material is subsequently used in the process of the
therapy. For example, a therapist made an emergency visit to the dentist
and had a tooth removed. Prior to the completion of the procedure, he
was asked to wait in the waiting room with a piece of gauze stuck in his
mouth, limiting his ability to speak. Much to his surprise the one other
patient in the waiting room was a new patient of his whom he had seen
about four times at that point. He had had no idea who the patient's
dentist was and certainly no prescription for the possibility of meeting
her there. Whatever idiosyncratic formula he might have had for such a
situation was definitely restricted by his physical discomfort and speech
restriction. The patient seemed surprised to see him, but glad. He
mumbled that he could not really talk and pointed to his mouth. She
appeared relatively oblivious to his embarassment and made a comment
about how interesting it was that they used the same dentist and that
must mean the dentist was indeed good. He nodded his head in assent
and wished either he or she would get called by the dentist. She stated
that she had been waiting a while, and he realized his emergency visit
must have delayed her and sensed she realized that too, although she did
not seem to mind. At this point, much to his relief, she was called into
the inner office.

When the therapist saw his patient for her next session, she com-
mented on how nice it was to have seen him in the dentist's office, that it
made her feel more secure in a place where she often felt anxious. He had
not expected that response, since he had felt uncomfortable and deposed
from his more customary position of greater ambiguity. She appeared to
have missed both his mental and physical discomfort and instead focused
on the positive nature of his presence for her. This clarified her state of
initial responsiveness to the therapy, although the therapist kept in mind
that the other side of her ambivalence had yet to appear and that this
incident in the dentist's waiting room could still provide material related
to his state of actual discomfort. The opportunity for an idiosyncratic
defense pattern remains here, however, if the therapist fails to notice or
represses the patient's range of possible feelings about the incident. The
immediate probable narcissistic injury to the therapist was averted by the
patient's narcissism and her narcissistic alliance with the beginning of
therapy, but the therapist needs to remain alert to the unraveling of the
patient's narcissism at the risk of threatening his own.

The frequency and impact of this type of occurrence have an important precipitant that can be of great assistance in helping to explain and manage the idiosyncratic response. This is the therapist's choice of patients, which in turn can be predictive of the likelihood of having extrasession contacts with patients. Since contact outside the session increases the possibility of influencing the transference in an unusual way, there is a general inclination to choose patients with whom the therapist will have contact only during sessions. Such an approach preserves the therapist's relative ambiguity, and this can create greater opportunity for interpreting patients' reactions as projections connected to unconscious wishes and fantasies. The introduction of reality can limit the projective aspect of the patient's associations, or emphasize one type of projection and obscure another. The free field can become cluttered. However, free association and therapist ambiguity are concepts of degree, so the question is to what extent reality may intrude to make the therapy ineffective. Some reality is inevitable such as fee, time, office, location, age, and physical appearance of the therapist, and these may well be considered useful boundaries that provide a requisite amount of structure to balance the considerable ambiguity and uncertainty of therapy sessions.

When a therapist chooses to see a patient, the therapist is agreeing to operate within certain limits that are supposed to exist for therapeutic reasons. These can and do vary from person to person. It may be that a therapist and a potential patient have met in a social situation, or meet for a time in another setting such as supervision. The person may feel that he or she is impressed with how the other person is perceived to be as his or her therapist. It is possible that in this particular situation, the potential patient could better work out the concerns associated with the outside contact than personal feelings about a therapist with whom the patient had no contact.

The student in supervision learns a great deal about the supervisor as a therapist, such as style, theoretical orientation, interpretations, and relatedness and so can make a relatively informed judgment about the potential for a therapist–patient relationship. However, the supervisor also learns about the supervisee and must decide if the current relationship, which is evaluative, will in this case facilitate or hinder a therapeutic relationship.

The boundaries of the therapy must facilitate the therapy. This really translates into a situation in which transference, countertransference, and resistance are well managed. The guidelines developed to do this aim at increasing projections for the patient and decreasing them for the therapist. The responsibility for determining what the therapeutic situation shall be rests with the therapist. The idiosyncratic response as we have defined it—habitual, automatic, and unscrutinized—can well get in the way of the therapist's responsibility. Certainly the therapist should not get involved in ostensibly therapeutic situations that are causing the therapist discomfort. At the same time, the therapist should not assume that past comfort is a guarantee of either present or future reactions. Every new possible course of therapy has to be evaluated for its novel as well as familiar probabilities, and the patient can be informed of what the therapist sees as lying ahead in terms of trouble spots. It is very likely that if difficulties arise from extratherapeutic contacts of the sort we have mentioned they can be resolved if the therapist has undertaken the therapy with an awareness of these possibilities and is open to dealing with them. Added to this has to be that the therapist is capable of working with them, which means a realistic assessment by the therapist of the situation when it originates, as well as continuing reappraisal as it develops.

COUNTERTRANSFERENCE

The origins of idiosyncratic responses can better be understood by viewing each response as a type of countertransference that is particularly reluctant to surface and bear examination. This is unnoticed material and, as such, can make an also unnoticed contribution to the treatment that operates as a source of confusion for all involved. Although there has been a marked increase in literature about countertransference (Epstein & Feiner, 1979a; Meyers, 1986; Slakter, 1987), most of it is concerned with definition and utility rather than discovery.

For example, Rawn (1987) indicates that countertransference has been defined broadly to include the total response of the analyst, as well as more specifically. In the latter instance, distinctions are made between realistic responses, reactions to the patient's transference, and the therapist's displacements of the past. Controversy also exists about its value. Reich (1951) emphasized that countertransference is not a therapeutic tool, whereas Searles (1958) stressed its potential utility. The controversies about what countertransference is and what to do with it are still current. However, there is agreement that there are unconscious therapist reactions to the patient that may affect, positively and/or negatively, the therapeutic process. Idiosyncratic responses have gotten some attention in that regard, though not much. Balint and Balint (1939) mentioned the effect of the therapist's style, which they appear to minimize but consider it part of countertransference. Winnicott (1947), in his discussion of the analyst's hate, noted the idiosyncratic aspects of countertransference. Bleger (1967) and Langs (1978) emphasized the use of the frame of the therapy that included both the style of the therapist and the tendency to ignore its impact.

The inclusion of the idiosyncratic response within the concept of countertransference provides an historical context. The patterned nature of the response indicates how set in advance it is, and so in need of a longitudinal view in order for the therapist both to understand it and be flexible about it. The particular patient contributes to it, but the stimulus is actually broader—the therapy situation itself, and what it means for the person to self-define as a therapist. There is a mixture of healthy and pathological narcissism entering the idiosyncratic mode. On the positive side, the ego desires mastery and competence in service of the patient and the therapist. The latter wants the therapy to be successful and in turn develops automatic sets that process data and often eventuate in timely effective behavior. The patient shares in the therapist's point of view, but sometimes it is tunnel vision. Then the negative aspect of the narcissism has invaded the process, and the response patterns are protecting the therapist from possible narcissistic slights while the patient is left to suffer or even be the therapist's victim. The avoidance of this can be facilitated by consistently reviewing the elements and antecedents of the therapist's style and remaining aware of how easily all this becomes not only countertransference but a type of countertransference that reinforces already existing repressions and denial.

A therapist was told by the patient at the beginning of a session that she had been angry at him since their previous session. He asked why, and she said he had been yawning during that session. She saw this as a reflection of her not having an interesting personality. She felt she was a dull, boring person, and his yawning was the validation. The therapist was surprised because he did not remember yawning. In fact, although she was often depressed and in turn quiet and lacking in energy during sessions, in the previous session the patient had been quite lively. The therapist remembered feeling engaged rather than bored or tired. She backed away from the accusation by stating that since the session was in the early afternoon the therapist may have just been fatigued, but it was clear that she felt the original belief on her part was correct, although she was ambivalent about having the therapist verify it. His style was to delay since he could not recall the yawning, but he did acknowledge that it was certainly possible he had behaved that way, and if so, he was sorry, that he believed she should certainly have his full attention. If his idiosyncratic response had been to assign the projection to her and admit nothing, she probably would have accepted that since her anger was ebbing as she talked, but it could have reinforced her negative self-image while it protected the therapist's narcissism. As the therapist thought about it more, he realized he had been working hard in the previous session, and experiencing relief that she was providing material. She had created some ambiguity for him, part of which was a doubt that there would be any consistent reality to the lifting of her depression. He still doubted her perception during the session she described, but he was conscious of having yawned in other sessions with her. She was fatiguing, and it became more apparent that they both knew it and that he had been unsuccessful in trying not to show it. Also, he hypothesized that the previous session, which he had believed was positive in tone, had made her feel tired. She had to work at it, but she assigned the fatigue to him and doubted the value of her efforts. Her accusatory reaction to him caused the therapist to reevaluate his usual method of dealing with her which really had more a quality of endurance than of interest. He had been suffering her, and she had probably sensed it, but he had waited for the one session in which he had not felt that way and tried to use that to let her know. Perhaps she needed him to be negatively reactive to her, and when he believed he had not been, she tried to put life back into what was normal for her.

As his whole manner of dealing with her came into question, the therapist also asked himself about his apology. She seemed embarassed by it, and her anger was deferred. He might have kept the focus on her staying with her feelings of how she believed he perceived her. He realized there were ways to do this without appearing as if he had played no real role in what eventually happened. He began to realize that the purpose of his delay, to figure out what was happening, which he considered his style, was diluted by what was really more his style, namely to appear fair and open in both his and her eyes. His motive may have been positive, but he was protecting the images of himself when the patient may have been interested in a different projected image, the reflection of her own bad self and object images. Their therapeutic alliance was strong enough that he could have fostered more exploration without either exonerating or blaming himself, but his idiosyncratic style obscured this.

LIVING DANGEROUSLY:
CREATIVE IDIOSYNCRACIES

There is a usual, customary, yet special way for any therapist to operate, and then, there is not, for nothing works all the time or forever. Yet many ways often work. A therapist said to a patient, "You hate the you that you see in me." The patient fell silent, overwhelmed by the truth of the statement.

Six months later the therapist repeated the statement in a different instance, and the patient denied it. The patient became angry and said, "You're wrong. You were right when you said that before, but not now."

The therapist nonetheless felt he was correct. He liked the concept, his phrasing, and even the intense reaction, which in the latter case the therapist decided was resistance. A week later, he sensed the same projective mechanism in another patient and said so, reusing the phrase. This patient said, "I don't understand what that means."

The therapist elaborated. The patient said, "sounds like some kind of meaningless psychological talk to me," and dismissed any further consideration of it. Three months later that patient said to the therapist, "you know, I think you hate the you that you see in me."

Then there is the viewpoint of Winnicott (1947). He talked about the therapist's need for patience and reliability, for truly understanding the patient's wishes, and for focusing the therapy on the patient's needs rather than on the needs of the therapist. In this vein he was able to tell a patient, a young boy, that he hated him and in fact used this approach more than once. He knew how to do it and when to do it, and he made it work, but the technique is probably not for duplication, and he certainly tried to be very aware of every aspect of what he was doing.

The practice of therapy is an incredibly demanding job. As such, it is expedient to find personal ways to just make it easier. However, without sacrificing one's creative style, it remains imperative to recognize that at best the therapist can have relative ease. Neither complacency nor self-doubt are going to be useful, but evaluation and reevaluation of what one does as a therapist really needs to be the usual way of doing things. What we have described as the idiosyncratic response is a case in point and part of a theme that is explored throughout this volume.

8

Changing and Unchanging

The changes receiving the most notoriety in the process of psychotherapy seem to belong to the patient. To the extent that the therapist is a participant in the therapeutic relationship and a facilitator of patient changes, the therapist changes the patient. At the same time, therapy is a reciprocal process in which both parties influence each other, so that both patient and therapist can change during the course of therapy. This model has its origins in the early mother–child relationship (Blanck & Blanck, 1986) and continues throughout the development of family structures. The mutuality of influence is discernible in every psychoanalytic theory in terms of the transference–countertransference interplay as well as in the works of contemporary writers on the clinical theory of psychoanalysis (Gedo, 1984; Levenson, 1983). Perhaps the most dramatic example of these phenomena is illustrated by Searles (1975b) in his papers on the patient's efforts to therapize the therapist.

Our intention is to elaborate this seminal material into an illustration of the variety of ways that patients and the therapy process change therapists. We also will discuss how therapists "unchange" some of these changes and in other ways remain constant regardless of patients' attempts to change therapists. This issue concerns the narcissism of the therapist as contained in the good therapeutic self, particularly the facilitative qualities of attentiveness, responsiveness, reliability, and durability (Winnicott, 1958). Our focus is on the changes that may occur, how and why they would occur, and what may be made of them in service of the therapy. We consider this an issue that has been given less attention than it deserves based on its possible impact on the therapist. Consequently we are emphasizing the change process from the therapist's perspective, with particular concern paid to the development of anxiety, boredom, anger, eroticism, and confusion.

ANXIETY

A therapist was referred a female patient by a former male patient, who had at times mentioned this woman as a friend for whom he felt a great deal of affection and concern. The prospective patient called the therapist for an appointment and indicated she was having difficulties in a current relationship with a man. She expressed an interest in an appointment for herself as well as for both of them and preferred that the initial appointment be with them as a couple. The therapist felt some confusion as to just what the woman wanted but decided to begin the clarification processing by agreeing to her request to see them together.

He did this and, although it was apparent that they did not get along, their individual problems were so striking that treating them as a couple seemed neither feasible nor appropriate. The therapist saw each of them individually a few times and saw them as a couple again as well to give them his impressions as to the best way they might proceed. The woman seemed willing to be in both individual and couples therapy, whereas the man seemed not very interested in either possibility, although he was more willing to be in couples therapy. Both had a series of failed relationships, including two previous marriages for each of them. Both seemed very narcissistic, the woman primarily histrionic, the man primarily paranoid. The man had had some previous therapy, mainly couples work in regard to his marriages. The woman had had several courses of individual therapy with different therapists, and had been dissatisfied with all of them. They appeared as two very desperate, angry, self-involved people who did want help but were going to be very demanding, resistive, and difficult to work with.

The therapist felt comfortable in his initial appraisal. He explained the value of individual therapy for both of them as a priority, with couples therapy at some later date if it then seemed workable. The therapist indicated a willingness to work with one or both of them, or to refer if either so desired, with his emphasis being on the fact that they were suffering and that they really could benefit from therapy. They both agreed to their need for some help but put off committing themselves to any course of action. The therapist indicated they could call him, and he could make some time available. They parted with the therapist feeling he had been useful but that they were not about to follow through. He had indicated their therapies would probably be lengthy, and they seemed more interested in something quick, convenient, and relatively effortless.

A few months later the therapist heard from the woman and arranged to see her. They had a session, and again it was clear that the woman could use therapy, but she was hesitant. She feared dealing with all the anxiety-provoking material that they both recognized was there.

She put the therapist off on logistical grounds—that his office location was not convenient, that the time he had available was not the best for her, a common type of resistance. He was patient about it and simply reiterated both her need and his willingness to work with her. She mentioned that she had stopped seeing her last therapist because that woman had made "too big a thing" about the patient missing appointments. This therapist did indicate that regular appointments were necessary and that he would have such expectations if they were to meet for a course of therapy.

A few telephone calls followed in which the woman would try to make appointments but could never agree on the time. The therapist still felt comfortable in his position, hoping she would commit herself but not anxious about it. Eventually she did, following one session with another therapist whom she said she chose out of convenience but decided did not understand her. Since the current therapist felt she was not hard to understand, although certainly she could be hard to work with, he agreed to see her on a weekly basis. Just prior to this, her male partner had called the therapist and asked for an appointment. However, he wanted a lower fee than had originally been charged, and the therapist refused. The man sounded annoyed about this but asked about the possibility of a referral to a therapist who would be willing to take a lower fee. The therapist asked what fee the man was willing to pay and said he would see what he could do. It struck him that considering the man's paranoid nature it might work better if the therapist were not seeing both the woman and her male friend concurrently. The therapist was able to locate a therapist who was quite competent, interested in seeing the man, and willing to accept the fee indicated. The therapist contacted the man and told him about the possible new therapist. The man took his number but was curt and not receptive. Nonetheless, the therapist felt things were being put into motion in a way that could be useful to all concerned.

At no time during all three preliminary negotiations did the therapist feel anxious. He had seen the people initially because someone he had known and liked referred them, and he had followed through in a professional manner. The man eventually went to the other therapist, and the woman started with this therapist. Only then did the therapist notice that she made him anxious. As long as he had been at a certain distance from her, her unwillingness to commit herself had little effect on him. Now that she was supposedly into the process, he really cared about what was going to happen. The need for a real therapeutic alliance was now very striking, as was the fact that this patient was prone to an "as-if" alliance. First, she brought to most sessions a statement of how emotionally difficult therapy was for her. The implication was, "this may be too hard for me," but this was coupled with a willingness to talk freely. She did not avoid painful topics, but she seemed to be trying to make the therapist feel as uncomfortable as she did. He felt at least some of it, his anxiety eventually centering on a need to keep her in the face of an implied threat that she might leave at any time, even though she really did not want to leave. He attempted to explore this with her, and she acknowledged her tendency both to use and abuse significant others, but he was feeling pulled into the possibility of some extraordinary effort to keep her. He felt as though a part of him would be lost if she took herself away and that from session to session his intactness was threatened by not knowing when she would say, "I can't bring myself to come here anymore."

Added to this sense of turmoil was the patient's schedule. She had an active career, and it interfered with their usual meeting times. He knew this from the start and was able comfortably to exercise some flexibility. However, the patient seemed to stretch the comfort zone, and it was a difficult resistance to evaluate. She was always apologetic, always open to some other time, but never really followed their original schedule. The pattern of variability reinforced this notion that if he became insistent for consistency's sake, she would find it impossible to continue. The therapist knew that really being somewhere, fully participating, and keeping the contract were problems for her. He saw a very firm stance on his part as likely to cause her to stop attending, yet was she really being a patient as things now stood?

The answer had to be a qualified one. She was not the ideal patient, but therapeutic things were indeed happening. She was trying to do what she could at the moment, at the same time that she was resisting, a relatively common pattern except that the particulars of it made the therapist anxious. He realized that he must have wanted her more as a patient than he had admitted to himself in the first place and that now he felt a great desire to succeed where others had failed.

Waiting for her to arrive for a session he got a telephone call instead. She said she was ill and could not make that session. She turned down the first substitute he offered her, but they did agree on another time. When she arrived for that session, he was apprehensive, and she did complain about how difficult it was to come at any time other than her regular time. The implication was that somehow the therapist had caused the session changes. As she said this, the therapist found his anxiety disappearing to be replaced with a slight amusement at the predictability of her response. She needed to complain, but once having done so, she dropped the complaint and got very involved in the session. He knew he would have numerous opportunities to explore this style of hers, and he also sensed that she needed him to be able to allow her to express it in her own way. Probably most of the time he could be flexible, as he had been, and he could continue to explore the issue from time to time, as he had been doing. Possibly at the same point, it would indeed take, and she would express herself in a way that fitted the therapeutic boundaries better.

Primarily, he did not have to feel anxious about what she was going to do with the therapy. He would do what he could, and he would see what happened. He might succeed where other therapists had failed, but he might not. If anything, being anxious would probably increase the chances of failure. So, he changed, relaxing into an appropriate therapeutic stance. He did not behave differently with her, still maintaining an attitude of flexibility within limits, but he felt a lot better about what he was doing. He had stayed competent, but the trip from competence through anxiety and back to congruence of feeling and action had indeed taken place and posed the risk of incompetence as well as having caused the therapist considerable discomfort.

BOREDOM

A woman therapist had been seeing a bright, articulate female patient for about 2 years and had enjoyed working with her. The patient had from time to time discussed a woman friend who seemed very similar to the patient and was in therapy with another therapist. The present therapist developed a favorable impression of the friend, and when the friend's husband contacted her for an appointment, she anticipated another person similar to the two women. Her anticipatory set was based on knowing the one woman directly, the other indirectly, and also having heard a few things about the husband as well. These comments had been positive.

The man's presenting complaint was sexual impotence, which apparently had been a problem prior to the marriage as well. At the time of his first contact with the therapist, he had been married about 6 months, and both he and his wife had attributed the problem originally to some premarital anxiety and possible guilt about sleeping together before they were married. However, the impotence had continued, and he had chosen the therapist based on his wife's positive impressions gleaned from her friend, the therapist's patient, although they had not told the friend just what the problem was, attributing it to some possible work-related issues of his.

All this seemed understandable to the therapist, and she found the man pleasant and strongly motivated to solve the sexual problem. He seemed very attached to his wife and very interested in pleasing her, but not as psychologically minded as the therapist imagined his wife to be.

His sexual difficulty cleared up within a matter of a few months, but in exploring its possible origins, it became clear that impotency was an issue in most areas of his life and was related to his having a very controlling mother. His wife was very assertive, a trait that he admired, whereas his mother was passively restrictive, manipulating him by her supposed weakness and neediness. He was a person who was really intimidated by the world, and he seemed increasingly interested in mastering the world. However, it quickly became apparent that his therapy would be a long-term undertaking. He was willing to commit to this, but frequency was another issue. He had difficulty talking, so that making it through one session a week became a chore for both the patient and the therapist.

She recognized his anxiety and realized she would have to play a more active, stimulative role than was her usual style. However, it was more than that. The patient appeared to lack imagination, to be unable to generalize insight, to avoid feelings, particularly anger, and to be almost as afraid of the therapist as he was of other women in his life. He was pleasant, appealing in his sincerity, but uninteresting. In contrast to the previous patient–therapist situation we described where the therapist was anxious to retain the patient, here the therapist began to hope the patient would say he did not feel the need to come any longer. Although she knew that even if he did state that, his anxiety level and background would not support it, she still felt tempted. She imagined he would say he felt better, which was true to some degree, and she would confirm this and therapy would end. He did not offer to stop, however, and she became guilty of clock watching, as well as of stifling yawns and fantasizing about how she could possibly make the sessions interesting for herself.

She thought about Michels' (1988) comments about the applicability of psychoanalytic conceptions and methods, as well as the case descriptions by Gedo (1988) of apraxias, essentially deficits, in this case a learning block. She wanted to make her problem a technical one, find the method, and make the case fascinating.

Yet despite her boredom, she was providing a basic holding environment for her patient that could serve as the basis for interventions that could help him take care of his deficit. She did not seem to really want to do this, but, rather, she wanted him to do it by himself. He was not being the way she wanted him to be, and beyond that, he was not being what she expected him to be. He never had been. Based on her preconceptions, she thought he would be someone else, and she was not really accepting of who he was. To her way of thinking, boring patients were for boring therapists, whereas interesting patients were her domain. He was to have been the male version of the female patient she already had and found interesting. The narcissistic image of herself as the therapist for the fascinating was very much her style. Once she admitted that to herself, she could begin to get interested in the man as a patient. She went from the heady anticipation of a new and exciting patient to boredom and restlessness with the reality of this patient in the sessions, to the fascination of the challenge of this type of patient. Her narcissistic image shifted from an emphasis on her own sophistication and selectivity to the desire to be an effective psychotherapist capable of responding to an unexpected and labored uniqueness as well as the more familiar personality patterns that had comfortably intrigued her in the past.

ANGER

One therapist's patient had always struggled with a great deal of disorganization in her life. She existed in a chaotic pattern that disturbed her, yet her efforts at mastering it generally invoked resentment and disinterest in terms of sustaining self-discipline. She felt more victimized than responsible for her problems, so that even when she would acknowledge her role in any particular troublesome situation, this would depress her and she would want to flee from the issue. The therapist understood her sensitivity and tried to respect her pace of both gaining and using insight. He saw her self-indulgent yet self-destructive style as an integral part of her pathology and attempted to ease his own frustration by agreeing on certain boundaries for therapy to take place. She particularly resented rules of any sort, so even agreeing on procedures took some doing. Getting her actually to follow them was still another project, and even discussing her problems in this regard was not an easy matter.

In some ways she could have been considered unworkable as a patient. Is it even reasonable, however, to expect that a person who manages to displease most people in her life, and be displeased by them, should make the therapist an exception? The patient was bright, quick, imaginative, appealing in many ways that probably could be considered eccentric, and overtly wanted to be in psychotherapy. Although she was negligent about time, kept secrets from the therapist, acted out, forgot sessions, and repeatedly failed to pay her fee when she was supposed to, the therapist was remarkably consistent in his manner of dealing with her. He kept trying to work with her, interpreting the frequent resistances and definitely being there for her. She responded positively in a number of ways, making significant personal and professional changes in her life that were positive for her, but she remained always in trouble with somebody, either not paying her rent on time, or getting speeding tickets, or locking herself out of her house, etc.

This patient had gotten divorced, and although not regretting the loss of her husband the person, she was lonely and found herself unable to make permanent contacts. She focused a lot on externals, got a face lift, participated in diet and exercise programs, but avoided intrapsychic issues. She also began to blame the therapist for her depressed feelings, and he began to feel annoyed. He suspected she was setting him up to reject her, and he explored that possibility, but she seemed to be involved in so much chaos, particularly with men, that it was difficult to focus on what was happening between the patient and the therapist. He wanted to talk about it, she did not, and she flooded him with other problems that indeed were pressing. Her suffering blunted his anger, but he could feel the shift from sympathy and empathy to hostility as she frustrated his best efforts.

His angry feelings peaked around a relatively minor breach of contract on her part. She had agreed to pay him $400 at her next session, but on arrival stated she would only pay him $300. He felt annoyed, seeing this as symptomatic of her typical mode of operating, and he questioned the discrepancy, albeit in a mild manner. The patient stated that she did not want to discuss it, that she would pay the balance soon, and that she was feeling too vulnerable that day to spend time on something that was more important to him than it was to her anyway.

Despite her angry comment, he usually would have focused on the issue of her vulnerability and reminded himself that indeed she always eventually did pay. However, the therapist felt angry, and he expressed some of his anger. He insisted they discuss why she had not kept to her contractual arrangement with him, and he pointed out that from her viewpoint there never was a good time for such a discussion. She became angry also, stating she would discuss it, but it would of course take valuable time away from what was really bothering her and really waste the session.

Now that he knew what the direction of the session was going to be, he felt less angry. He was able to indicate that although it was often difficult for her to meet her obligations, this procrastination created further anxiety for her. He did not wish to be the cause of pain for her at the moment, but playing out a lifelong pattern of self-inflicted pain by drawing others into it was scarcely helpful, and it would do her little good to get his cooperation. Her major task with him was to tell him what was going on with her, not just talk about what she felt like when she felt like it.

She became tearful, acknowledging the accuracy of the therapist's comments, but indicating that having failed to live up to her contract with the therapist was just another painful reminder of how bad a person she was. She could not stand thinking about it.

The therapist responded that he understood how painful it was for her, but that the thoughts of her badness were strong and needed to be discussed, and that they could deal with it together rather than leave it alone to continue to fester and disturb her. In essence, the chances were that she would feel better by talking than by avoiding, and the payment issue was the concern of the moment. The therapist's presentation was calm, and the patient began to respond in a more organized manner. She proposed a solution that was reasonable for both of them, and rather quickly, the specific concern was resolved.

However, although the therapist had moved from feeling angry to feeling calm, he was aware that the patient's style was such that provocation would be repeated. Her intentions were as stated, but the chaos of her life was such that, at best, limited organization was probable. The concept of structural deficit again comes into play, as it did in our example of the boredom reaction by the therapist. In the present instance, disorganization was the patient's way of life, so that over time, the boundaries of the therapy had always been fluid. Such a flow was in response to the patient's limited internal controls, and it certainly was doubtful that any rapid resolution would be reached considering the magnitude of the problem. The therapist's recognition of the inevitability of subsequent confrontations resulted in a further feeling shift to a more depressed affect, but one tinged with anger once more. He felt as though the patient was entrapping him so that he would always be angry at her because she was incapable of moving at a pace that would accommodate his need for her to make progress. He suddenly thought, she is a bad mother, and he knew he had thought of her as his own mother who would never really soothe him. What was really making him angry was the image of this deceptively promising maternal figure who he could count on to fail him in their relationship. She could not live up to his expectations for her, and he, in turn, was not consistently able to use his understanding of her disorganization to temper his own frustration. As he recognized his own limitations, so he saw her as lacking what Geist (1984) has described as empathy with the self that provides for the internalization of structure through the soothing mechanism. Indeed, the therapist was having some of the same trouble himself, but he was now able to disengage from it. He suspected that he would feel angry and frustrated with her in the future, but that these feelings would be less intense, and that he would work with her more evenly to provide an atmosphere for the development of her self-empathy. In this instance there were movements from relative calm based on a positive expectation through a variety of angry feelings and returning to a more realistic calm based on better understanding of the therapist as well as the patient.

EROTICISM

The therapist's patient, an attractive, articulate male in his early 40s, was developing an obvious attachment to the therapist. The manifestations of an erotic transference were apparent in both overt associations and dream material. At the time he was recently divorced and spent considerable amounts of each session talking about finding the ideal woman for himself. This woman always looked like the therapist, and the patient made it clear that his image of the therapist was the image of the perfect woman. He was embarassed by sexual material relating to the therapist, although he reported it. His primary emphasis was on how wonderful she was, warm, caring, giving, a beautiful woman who any man would want, but was of course beyond his reach. He made it clear that he hoped he was not offending the therapist by his desire for her, that he knew she was not available to him in that way, but that he hoped he would ultimately find someone as much like her as possible.

The therapist found his erotic interest both timid and flattering, but she was puzzled by her own lack of responsiveness. Generally she found that with a strong positive transference she could in fantasy feel her possible role as the patient's partner. So if the patient described a sexual act with her, she would be able to imagine what that would feel like for her as well as for him, and she found her own fantasies useful in understanding the projection and transference of patients. In this case, she could not imagine having sexual relations with this patient. He seemed to be a child to her, and she could only imagine comforting him in a very maternal way. She realized that his style promoted such a response from women, but he was sexually active and obviously women's responses to him were not solely maternal in the way her's were. She began to wonder if the limit on her fantasy was not designed to block a stronger countertransferential reaction. She saw the patient as weak and immature in many ways, with his idealization of her symbolizing the avoidance of a strong male role. She had a contempt for him that she was expressing by being sexually neutral in her own fantasy. She was really saying, "You can try and seduce all you want, but I'm not going to respond." The patient had taken a masochistic position in his adoration, and her feelings became sadistic and were represented as withholding in her fantasy.

When she realized this, she was able to exercise her own fantasy about sexual relations with the patient. In her mind she let it become his kind of sex, and she found herself with erotic feelings toward him. He became a stronger figure, and she had several dreams in which they were sexual partners. In the therapy, she found herslf more interested than she had been in his sexual fantasies. He looked, sounded, and in her feelings became more attractive to her. She felt she could now really sense him as a sexual object and feel his sexuality. She was excited about this, but she also noticed that he was not really different. She began to wonder if what she could not connect to before was not now something she had created. She had transformed their positions so that his insistent adoration became a powerful command. His was now the strong, respected position, whereas hers was the masochistic compliant one.

Then she began to get the transference–countertransference relationship in balance. His masochism had threatened to stimulate the emergence of her erotic masochism, and to prevent this, she utilized detachment in fantasy. She felt anger at this threat, and she transformed the anger into erotic fantasies about the patient. In so doing she also changed the patient, but if she conceptualized his changed role as representing the aggression he was not displaying in his sexuality, then she had a more accurate picture of him. He hid his aggression, withholding, as she had been when she had blocked her sexual fantasies about him. The possibility of an erotic identification with the patient had disturbed her to the point of mobilizing aggressive feelings against him and neutralizing her own sexual feelings. Once she allowed herself to entertain the range of sexual fantasies that this patient stimulated for her, she could then begin to understand the patient's sexuality. She had to give herself the same freedom of fantasy that she encouraged in the patient, although he would verbalize it. At first she had restricted her fantasy and had felt anger at a patient who overtly respected her. From her discovery of her anger, she was able to develop her erotic fantasies, and from their distortions, she was able to discover more about herself and the patient. She moved through the apparent absence of erotic feelings, and finally to a comfort level of feeling responsiveness to whatever his erotic feelings tended to be. Throughout, she retained a spirit of inquiry important to any therapeutic endeavor and probably rooted in voyeurism, so that in a sense, she always had an erotic investment in the therapy.

CONFUSION

Thus far we have been describing instances of changing and unchanging feelings as well as a relative constancy of behavior by the therapist regardless of the feeling ranges. All the examples used have positive endings in the sense that the therapists worked with their own feelings and were able to be more effective in the therapy because of their work. We have aimed at illustrating the range of feelings possible, and although we have focused on a particular feeling in each section, it is also apparent that many feelings will be involved even when one is primary. Therapists need to be prepared for the emotional shifts that will often occur and accompanying ideational shifts. Changing and unchanging are common probabilities, and they have striking consequences for the progress of the therapy. In our examples, we always provided solutions, but that may not always be the case. In addition, when solutions do occur, the resolution may not be positive. The therapist's feeling and ideational shifts, or reactions against them with inflexibility, can put the therapy at risk. At the same time, the recognition of what is happening can lead to resolution and improvement in the effectiveness of the therapy. We have stressed the latter, but we certainly also wish to acknowledge the therapist's vulnerability and the potential dangers intrinsic to the process of changing and unchanging. The therapist will experience at least the possibility of emotional change, and accompanying ideational shifts, with all patients and has to be aware of this and then work with it. At the same time that the therapist is flexible, he or she is unchanging in two ways. The first is part of the flexibility, requiring movement from one feeling and understanding to others. The second is retaining a constancy for the patient and thus being unchanging in regard to a reliable therapeutic stance. The therapist's narcissism is threatened during this process by the acknowledgment of vulnerability and by the insecurity generated by changing.

A further source of insecurity for most therapists is the confusion that can occur personally in regard to the theoretical and technical uncertainties in the field. To illustrate this, we want to pose a number of questions the answers to which can certainly affect the conduct of therapy. These are questions without definitive answers, so that therapists are essentially testing them in clinical situations, and changing answers. Although we discuss the importance of theory in another chapter, some theoretical questions are raised here to show their impact on the therapist's changing and unchanging process. Psychoanalytic theory will serve as the model since we are most familiar with it, but the questions are applicable to other theories as well.

Patients frequently ask about the reasons for behavior, so certainly a basic question is the issue of motivation. The original psychoanalytic theory of motivation was a drive theory, primarily libidinal and subsequently aggressive as well. Ego psychology developed from the original drive theory, but remained quite connected to it, possibly adding a third drive such as adaptation (Hartmann, 1939). Object-relations, interpersonal, and self-theories have been subsequent additions and have attempted to move away from the original drive model. Greenberg and Mitchell (1983) have proposed the broad divisions of psychoanalytic models into drive/structure and relational/structure. In the drive model, relationships are secondary to the instincts, whereas that position is reversed in the relational model. Although the second model stresses relationships and attempts to distance itself from drive theory in its original version, the need for relatedness emphasized by object-relations theorists such as Fairbairn (1952) and Winnicott (1958) becomes an object-seeking drive. In essence a force of some description, with a driven, needful quality about it, appears as a motivational core. In theorists not as easily categorized as those described so far, such as Gedo (1988), repetition is a major force. Hedges (1983) describes self-psychology as without a "prime mover," but that really refers to conflict or mental content. There is a need for the developing person to maintain equilibrium, defined as a cohesively functioning self.

Thus, the tendency is to choose a major motivational force of some sort, give it a name, and include a variety of constructs within it and then to view it as the answer to the "why" question. This in turn provides a focus for the psychotherapist. For example, is a particular problem to be seen primarily as difficulty in libidinal drive expression, or relatedness to others? Although the either–or possibilities here include each other to some extent, they do so by subordination. The expression of the libidinal drive has a person as the target object, whereas the expression of relatedness has the affective quality of the libidinal drive. However, in one case the therapist would emphasize the qualities of the drive, in the other case, the qualities of the relationship.

If the therapist's adherence to a specific primary motivational focus were to shift, so would the content and style of the therapy. The awareness of the therapist in regard to clinical and theoretical developments raises the possibility of changing how one practices psychotherapy, even within one school of psychotherapy such as psychoanalysis. It is crucial to be open to new developments, which also implies a willingness to test them out and, in turn, requires integrated shifts. The patient is not in therapy to be taken for a roller-coaster ride of the therapist's making, nor is the patient to be neglected in regard to new developments as a result of the therapist's timidity or rigidity. Having a definite approach can certainly be narcissisticly supportive, but the changing and unchanging of viewpoints and methodology need to remain options.

For example, we would be reluctant to classify ourselves as either drive therapists or relational psychoanalysts, but we probably approach one more than the other. We are not even convinced of the existence of a single main motivational force, although we certainly see the existence of a number of major motivations. Libido, aggression, relatedness, intimacy, self-cohesiveness, repetition, even anxiety, are certainly significant movers that we observe in our patients. However, the individuality of each patient results in different patterns of motivation and different responses on our parts. In one sense we probably mix models, depending primarily on the patient, although the actual determinant is our perception of the patient and that is certainly colored by our own assumptions or metapsychology. We suspect that is what most psychotherapists do, although to varying degrees with some more tied to their assumptions than others. In this regard, one might contrast George Klein (1976) and his attempt to abandon metapsychology in favor of a clinical theory of psychoanalysis with Brenner (1982) and his addition of depressive affect to anxiety as a stimulus for psychic conflict.

We do not know the definitive motivational source, or sources, for human motivation, although we have a number of fairly certain possibilities—all of which we accord respect and look for in our patients. Our approach is similar to Hedges's (1983) and his use of four listening perspectives based on the levels of self- and object experience being expressed by the patient. These include the internal perspective for neurotic conflict, the self-object perspective for narcissistic disorders, the perspective of the merger-object for borderlines, and a perspective focused on part-selves and part-objects for more primitive mental states. This is essentially a developmental approach based on dominant levels of personality structure, and we have a similar conception, although it is not organized the same way as the one of Hedges. Other types of differential conceptualizations and approaches to patients have been suggested by Blanck and Blanck (1986) and Gedo (1988). In all these models, attempts are made to understand the dominant developmental levels presented by the patient and the interaction of psychic structures. The patient is seen as unfolding and changing as the therapy progresses, and the therapist must do the same as it is warranted, including accepting theoretical reformulations and technical shifts. For example, Gedo (1988) suggests three types of interventions other than interpretation. These are procedures aimed at overcoming persistent illusions of childhood, and at developing a clear set of motivational priorities and activities designed to promote regulation of stimulation.

These by no means limit the list of possible interventions, although the associative process remains our basic technique, and our metapsychology contains familiar constructs such as repetition, overdetermination, dynamics, separation–individuation, and holding environment, along with, of course, narcissism. Our concern in this chapter is that the shifts required to conceptualize and work with a particular patient even within the framework of a specified theory, such as psychoanalysis, can cause emotional confusion and insecurity on the therapist's part. The dialogue with the patient in which both patient and therapist are listening also can result in an inner dialogue for the therapist. The inner dialogue raises a narcissistic threat to the therapist's knowledge and competence.

The therapist needs to live with this and learn from it, which can certainly include making mistakes and changes. More defensive possibilities are erratic approaches reflecting excessive anxiety, or shutting out alternatives to preserve an approach that maintains the therapist's security. With these, the patient can become the confused person instead of the therapist.

A second question we pose is "How does therapy cure?" The word "cure" is used here in a relative sense to mean the attainment of some positive result. One way to respond to this would be to consider the number of possibilities suggested by major analytic schools. For example, a traditional psychoanalytic view would be that with the revelation of an oedipal transference through defense analysis, interpretation, and working through, there will be successful resolution of a developmental conflict, such as genital primacy. Other analytic possibilities have been overcoming archaic rage, attaining object constancy, or for self-analysis, a structurally complete self (Kohut, 1984). These are ideals of course, dependent on particular patient–therapist matches and a host of other variables, but even when these terse statements are filled out with detailed examples, they just do not quite answer the question we posed. Levenson (1983), who writes with both clarity and wit, describes successful therapy as interpersonal competence based on semiotic skills, with the therapist and patient expanding an infinite regress of material.

That description still does not explain the curative power of effective psychotherapy. Gedo comes closer at the end of his comments on learning in psychoanalysis when he states, "I must admit I am not yet prepared to offer a definitive statement about *how* learning takes place in psychoanalysis" (1988, p. 225). The implication is that he does not know, and that is the issue as well as the answer to our question. We do not know. Sometimes we know, or think we know, but sometimes we do not, and the times of certainty are not predictable, so confusion occurs for the therapist.

Levenson has said, "Clinical experience suggests that when a patient has elaborated a network of perception . . . recognized the richness of his own associative processes, he *does* make decisions—usually satisfactory ones" (1983, p. 120). Thus we know that if we do our part, patients will learn to do theirs, but we do not know with certainty or exact predictability how they will accomplish this learning, or exactly when, nor can we be sure who did or did not do his or her part if all does not go well.

An example of the mystery of patient learning is seen with a therapist who, through a series of drive-oriented interpretations, was achieving success with the elimination of a serious addiction. Attempting a verification of his method, he questioned the patient as to why she had given up the addiction. At first she was hesitant, then said, "Well sometimes you say something that really sticks with me, that I really think about, and that does it."

The therapist then asked, did the patient recall just what it was he had said in this case? She said, "It is something like that other time when I was living with Jim, and I hated it, and we both knew I ought to leave, and I even was spending most of my time with Tom, who wanted to live with me, and I couldn't seem to do it."

"Yes," said the therapist, "I remember, but then you did leave and now you're happy living with Tom."

> Yes, [she said] well what got me to do it, really, was when you said, "Tom seems to be able to do something you can't." We had been talking about Tom. I mean, I had actually been criticizing him, seeing him as maybe not being as strong as I was, and you said that. It made me feel, like hell, I can do whatever he can do. He had already left his wife and moved into his own place, and then I moved in with him. I'm sure you challenged me before, but that time did it. I wasn't afraid anymore, and it was as though you were my father telling me I couldn't do something, wasn't able to, and I showed you, and myself, and Tom, and Jim, and everybody, but I suppose mostly myself, that I could.

The therapist was taken aback. Although she had not answered his original question, which was subsequently answered in line with his expectation, the example his patient had described surprised him. He had not intended to challenge her, nor to try to get her to learn she had enough strength to move when he made the remark she cited. He had been attempting to get her to look at Tom's strengths in a realistic way, and instead she had learned something he had not expected or intended.

This type of "surprise" learning is not unusual, and it certainly tempers our grandiosity. We have to expect that clinical material will raise questions about what we have done as well as what we are doing. Our self-images need to embrace the idea and feeling of relative uncertainty. We remain attempters, experimenters, somewhat sure and learned, but at the same time, learning as we go.

The last question we are going to pose in this section is "To what extent do the therapeutic and real personalities of the therapist have to match?" We know they can be different and usually are, but *how* different without the therapy being affected? Changes in the life of the psychotherapist outside of therapy have an effect on the therapist's personality, which in turn can shade over into the therapy. The type of changes we are considering refer to personal stress and adversity, such as divorce, physical illness, loss, and/or financial reverses. These types of external situations pose a threat to the therapist because they are distracting and provoke both anxiety and depression. Generally therapists will both work on them and continue to do therapy at the same time, believing they can contain their personal issues and still perform effectively. In fact, the work may often operate as an antidote to the personal pain. However, the work may also be interfered with because the therapist's thoughts and feelings are elsewhere. Confusion can occur as the therapist struggles with the possibility that he or she is not doing the best job, that the therapy itself has become too demanding for the therapist.

There is no definite answer to this question either. It is a very personal, subjective issue, but it is important to know one's limits and not be so narcissistic as to consider the probability of invulnerability and invincibility to external stress. Changes in the therapist's competence can occur this way, and it may take time and efforts at personal resolution, such as therapy for the therapist, to unchange the deleterious effects. Therapists need to be aware of this possibility, to be attuned to their confusion at such a time, and to make prudent decisions about how they can practice them. Therapists have literally died in their therapy chairs as patients continued with them because the patients were sympathetic to the therapists' struggles to be helpful regardless of changing personal conditions. Yet were these therapists really helping their patients? In some cases it appears they were not, for subsequently the patients reported very mixed feelings about continuing. The patients did not want to upset the therapists, or to lose their therapists, but they felt trapped by the therapists' own unwillingness to face up to illness that was increasingly debilitating. Narcissistic denial on the therapists' parts gave them no choice, but it also restricted the choice of the patients. As therapists we have to learn to be comfortable enough with our limits to make appropriate changes in our practices, including suspension or cessation of practice if needed, as well as to help patients accept those limits when they do occur.

CONCLUDING COMMENTS

In this chapter we have considered the process of change within therapy on the part of the therapist. We have used anxiety, boredom, anger, eroticism, and confusion as examples of these alterations. We have talked about what can occur as changing and unchanging, the latter having the dual meaning of changing what has already been changed, and retaining a consistent, reliable stance. Therapy is a vehicle that stimulates change in the therapist as well as the patient, and in most instances the therapist can learn from and use such changes. However, the therapist has to be aware of the possibilities and remain flexible enough to appreciate them. This means a narcissistic structure that can accommodate uncertainty and continued self-exploration while being appropriately consistent. If a therapist stops changing and unchanging, then it is likely that psychotherapy has also stopped.

9

Listening with
the Right Ear

The centrality of listening in psychotherapy is acknowledged by all schools of therapy; the distinctions arise around how the therapist listens, what is listened to, and what the therapist does with the material. We are approaching the listening process from a psychoanalytic perspective, but, as Hedges (1983) illustrates, the various psychoanalytic theories also have their particular listening approaches, so uniformity will be relative. Our interest is not so much in the validation of specific theories in terms of their listening and communicative properties, but in listening in such a way as to be able to hear what the talker is saying. This includes both hearing and observing as listening media.

The understanding of what is heard is of course subject to the set that the listener has brought to the process. For example, in demonstrating the complexity of listening, Langs (1982) provides a schema for what to listen to, then how to organize the material, and finally what to do with it. The listening takes place on numerous levels, particularly the apparent and the concealed, but subjectivity is immediately a variable as soon as such a distinction is made. Actually, the personal element in listening is always there, but it is easier to develop a consensus about manifest content. However, it is clear that all listeners will have their personal hearing experiences, with degrees of variation, regardless of the obviousness of what they have observed. Listening to latent content provides opportunities for greater variations based on the theory and countertransferences of the listener. At the same time, a psychoanalytic listener of whatever persuasion does believe in the presence of latent content and will always be listening for hidden meanings.

Langs (1982) links listening with intervening on the grounds that the practical value of listening is to get material for subsequent interventions. He presents a three-part listening–intervening program and a six-part observational one. The first schema includes adaptive and maladaptive reactions on conscious and unconscious levels, whereas the second program focuses on therapeutic boundaries, the patient–therapist relationship, mode of cure, mode of communication, and dynamic and genetic implications of material. At this point, greater disagreement appears as to the appropriateness of the model, and the disagreement increases if one moves on to what to do with the results of the listening process. In this regard, Langs suggests that the goals of the listening process are comprehension of the therapeutic relationship, the patient's emotional problems, then interpretation and maintenance of the therapeutic environment. He adds that the therapist listens through observation, empathy, intuition, and the experience of relatedness, and he goes on to describe a detailed network of communication that takes place in an adaptive context that is psychotherapy.

We have mentioned the work of Langs because he has devoted considerable attention to listening and because much of what he describes as part of the process would be noted by others as well, even though they would probably disagree about priorities or usage of the material.

Freud (1912/1958) started the emphasis on the listening process with his suggestion of listening with "evenly-suspended attention." He did understate the complexity of the process, a fact which has become more apparent over time. Being attuned to that complexity is part of our concern, and in such an endeavor, we note the influence of Reik (1949). He stressed the "third ear" in listening, which is used to hear what others felt and thought, but did not state. Beyond that, the third ear listens to the inner voices of the therapist, and in that sense, it is our avenue to the narcissism of the therapist as it operates in the listening process. Thus, self-listening is our major focus. Also, since the listening process has been most addressed as it occurs in psychotherapy, we will consider it in a very important area where it has gotten less attention, namely supervision. The impact of the supervisory process in the actual practice of psychotherapy can be very powerful so that it can be very useful to focus on the listening process from the perspective of the supervisor. There also seems to be a great yearning on the part of most therapists to supervise, and at least a fair number do become supervisors, many without any specific training in supervision. This is an additional reason for our comments being made in the context of supervision.

There is a growing body of literature on the supervisory process, both general (Hess, 1980) and psychoanalytic (Caligor, Bromberg, &

Meltzer, 1984; Ekstein & Wallerstein, 1972; Fleming & Bendek, 1983; Wallerstein, 1981), the latter being our focus. All the literature attests to the complexity of the process. The value of supervision is taken as a given, although its essential components and the nature of the supervisory relationship are open to questions. It is clear that the supervisory situation can be rewarding and/or troublesome for both supervisors and supervisees. We are going to examine some of the trouble spots and consider how the narcissism of all the parties involved may be a factor in disturbing or facilitating the listening process that is essential to effective supervision. First we will consider the concept of supervision and then look at the supervisor–supervisee interactions.

SUPERVISION

Supervision in psychoanalytic approaches appears to have formally originated in the 1920s (Eitingon, 1937) as one of three major components of the training of psychoanalysts. It was called a control or supervised analysis, with the other two components being a training or personal analysis and the theoretical and technical curriculum. The distinction between therapy and supervision was not very clear, although usually the training analysis preceeded or at least accompanied the supervision and formal course instruction. The basic idea in supervision has been, and remains, that the supervisee is working with patients and in turn discussing this work with a more experienced therapist, the supervisor. The supervisor is there to help the therapist help the patient. There are many different ways to do this, but it is clear that supervision itself is intended to be an instructive process with the supervisor as the teacher with an emphasis on improving the supervisee's skills as a therapist. In this teaching role, the supervisor is also an evaluator of the supervisee and may have interactions that are therapeutic for the supervisee without at the same time being the supervisee's therapist. Thus, one unresolved controversy in regard to supervision is the degree to which both participants agree to make it therapeutic. It is understood that it may be incidentally or adjunctively therapeutic for either or both parties in that satisfaction and personal growth may occur based on the learning that occurs as well as the relationship itself. The experience is designed to be a positive one, although that is not always the case. However, since the person of the therapist is a key variable in the whole interactive sequence of supervision and therapy, the supervisor is faced with the supervisee's attitudes about both the therapy being practiced by the supervisee and the supervision.

Two types of supervisee countertransference are apparent, one toward the patient and the other toward the supervisor. To whatever extent either type or both types interfere with the therapy and/or the supervision, the supervisor needs to address them. The question is, how? Some supervisors make short shrift of the supervisees' countertransferences, basically noting how they interfere and recommending they be taken care of but assigning the work of that to the supervisee's therapist or potential therapist if the supervisee is without one at the time of supervision. Other supervisors focus on the countertransference, including its origins, and attempt to assist in alleviating it. For example, Grotjahn (1955) proposed an active supervisory role of interpreting the countertransference. Recently Issacharoff (1982) suggested a supervisory model stressing countertransference exploration when the supervisee has trouble learning about the patient. DeBell sums up the state of the question as follows: "To state the matter in extreme terms, everybody appears to oppose 'treatment' of the supervisee, and yet everybody does it" (1981, p. 42).

Thus, it is clear that supervision is not to be a substitute for therapy, but the probability of it being "therapeutic" is strong. How therapeutic and in what manner is undecided and would appear to be reflective of the particular styles of the supervisors and supervisees. Both participants in the supervision will be influenced by their personalities and their theoretical and technical formulations and interventions. Confrontation and clarification in regard to the supervisee's personal problems will most likely occur when these appear to the supervisor or supervisee to be interfering with either the case under discussion or the supervision itself. The intent of such activity, however, is mainly to educate the supervisee, improving self-reflective capacities and facilitating learning. Our impression is that if a learning alliance, analogous to a therapeutic alliance, has been established, supervisees appreciate supervisors' concerns with countertransference. The manner in which this is carried out, however, is crucial. The learning alliance means the relative absence of defensiveness by both parties. The supervisor is appropriately certain that the countertransference problem exists and is not concerned about being seen as intrusive or critical. The supervisee in turn is accepting of the probability of the problem and the value in addressing it.

Then there is the question of who should adapt to whom in regard to style. Supervisors have preferences, such as being active or not, focusing on supervisor–supervisee or supervisee–patient interactions, or being patient- or process-centered. Supervisees also have preferences, which may not fit those of the supervisors. Since the supervisor is the evaluator, it is frequently the task of the supervisee to fit in. The style of the supervisor also offers a model in terms of supervision, and by both implication and direction, practicing psychotherapy. This would suggest that, much as the therapist has flexibility in regard to approaching each patient, the same conception would apply to supervision. However, the supervisee is usually more of a captive in respect to the supervisor than a patient is to a therapist, and our impression is that supervisors are more careless with supervisees, and more grandiose, paying less attention to the supervisee than they would to a patient. The needs of the supervisee are often subordinated to the needs of the supervisor. Since the main need of most supervisees is to get a good evaluation, or at least, not get a bad one, they may forsake an insistence on learning for supervisory approval. In essence, many supervisees try to figure out what the supervisor wants and then do it in supervision. There are also supervisors who have a great need for approval, and they reverse the process, always trying to please the supervisee. Since supervision is supposed to be a teaching–learning situation within the context of a relationship of mutual trust and respect, there really ought to be an adaptive balance. A learning core needs to be transmitted if at all possible, but the supervisor does have a responsibility to discern how best to do this for each supervisee. In turn the supervisee has a responsibility to work to get at least the learning core while trying to adjust to the different ways various supervisors offer it.

The presence of this learning core suggests a relatively formal structure following the belief that within a tolerable range there is an expectable, usual treatment course involving a cooperative therapist–patient relationship. The general outline includes the supervisor's and the supervisee's impression of the case under discussion, followed by conceptualization of appropriate treatment procedures. Then the supervisor would evaluate the supervisee's defensive and adaptive strategies, and consider the need for altered strategies as well as how to teach these (DeBell, 1981). The teaching mechanics are in turn related to the student's learning capacities, such as experience, knowledge, and countertransferential reactions.

A variation on this procedure would be to focus on the student's problems in conceptualizing, understanding, and working with the patient. The supervisor focuses on treatment procedures designed to fit the capacities of the supervisee. Whereas one approach is more specifically adaptive than another, there often tends to be a blending of formality with impressionism that still follows general guidelines of teaching and learning to do psychotherapy. For this to be effective, both parties have to put aside preconceptions and narcissistic threats and attempt a selective, purposive listening process.

Friedman (1988) approaches the ingredients of supervision from a different perspective, namely that therapy is an abnormal relationship that is difficult for therapists and gives them problems. Thus, he begins by asking the therapist if he or she has problems. If no problems are reported, then the supervisor shifts to expectations, followed by exploring the supervisee's reactions to the patient's response to the therapist's reactions. The questions about the patient and about what was happening in the session are set at the same time in the context of the therapist's hopes, theory, and techniques. Technical terms are also developed out of problems, such as resistance and regression, which appear as avenues to problems rather than as answers. Supervision operates in a tolerant, safe atmosphere, keeping evaluations to an intrusive minimum. Creative receptiveness is taught in the context of theory, social schemas, and interpersonal desires. The theory of therapy and the theory of the mind are intermingled with the practice of therapy and its naturally problematic essence.

Schlesinger (1981) offers another look at the essentials of psychoanalytic supervision. He describes the task of supervision as enabling supervisees to integrate what they have learned about themselves with didactic material from the curriculum. The supervisor needs to listen in such a way as to be attuned to what the supervisee's particular needs are and to facilitate appropriate clinical experiences to meet these needs. The supervisor utilizes an interior dialogue to be in tune with the supervisee's development and supports the pursuit of learning. The supervisor starts where the supervisee is and works to develop an alliance of learning that encourages self-evaluation and personal growth as well. The supervisor is a teacher, a model, and to whatever degree necessary, an explorer of the supervisee's problems, both learning and personal.

The supervisee has certain learning objectives that make the fit for the useful learning alliance. These include learning how to let the therapeutic situation develop, to conceptualize tentative genetic-dynamic formulations, to develop the capacity for self-analysis, and to learn more about clinical theory and metapsychology. The supervisee and the supervisor can also be partners in specialized techniques, such as reciprocal free association (Lothane, 1984) supervisee's dreams about supervision (Langs, 1984), and the concept of parallel process.

Searles (1955) appears to have been the first to notice the parallel process, which was in turn elaborated on by Ekstein and Wallerstein (1972). The supervisor uses interaction replicated in the supervisory relationship to clarify problems the supervisee has in the patient–therapist relationship. Thus the therapist's problems in supervision and in psychotherapy are related, and the supervisee can use the supervision problems to learn how to work with the patient. This borders on psychotherapy for the trainee, but it aims at being distinct by a focus on learning in relation to the patient. Caligor (1981) sees the parallel process in supervision as omnipresent, though in varying degrees. The supervisor and the supervisee are pulled to participate in the same way, each to the other and then to the patient. That it happens seems valid, but why and how it happens is less clear. There is cognition, and empathic responsiveness, and a certain resonant repetition. What does seem clear is that, for the parallel process to be useful, the supervisor must be aware of it and deal with the transferences and countertransferences that are part of it, as well as the reciprocal processes that are stimulated.

The negatives of parallel process have also been mentioned, as for example defensiveness by the supervisor. There are two major questions involved. One is why the supervisor gets drawn into treating the supervisee the same way the supervisee treats the patient. A benign answer is empathy, whereas a more disturbing answer is discomfort on the supervisor's part with the way therapy is being conducted. In essence the supervisor has a need to treat the supervisee in a disturbing way for the supervisor's own narcissistic reasons. Dealing with that question is still problematic. It can be a teaching device, but there are those who simply see it as an impediment to supervision. More attention has been paid to the second aspect of it, namely really learning how the supervisee operates because it has now become how the supervisor operates. However, a change on the supervisor's part is suggested since parallel process tends to arise around problems. The implication seems to be that parallel process is a kind of countertransference that needs to be noticed and worked on if both supervision and therapy are to become effective.

Our overview of supervision suggests that the supervisor is primarily a teacher, and in this role, he or she also provides a model for how to be both a supervisor and a therapist. The supervisor also operates in some fashion as a therapist for the supervisee, albeit to an undetermined degree and with the focus on improving the student's functioning with the patient. Supervisors thus tend to be therapeutic with supervisees without being therapists, their emphasis on teaching rather than therapy. The degree and mechanics of this are not fixed, nor are the various possible supervisory styles of the supervisor. An interesting example of the possibilities was offered by Levenson (1982). The first category he described is holding, in which the supervisor is a clear listener, obviously present, but responding only if asked. Her presence is what is notable. In the particular example he gave, the supervision had no particular structure, but there was a holding atmosphere in which the supervisee was essentially left to explore, to make it or not to. Such an approach appears to require a supervisor of considerable experience and expertise (in this case it was Clara Thompson) and supervisees who already are fairly knowledgeable and experienced as well (in turn they were Levenson and Erwin Singer). This kind of holding would probably result in frightening the less competent.

A "by the numbers" approach is next on the list; this is basically an instruction manual of how to proceed, an authoritarian metapsychology that is both reassuring but unforgiving. A tight fit between theory and practice is the objective, with the metapsychology determining the therapeutic intervention. The value of all this rests on the accuracy of the metapsychology, derived second hand and open to question without being very open to imagination. As with many dogmatic approaches, the value is also the flaw. When it appears to work, all's well and the sun shines, but when it does not work, as can happen, the clouds gather, and it is easy to blame the supervisee for improper implementation or inaccurate description that provided the original metapsychological construction. If the supervisee is not prone to accepting the blame, he or she may denigrate the supervisor for not really knowing metapsychology and so lose confidence in the supervisor. A more tentative approach, with more room for exploration, is neither as initially nor as continually reassuring, but it does alleviate the repetition of doctrinaire mistakes and provides essential growth possibilities.

Levenson's favorite approach seems to be the algorithmic method, which is a systematic series designed to lead to a solution but not because it explains or is specifically a theory of the problem. It sounds a bit like chance metapsychology, personally developed relevance, with the causality of success a bit of a mystery. The unsettling aspects are partially offset by three major operational steps. The first of these is setting limits, which includes the customary arrangements of therapy, as length and frequency of sessions, but there is a less direct structuring of what is going to be possible for both patient and therapist. The second step is a detailed inquiry, which can be carried out in the customary Sullivanian manner or other approximations, including some guided associations. The aim here is to understand the life story of the patient, including the discontinuities. These serve as focal areas for patient and therapist and reflect the transference, with real and fantasied interactions between the parties.

A lot of room is left for implementation of these steps, particularly the transference. Although most theories of transference, including our own, stress projection as the essential ingredient of transference, Levenson stresses a complex exchange between therapist and patient. This is defined as "a dialogue of two real people who are interacting in a real way out of their own particular interests and experiences and investments" (1982, p. 11). Thus what one gets is a mixture of real and projection, probably what one always gets except that Levenson is a bit more open about the real. We will call it "authentic distortion," as opposed to when one or the other of the participants is dedicated, with or without awareness, to lying.

Based on the algorithmic approach, Levenson aids the supervisee with structuring, learning detailed inquiry, honing an awareness of omissions, and remembering that whatever is going on there is always an interaction. The possibilities of parallel process are also considered. The point is made that interpretation is a process of numerous viewpoints, none naturally definitive, and finally, emphasis is given to the therapist's realistic interaction with the patient. There is something quite appealing and definitely imaginative about all this. However, we still find ourselves drawn toward the search for the theory that works, a theory of logical formality that at the same time breathes enough life into itself to keep evolving but in a purposeful, defined and defining, goal-directed manner.

Levenson mentions three other models, the first emphasizing the supervisor working with the countertransference of the supervisee. That some of this is inevitable in most supervisions has already been established, although Levenson is not too impressed with it as a supervisory method. It also of course raises the difficult question of developing the "useful border" between supervision and psychotherapy. The two other methods described include harassment as a loosening technique, apparently designed particularly for the obsessional but definitely a strain on the supervisee's narcissism, and parallel process where the supervisor and supervisee unconsciously (or in some fashion that appears to have less than discernible roots) play out the supervisee's interaction with the patient.

As Levenson has pointed out, this is not an exhaustive list of supervisory methods, nor are the methods independent. What is striking in Levenson's account and the Caligor et al. (1984) book is how everyone proceeds a wee bit differently. Supervision remains a personal process, even within particular schools and general guidelines. Our concern is being able to listen in a way that will make us enablers. As supervisors, we want to leave the students with the feeling and belief that we have heard them. We have already credited Theodor Reik with the "third ear" phrase, which he admitted to borrowing from Nietzsche, and we add our admiration for the chapter by Bromberg (1984) called "The Third Ear." Our variation is the "right ear," since the multitude of listening perspectives makes it only too easy to use the "wrong ear."

As one of our fathers used to say, "Stand on this side and talk to my good ear," as an explanation for his partial deafness. In this case, we must have that good ear open to the supervisee on both sides. We offer some guidelines that have a basic theme, namely to give the supervisee what he or she needs as opposed to a rote approach of any sort. This has to begin with listening to determine what the needs are, and if it turns out that the supervisee ought to be something other than a psychoanalytic therapist of whatever stripe, or perhaps no type of therapist, he must be prepared to accept this fact. Supervision offers the possibility of teaching the trainee how to work with patients and an opportunity to decide whether or not he or she wants to do such work. The evaluative function is there of course as a screening device for competence, but the question of degree of interest also is part of the exploratory process.

In our discussion we also use supervisor–supervisee dyads representing a variety of experience from both sides. Our purpose in doing this is that a large amount of supervision takes place within differential experiential levels. For example, psychotherapists are trained in particular disciplines, such as social work, and during that training, their experience is usually limited, whereas the experience of their supervisors may be more extensive. Students in postdoctoral training are usually more experienced and so are the supervisors, but as the gap narrows, competition may increase. Also, orientation differences occur, sometimes subtle, at other times more masked. Then there are psychotherapists who seek supervision, not as part of any formal training program, but perhaps because of difficulty with a particular case or just a sense of wanting to learn more in the way that supervision can teach. The supervisor over time is faced with a number of students who are not the supervisor. This would seem obvious, but the uniqueness of both parties is often forgotten, and certainly some resentment could accompany this. Some supervisees might like to be the supervisor, others just try to make it appear that way, and still others are very intent on being themselves. Supervisors get drawn in too, sometimes wanting to show off, or to please, or to vent some aggression, or to "purify" the profession. There are a stream of motives entering into the supervision process that have limited connections to the more obvious learning situation, and they require recognition and sorting out as to their teaching–learning value. It is also useful to keep in mind that although the supervisor usually has the greater amount of experience and exposure to patients, the supervisee is in closer proximity to the particular patient being supervised. This patient may provide some new learning possibilities for the supervisor and so might the interaction with the supervisee. Discounting any evaluative institution for the moment, there are three major players—supervisor, supervisee, and patient—all with rights, desires, hopes, and interests that are to be respected throughout the supervision. Again, such logic seems obvious, almost as obvious as stating that the patient is indeed a person, but often the most basic of facts needs to be reiterated.

WHAT DOES THE SUPERVISEE KNOW?

This is a two-part, connected question. The first part asks what the supervisee knows about this patient under supervision, and the second part inquires about the supervisee's overall knowledge in regard to practicing therapy, including assessment, theory, technique, and ability to benefit from supervision. Both questions are asked and at least partially answered over time as the student describes the patient–therapist interaction.

Most students appear to want some guidelines for how to describe what is happening in therapy. In this vein, we generally advocate providing something to serve as an outline that we have learned from the past is a useful learning tool. Thus, the supervisor can indicate a psychoanalytic orientation and further specify that this means development of a genetic-dynamic view of the patient's concerns; the attribution of unconscious motivations; discernment of the formations and presence of transference, alliances, resistance, and countertransference; creation of a therapeutic dialogue; and use of such techniques as ego-building, clarification, explanation, interpretation, and working things through. Even writing this necessitated the formation of a very long sentence, so it needs to be said aptly, when the examples arise. In essence, we believe the patient has a limited awareness of the causes of his or her difficulties and mixed feelings about both learning causality and learning methods of change. We expect the supervisee to provide a setting in which the patient will feel safe enough to talk, to trust a stranger, and to use transference and various alliances to turn that stranger into an unusual kind of friend.

It is helpful to find out how the therapist and patient talk with each other, as for example the degree of ritual as opposed to spontaneity, the degree of formality, the use of humor, comments about incidentals, etc. The supervisor wants to get a sense of the trouble spots and the points of ease existing between therapist and patient. Both people have roles, and it is of importance to see how they are played out.

Thus, the supervisor may ask, "How did the session begin?"

THERAPIST: Well, the patient, Tim, talked about some trouble on the job.
SUPERVISOR: Could you describe it a little differently? What did you and the patient say to each other when you first met for the last session?
THERAPIST: Oh, you mean, hello, and that sort of thing?
SUPERVISOR: Yes, was it hello, and who said it first?

Of course, this is one of many variations on the same idea, namely what actually happened. Some therapists report it automatically, some if they feel it is unusual, some ignore it, but most supervisors have an interest in it, as they do in endings. The beginning of a session sets the tone, and it provides opportunities to deal with some important issues in what sometimes seems like unexpected rapidity. Therapy is usually some type of detective story, and the clues are all about.

THERAPIST: I said to her, Ellen how are you today? Although she
had greeted me when she entered the room, she seemed perplexed, almost annoyed by my question. I felt as though I had
done something wrong, but I didn't know what it was.

The supervisor has a choice here of following the possibility that
the patient, Ellen, did not immediately want to talk about how she was,
that she wanted to control the pace, or that she wanted to avoid something. Or the supervisor can explore none of that and, instead, ask about
what came first, how did the patient greet the therapist, which is what the
supervisor asked:

THERAPIST: She said, hello.
SUPERVISOR: Just, hello, not your name?
THERAPIST: She never uses my name, that I've noticed, but I do use
hers. I mean, we are really on a first name level, I would have
thought.

In a subsequent supervisory session the therapist explained what
the patient had experienced. When he had greeted her with the use of her
name she felt chastised. When her mother had been angry at her she
would start by saying, "Ellen," and then continue with some critical
comment. Thus, the patient was disturbed not by the therapist's question, but by the use of her name which in that particular context evoked
unpleasant transferential associations.

Our point then is that, given an array of data and an interpersonal
situation, the supervisor should help the supervisee sort it out by starting
with what it seems to be, the basic, the obvious, and work from there.
We are definitely believers in hidden meanings but also in levels of
meaning. If the therapist and patient both start with what appears to be
happening between them, the whole process appears sensible as well. The
patient can be and feel understood, and so can the therapist. Although
the process by no means stops there, such communication provides a
context for further exploration.

Other basic questions of concern are whether the therapist likes
the patient, and whether the patient likes the therapist. Therapists in
supervision are not prone to saying they dislike a patient, but they
will admit to being uncomfortable with a patient, or angry, or even rank
their patients in terms of appeal. The result of this social desirability
factor in supervisory presentations is that the supervisor has to consider whether or not the supervisee acts overall as though he or she
likes the patient.

SUPERVISOR: The patient was late for this session and had cancelled the previous one. Was there something you had suspected might be giving rise to such a reaction?

THERAPIST: Yes, although it puzzles me because I really like this patient, but I had been late for the session she was late for as well. There was traffic, I got held up, my resistance I suppose.

SUPERVISOR: Both of you were late, after she cancelled the previous session. What do you think that was about?

THERAPIST: Well, she said her car wouldn't start, and then it was too late, but I think she was angry at me because perhaps I had been a bit distracted the previous session. I think she just took it a step further and was unable to come at all.

The supervisor has several choices here. The supervisee is labeling his behavior as resistance, although he sounds more guilty at what the patient ended up doing than convinced of resistance. He also appears angry at both himself and her. The supervisor does not choose to follow the resistance theme, or even the feelings that could be connected to it, nor does he suggest what the patient was doing. Instead, he goes back to the beginning.

SUPERVISOR: Although you were late for this last session, so was the patient.

THERAPIST: Yes, but, well see I was relieved because we sort of arrived together, but late. She remarked about the traffic, and so did I, and, well, I didn't do any more about it. I mean I realize the content of past sessions could have upset her, but I am not convinced. I went over it, and I don't know. I mean, what do you think?

SUPERVISOR: Do you feel this woman likes you?

THERAPIST: I did.

SUPERVISOR: How about a conspiracy to both be late?

This last comment is said somewhat humorously, but the supervisor is trying to develop a picture of the feeling motivations between the two people, and he is concentrating on the stated probability that they like each other, despite their conflict about being together.

SUPERVISOR: It is possible that you and this patient both sense that therapy is difficult for her. She is burdened, and she is burdening you. Although you both know that is the deal, you want to ease up a little because you like each other. The result is you

are both late. Since you were late you made up the time for
her, but the lateness did occur. Actually the previous time she
tried to help you out even more and not come at all, but that
didn't feel so good to you, or to her I would guess.

THERAPIST: I really do believe I like her, though it made me angry
that she cancelled, and in fact I didn't like her being late in the
next session. I think I wanted to look at my resistance, not her
resistance.

SUPERVISOR: All right, so what is this resistance of yours? Is it that
you like her and she likes you?

THERAPIST: (Laughing) Maybe it is. I mean, I know I don't want to
make her feel bad, and I want her to keep liking me, and I felt
hurt, and angry, and guilty, and probably in trouble with you,
and I even thought, maybe I've lost her. So, it was mixed. I
mean, I was glad she was there, but I would have liked it better
if she had been on time.

SUPERVISOR: Let's think more about what's happening to her, how
frightened she is, how she does and doesn't want to see you,
and I would guess the same for you. At this point we don't
know what the issues are, I mean, what type of relationship is
hinted at here that disturbs you, or even if you both are
uncomfortable in the same way. We have a lot of lines to
follow. Let's see where they go.

The supervisor is also beginning the process of clarifying liking and
not-liking, particularly taking the absolutism out of these terms. The
positive and negative impressions are relative and shifting, although
coalescing to some constancy, usually positive if the therapist is going to
continue with the patient. So if the therapist likes the patient, this
translates into most-of-the-time good feelings, although as we have just
seen, liking the patient can also result in protective avoidances. Supervisors can certainly have empathy for liking a patient too much, for erotic
transferences and countertransferences, and for discerning what feels real
as opposed to artificial in the relationship.

The emphasis is on first getting a sense of the patient and, through
this sense, learning to establish a working contract, including arrangements, a key one of which is that the patient is going to try to tell the
therapist all about himself or herself. Two issues arise here, and we will
take the easier one first, which is that "all about" is another one of those
relative terms. It is more probable that the patient may tell the therapist a
"lot about" personal matters, and if the therapist listens carefully, separates the wheat from the chaff, the therapist will hear what is important,
and get inklings of what is missing. The supervisor's message might be,

insist the patient try, but understand the patient's limits. Work first with what you get, go after what more you think you need, and you will get some of that too. Patients seductively discourage or encourage therapists, and understanding who the patient is opens the way to sensing the character style and its tools of interaction.

The second question, the tough one, is, suppose the therapist's sense of the patient is that he or she is a thoroughly unpleasant person disliked by most people who have anything to do with him or her. However, that is not the biggest problem. The main difficulty is, the therapist does not like the patient either, raising the question of whether a therapist can work effectively with a patient that he or she does not like. Certainly there are many ways to handle such a situation, one of the most common being that the therapist discourages and ultimately, and usually quickly, gets rid of such a patient, who in turn is deemed unsuitable, unworkable, and unmotivated—not really a patient. There may well be people for whom there can be no therapists because therapists are too limited. However, we believe the number of such people who are really that unworkable is very limited. Another popular method is to convert such people into patients by reversal, reaction formation, denial, and similar sorts of operations. The patient really is basically good, just misunderstood. Such an approach creates two unreal people, the illusory patient and the foolish therapist, dancing until one of them drops. It is usually the patient, stating, "I don't really think this is doing me any good."

A third possibility is the therapist faces the reality of mostly not liking the patient and uses those feelings to help the patient, not to learn to like the patient. As an example consider a 50-year-old man divorced for 20 years and with no children. He is an attorney in a large city, and he has little interest in his work. He has a derogatory attitude toward women, all minorities, and himself, but he wants everything done for him. Although he ultimately passed the bar exam, he has no confidence in his knowledge of legal issues and wishes to avoid any decision making. At the same time he believes his age, time in the job, and apparently the very fact of his existence, should mean he gets promoted and paid well. Mostly he is bypassed, and people find him too hostile and self-involved to want to deal with him. He describes himself as, "not somebody you want to have a meal with." He is grandiose without a desire to work, and he is in pain. It is the last part that brings him into therapy—loneliness, bouts of depression, enormous self-doubt; and there is a great deal to pity about this man but not much to like.

The therapist has this patient in supervision in a training program. It is the only patient he has at the moment, so for pragmatic reasons he wants to keep the patient. He believes he should like the patient in order to avoid counterproductive negative reactions on his part, so he tries to like the patient. He begins by telling the supervisor that there is something likable about this patient, but both the therapist and the supervisor, and frequently, this patient, doubt it. The patient knows he is hard to be with, but he does not want to do what is necessary to change that. One conclusion, seemingly obvious, is that he is not a patient. In this case, let us reject that possibility and merely acknowledge that he is a difficult patient.

The supervisor focuses on two interconnected issues for the therapist. These are what the therapist does not like about the patient, primarily his narcissistic demands, and how these cause the patient problems. The therapist then works to develop an understanding of how such severe character pathology developed, and what might be accomplished. Perhaps very little, and probably not a great deal, but maybe enough so the therapist will at least like himself. He should not expect the patient to like him, however. This is not a reciprocal deal. The therapist is essentially going to negotiate with himself, and then with the patient, or probably a bit of both at the same time.

The therapist is going to tell himself, look you need this patient for a variety of reasons. He can be a learning experience, and he is certainly a challenge, and he is in pain, and it is your job to help unlikeable patients as well as professionals you can admire and can identify with. Besides, he is your only patient, so learn how to help him and do not worry about disliking him. If he is your patient, and he is interested in spending some time with you, and paying you (in this case he paid the clinic, but the payment was for services rendered by the therapist), you have got to like him a little, or some of the time. In this dialogue the therapist either sees enough of the positive side of his ambivalence to want to work with the patient or the therapy is terminated. Assuming the positive probability, the therapist must now move on to negotiate with the patient.

However, we want to note here that it is not the supervisor's job to get the therapist to like the patient, nor are we suggesting that this therapist has more than some positive regard for the patient. We rarely see anything approaching unconditional positive regard with patients and therapists, although we certainly see considerable warmth and empathy. In this case we are talking about some identification and probably a rather complete understanding of the patient. We are also indicating that it is possible to work with a patient the therapist dislikes more than he likes.

In this instance we have a patient who does not much like himself or anybody else but is pained by the way the world has treated him. He wants relief from his depression and his isolation, and he wants the therapist to provide the relief, not only by telling the patient what to do, but somehow by doing it for him. The patient is at best a reluctant giver, and as he and the therapist trace his history, much of which he states he cannot remember, it is clear that his mother was depriving and giving on an inconsistent basis, that she died when he was an early adolescent, and that he feels such a raw deal means he is owed plenty. The details of his life support the idea that not a lot was provided for him, but a fair amount was expected, and he did some of it. At this point, he has decided he has simply done enough.

The therapist has to point out that the patient still has to keep at it, although he understands the patient has no desire for this. The patient will accuse the therapist of being demanding, of not really understanding, of in fact not liking him. The therapist will eventually say, if you want to be liked you must do something. The patient will agree, but say he really cannot because he really does not want to, that it is not fair. The therapist will also tell the supervisor, this guy is impossible; but if that is true, is therapy possible? The dilemma appears, the non-patient patient.

How to pursue the therapeutic experience in this instance is up to the therapist. He may negotiate the patient into a working position, get him to do a little, help him to deal with himself even if the emerging self is nothing the therapist would want to own. The point is, it can be done, with the therapist's negativity put in service of persistence and constancy of presence. We can easily list all the things such a therapy is not and note the limits and frustrations. Such a patient is not sought after by therapists, not welcomed by therapists, usually not even tolerated by therapists. Yet toleration has its assets. Consider all the patients who tolerate their therapists, and good things still happen.

Thus far we have emphasized the supervisor helping the therapist get to know the patient, suggested some general guidelines, and provided some specific examples of trouble spots. The goal is to find out who this person is, and when the therapist discovers what he or she doesn't know, to ask. We are assuming tact, appropriateness, a sense of timing, and willingness to inquire about details, to discuss openly subjects that are often embarassing, such as sex and money. Certainly if the therapist has trouble with these points, the supervisor can take note and provide possible ways to solve the problems and thereby facilitate the building of a working relationship.

Assuming the therapist's knowledge of the patient as a person is established and the therapeutic boundaries then put into place so that the process is into more of a continual flow, the question then arises for the supervisor as to what the therapist knows about the material that is now forthcoming on a regular basis. Since as supervisors, we have made it clear to our supervisees that we expect a psychoanalytic orientation, even allowing for a loose version of such thinking, we are now interested in the conversions of clinical data to theoretical construct to clinical practice so that the therapist actually learns a working theory of the mind that is both derived from and translates into treating mental disorders.

For example, a woman therapist described to her supervisor a case in which the patient's presenting complaint was a fear of traveling, including relatively short distances, such as going to work. The fear would take the form of the patient having to go to the bathroom, but being trapped on a bus or subway, and losing control. Although this never exactly happened, several times the patient had to get off whatever transportation she was using and find a bathroom. As a result, she was frequently late for work, and she decided to handle this by telling her employers the general problem and stating that she was seeking therapy for it. Although the patient and therapist agreed to work together, and the patient was quite verbal in both describing her anxiety and its possible origins, the therapist seemed to have no idea as to the origins of phobias.

Again recognizing that each symptom has its special shapes and stimuli, there is still a large body of literature suggesting that phobias are related to unresolved hostility (Meissner, Rizzuto, Sashin, & Buie, 1987). In addition the anal-expulsive nature of the symptom and the need to be late pointed at hostility as a likely avenue of exploration. However, the idea that a person is apparently afraid of one thing because that is more tolerable than what the person is really afraid of, an unacceptable impulse, did not become congruent for the supervisee. She began with the most obvious, the fear, and just stayed with that, supporting the probability that work was stressful and that the patient was handling the symptom, and that she was getting a lot of assistance. They developed practical ways to minimize the impact of the phobia, and the patient seemed positively inclined toward the therapist for her help. The therapist saw no anger, and although the supervisor explained the theory, and raised the possibility of the therapist being diverted into possible collusion with the patient's symptomatic way of living, the therapist reported intellectual comprehension without translating any of it into practice where she mainly congratulated the patient on feeling better about herself.

There are of course questions here as to why the therapist was resisting the supervisor, as well as her countertransferential reactions to the patient, but our issue of the moment is what the supervisee did not know. In this case the lack of knowledge played at least some role in further difficulties with the patient. As she became more open with the therapist, the patient described sexual difficulties with her husband that had predated their marriage as well as a chronic eating problem. However, before any substantial consideration could be given to the theoretical issues involved in the new revelations, the patient also announced she was going away for about 2 months and was uncertain as to whether she would continue therapy when she returned, since she was feeling so much better. There were plenty of inconsistencies in what the patient was proposing, but a particular anguish for the therapist was that she was so unprepared and definitely felt rejected. The patient's anger as a motivating force against both others and herself was a recurrent theme, as was her fear, and her phobic disappearing act following her announcement of further serious problems.

One might assume that a supervisor could presume a basic theoretical knowledge proportionate to the level of training of the supervisee. Exposure to some knowledge is the more likely possibility, and much of it is not meaningful without pertinent accompanying clinical experience. Also, supervisees seem to divide in regard to theory, some embracing it and specializing in psychodynamic formulations, whereas others either find it difficult to grasp or are skeptics. We are talking about theory a bit as though there existed a great body of established facts just waiting to be learned and then neatly applied. This is not the case, however, there is a substantial amount of theory, particularly psychoanalytic, and the student needs to become familiar with it to try out the possibilities. The same principle applies to accompanying techniques, the "what to do when" approach, for certainly the best packaged theoretical formulations can go nowhere, or even be detrimental, if the therapist has limited application skills. At times, however, the threat to the student's narcissism in admitting lack of knowledge results in denial and pretense.

WHAT DOES THE SUPERVISOR KNOW?

Some of the supervisor's knowledge and skills have been demonstrated in the previous section, although the emphasis there was on the supervisee's knowledge. In essence what the supervisor needs to know is whatever the supervisee needs to know in a given supervision situation. The extent of that will not always be apparent to the supervisor because the situation is perceived through the supervisee. Even when that factor is reduced, such as with tape or video recordings, or even direct observation, the supervisor is still once removed from the situation, and so some of what could be given to the supervisee may not occur because the supervisor does not see the need. Then supervisees raise some questions, directly or indirectly, that go beyond the supervisor's range of knowledge, although usually these can be answered in time. There are also questions, such as prognostic estimates, which may be relatively unanswerable. Qualified answers are appropriate as well. The supervisor ought to be willing to admit to doubts and uncertainties, certainly a realistic glimpse of the position therapists are often in. Then, since the therapist has the most contact with the patient, the point can be emphasized that the supervisee is in the best position to know the patient.

Supervisors ought to have a thorough knowledge of the theoretical position they are trying to teach supervisees, as well as a command of technical procedures to give clinical meaning to the theory. Then they need a rationale for how they will attempt to impart their knowledge and skill to the supervisee. Supervisors have preferred styles of supervising. Some like to say little, let the supervisee work out the solutions, answer questions by raising questions. Others are more active, quick to fill in the blanks, provide possibilities. Variations certainly exist in what the supervisor will focus on, for example, in regard to countertransference. There is no definitive style, but whatever the supervisor's style, he or she should be able to justify it as an appropriate teaching method.

For example, if a therapist describes feeling at an impasse, and essentially asks what to do, the supervisor may not say. However, either way the supervisor should be able to indicate why the particular supervisory approach was followed. We believe supervisees ought to question their supervisors, find out what they know, and get help when needed, whereas the supervisors need to listen to each supervisee and consider what will be the best way to facilitate learning. As another example, a supervisor may sense that a particular patient will leave therapy prematurely if the therapist does not take certain actions. The supervisor can tell the therapist what to do, and the therapist may even do it and learn it that way. Or, the supervisor may simply listen to what the therapist is doing and question it, without offering solutions, and see what happens. Taking this a step further, the supervisor may just listen, and see if the therapist can come up with anything. Let us suppose in the latter two instances the patient terminates, and then an attempt could occur to make the learning retrospective. All of these methods can work, and the supervisor should try to figure out what method is best when and with whom. The supervisee, in turn, needs to question mistakes in therapy and to discern how they were handled in supervision as well as why particular methods were used.

Supervisees will often "psych out" supervisors, thus devising a way to get approval, such as presenting dreams, or stressing theory development, or being open about possible countertransference, depending on what they sense (or have been told by previous supervisees) the supervisor likes to hear. Just as flexibility of style is required, so is an awareness of possible supervisee manipulations. The supervisor could get to know the supervisee, regardless of whether they spend a lot of time on personal or countertransferential issues. Knowing the supervisee only enhances the possibility of the supervisor being able to teach.

All of us have had good and bad supervisors. The training of supervisors is often absent or haphazard, so it is hard to know in advance what the supervisee is really going to experience. Some empirical data is available that may provide some direction toward the development of better supervision. Nelson (1978) surveyed trainees from clinical and counseling psychology, psychiatry, and social work in regard to their preferences for goals and methods of supervision, and roles and characteristics of supervisors. The possible goals of supervision were therapeutic competence, professional confidence and independence, theoretical knowledge, increased interest in therapy, increased awareness of how a therapist functions, self-awareness, and positive outlook about being a therapist. The last goal was ranked last, whereas therapeutic competence was ranked first for supervisees in all disciplines. Self-awareness was considered more important for beginners than for more advanced trainees.

Supervisory methods were put into the two categories of acquiring information about the supervisee's therapy sessions, and teaching therapy techniques. Videotaping and direct observation were preferred by all groups except social workers, who preferred direct observation the least and ranked verbal reporting as their first choice. The favorite choice of teaching method for three of the groups was observing the supervisor doing therapy. In addition, the other possible choices were supervisor as cotherapist, which was ranked last by psychiatric residents, but second by the psychologists, verbal description of therapy techniques, listening to tapes, role playing, and source material. The preference for observation of the supervisor was stronger for beginners.

In regard to supervisor characteristics, psychologists and psychiatrists gave high ratings to interest in supervision, experience, and theoretical or technical knowledge, whereas social workers emphasized genuineness, ability to provide feedback, and self-awareness: There were 12 possibilities, and the remaining six were ranked by all groups in descending order and included flexibility, ability to guide and provide structure, empathy, warmth, easy accessibility, and permissiveness. Even though these last six characteristics were not considered as important, rankings of bipolar supervisor characteristics such as flexible–rigid, self-revealing–self-concealing, and permissive–prohibitive came out in favor of flexible, self-revealing, and permissive. In regard to role behaviors, allowing the supervisee to develop a personal therapeutic style and exploration of supervisee feelings toward patients were the highest ranked, with teaching therapy techniques about in the middle of the 12 preferences.

This study has a number of limitations. The sample is small, 12 from each of the four groups, and most of the trainees identified as eclectic, and, although the groups were divided into beginning and advanced, they all were relatively inexperienced. Also, as Nelson (1978) points out, preferences are not the same as evidence of effectiveness. It is clear, however, that the supervisees wanted to become competent therapists and wanted their supervisors to know how to teach them how to be more effective and how to develop an individual style. Although the trainees wanted to be shown what to do, they also wanted the freedom to develop their own styles, and they valued highly the supervisors' interest in supervision.

A larger study of retrospective evaluations of best and worst supervisors has been reported by Allen, Szollos, and Williams (1986) who sampled 142 doctoral students from 37 clinical and counseling psychology programs. They found that the best and worst experiences were particularly differentiated by the skill and reliability of the supervisors. The best supervisors were those who were seen as having definite expertise and being trustworthy; sociability was not a significant discriminator. Good supervisors respected differences between themselves and supervisees. They had theoretical orientations that were viewed as useful for understanding patients and taught practical skills. They appeared interested in supervision, provided clear feedback, and were open to it themselves.

Poor supervision was described more by the absence than the existence of specific characteristics, such as disinterest, lacking effective teaching methods, poor role modeling, including being authoritarian, exploitative, and subtly neglectful, and being deficient in communication.

There are some differences between these results and the findings of the Nelson (1978) study. The sample was larger, but it was limited to psychology trainees. They did not have a preference for direct observation of the supervisor, which may reflect the theoretical orientation distribution of about one-third each for eclectic, psychodynamic, and cognitive-behavioral. Psychodynamic supervision traditionally relies on the verbal report, and the supervisors were primarily psychodynamic or behavioral. Also, these trainees appeared to place more value on personal growth issues compared to technical skills, which again reflects the conception already noted of the variability in the needs of supervisees. However, as in the Nelson study, there was a strong emphasis on the supervisor's competence and interest. Also, the need for theory is emphasized in the dislike of atheoretical eclecticism where the supervisors did not put their clinical interventions within conceptual perspectives.

Hess (1980) has described six models of supervision: lecturer, teacher, case reviewer, collegial peer, monitor, and therapist. They overlap, and although any supervisor may prefer one or more over the others, or be called on because of the circumstances of specific supervisions to emphasize one or more, it is probable that supervisors generally need some capabilities in all of these roles. This can be illustrated by considering the goals attributed to each of these roles. Supervisors are expected to display a myriad of conceptual schemes and techniques (lecturer), teach content and skills (teacher), explore various ways of looking at cases (reviewer), develop a cooperative relationship (collegial), evaluate (monitor), and foster the therapist's personal development (therapist). However, despite the variety of skills that may need to be employed, the main function of a supervisor is teaching, and the main goal is to improve the supervisee's effectiveness as a therapist. There is limited empirical data regarding supervision, with most of it dealing with counseling and having to be extended to encompass psychotherapy and psychoanalytic supervision. There is no empirical evidence that would support the relative effectiveness of particular types and models of supervision in reference to the ultimate therapeutic effectiveness of the supervisee, although there are numerous opinions and possibilities.

With the understanding that it is probably easier to be definitive about psychotherapy, itself a concept not easy to define, than it is about psychotherapy supervision, the supervisor can help by clarifying with the supervisee what it is they both intend to do. These goals will probably shift as they proceed and are, of course, dependent on the type of patient, setting, and supervisory opportunities, such as direct observation or video-taping, that are available. Over a long period we have supervised a variety of people at different levels ranging from beginners to people with active practices, have been supervised ourselves at different stages of our careers, and have participated in peer supervision. As a result, we are aware that the supervisees' needs are different at different times, as are the supervisors'. Good listening by both supervisor and supervisee will enable attunement to these differences, but as the trainer, the supervisor is particularly responsible for knowing this. Once a plan is agreed on, the supervisor then has to display the competence needed to carry the plan forward.

Among other factors, the success of the plan depends heavily on the relationship between the supervisor and supervisee. This is our next area of concern, and again, there is limited empirical investigation. Kennard, Stewart, and Gluck (1987) report that there have been studies exploring similarities in attitude and gender, and they suggest consideration of theoretical orientation and behavioral style as well. Kennard et al. (1987) provide some preliminary data from 26 clinical psychology trainees and 47 supervisors of these students. Based on the supervisees' perceptions of the quality of supervision, there were positive and negative experience groups, with 10% of the supervisors in both groups. Thus, some of the same supervisors were identified by different students as providing a good or bad experience. Most of the participants were either psychodynamic or eclectic in orientation.

It was possible to find evidence for a "match" in supervisory relationships where the perceptions of the relationship were in relative agreement. When the trainees were interested in the supervisors' feedback about their attitudes and behavior toward supervision, as well as supervisors' suggestions about professional development, and perceived the supervisory experience as positive, so did the supervisors. Similarities in theoretical orientation and interpretive style were also contributors to positive experiences. Although Kennard et al. (1987) indicate the methodological limitations of their study, their work does support the importance of the relationship between supervisor and supervisee in contributing to a positive or negative experience for both parties and implies some degree of a similar effect on the patient.

THE SUPERVISORY RELATIONSHIP

Although there is no empirical evidence about the effects of supervision on the treatment of the patient, we hope that a positive supervision experience will contribute to the betterment of the patient as well as the supervisor and supervisee. As trainers, we follow the logic of other trainers that supervision is necessary to produce an effective psychotherapist. At the same time, we realize that just as one supervisor may be categorized as good or bad by different trainees, so one student may be seen as competent and incompetent by different supervisors. The fit between supervisor and supervisee is a major issue in determining the effectiveness of the supervision. A good fit appears when both parties agree that the supervision was of value to the supervisee in helping him or her to be a more effective psychotherapist. A bad fit occurs when either party disagrees with this idea, or when both people attest to its ineffectiveness. Bad fits may still have learning value, however, but our interest is in producing a good fit as often as possible.

We have a number of suggestions in this area that essentially epitomize listening with the right ear. Just as therapists bring their own needs to therapy sessions and need to learn to subordinate these to the work of therapy, so supervisors have the same task in regard to supervision. An added feature is that supervisees may have a resistance to the learning process. Depending on their self-perceived level of skill, they may view specific supervisory experiences as requirements to be endured rather than as essential learning possibilities. They then attempt to deceive the supervisor, and they sometimes succeed. So the supervisor's initial task in the relationship is to ascertain what the trainee really wants. The learning motivation needs to be there, or the trainee is misplaced as a possible therapist.

Assuming that it is in place, the supervisor needs to recognize that narcissistic threats are very possible for the trainee because mistakes, or certainly other views, are very probable. Thus we see it as important to provide a supportive environment for the therapist. This means encouragement, understanding, and freedom to explore ideas and approaches as a therapist. When criticisms are forthcoming, they can be phrased and timed in such a way that the supervisee retains significant self-esteem. The idea should not be to demean the supervisee in any way but, rather, to have a positive outcome. Although the supervisor ought to know more than the supervisee, the manner of transmitting that knowledge is crucial. The supervisor needs to get a sense of what will work with each supervisee and use that approach. For example, with some trainees, it is helpful openly to convey the supervisor's understanding of their difficulties before raising the possibility of a particular intervention. Thus the supervisor might say, "I sense you don't want to make the patient feel uncomfortable, but perhaps you could . . ." Or, "From what you told me about your own feelings in regard to mothering, this could be an issue of some discomfort for you. Still, it looks as if you explored . . ."

In contrast, some trainees handle a more direct approach quite effectively. Then the supervisor might say, "You haven't found out very much about this person's relationship with her father. See if you can get into that in more detail."

Of course the supervisor's style is also an issue here. Although any supervisor has favorite ways of approaching the supervision, there ought to be flexibility. Always doing the same thing, or the same three or four things, based on their previous validation is no guarantee of continued success. The supervisor can learn about supervising each time he or she supervises, and learning how to get results with each supervisee is a major possibility, and task. There is a need to be flexible, have a process, flow with it, and establish a learning situation for the supervisee that can get carried into the actual work with the patient.

What can a supervisor do with a bright student who is doing therapy as a training requirement but essentially does not believe it can be effective, feels overwhelmed by the patient's misery, does not wish to look at countertransference, has tried personal psychotherapy with a number of different therapists and felt it was of no value, and who distrusts the supervisor? Advise the student to go into research, or to get out of the field altogether, or abandon the student, or avoid the student, or get caught up in a hostile interaction? All these are possibilities, but just as it is possible to work with a patient the therapist does not like, so it is possible to do this with a supervisee. The trainee's feelings are respected, but he or she does not have a right to do therapy and to fail to try to be effective as a therapist. As long as the person agrees to attempt therapeutic work, the possibility of supervision exists. The supervisor already believes in the effectiveness of psychotherapy, so the supervisor's optimism has to substitute for the trainee's and dilute the pessimism. Although personal boundaries are respected, some confrontation will be necessary to address any issues the supervisor believes are crucial. The trainee is encouraged to keep at it, to accept difficulties, and is reinforced when some of the effort works, as it usually does. Some trust may even be established. Intelligence, awareness of personal struggles, sensitivity to the patient's suffering, can all be brought into play to help the trainee attempt to help the patient. The trainee may complete the supervision without a positive word for the supervisor, but the goal is not to get the supervisee to like the supervisor, or the patient, or anybody else in life. Instead the goal remains teaching a person to be a therapist, and in such a case, it involves imagination, accommodation, and perserverance; but it still can be accomplished. From an evaluative point of view, he or she may not appear as a good candidate for future work as a psychotherapist, but in certain situations a trainee may be backed into doing therapy and being supervised for a given period of time, and then the supervisor has the possibilities just described.

This brings us to the question of what would be our ideal supervisory relationship. As supervisors, we would tend to prefer working with someone who is in practice, has some experience, and seeks supervision to hone skills rather than merely to fulfill requirements. Mutuality is relatively easy here, and the experience tends to be stimulating and rewarding. Peer supervision can be close to this, but there is more of a possibility of competition playing an intrusive role. Other situations, such as training programs or supervising people who are meeting licensure requirements, are more evaluative and, in turn, less enjoyable. Particularly difficult is supervision in discipline training programs, such as clinical psychology or psychiatric nursing, where the students and supervisors may be assigned to each other and do not share similar theoretical orientations, so there is a "forced fit."

Since most supervision occurs in a training context and does involve evaluation, we will suggest concerns that we believe a supervisor ought to consider as components of an evaluation. The first is, does the therapist seem to have a good idea of who the patient is? This is a diagnostic impression, but in the broad sense rather than the attachment of a label. Then, is the therapist really interested in doing therapy with the patient, and by extension interested in being a psychotherapist? Also, does the supervisee have theoretical and technical knowledge about therapy that would be expected based on the levels of experience and training? Can the therapist make clinical applications? Is the trainee interested in and capable of learning from supervision? Is there an appropriate awareness of countertransferences and an openness to exploring them? Is the supervisee truly interested in being supervised? Can the trainee establish a relationship with the supervisor in which a learning alliance takes place? In the supervisor's opinion, will the supervisee make an effective psychotherapist?

This is not an exhaustive list, but it covers major areas of possible therapeutic effectiveness as well as the supervisor–supervisee relationship. Depending on the setting and situation, the supervisor might also make note of the supervisee's relationship to the broader structure, such as relating to other staff members and the administrative staff, as well as record keeping, fee collection, of whatever nature that is required of the supervisee. The supervisor may have a narrative format to describe the supervisee's work, or combine this with a more formalized rating scale. An example of the latter, developed by one of us, is described below.

The Supervisor's Rating Schedule (SRS) covers nine broad areas, rated on a 5-point scale, 1 being the lowest and 5 being the highest. Descriptions may accompany the numbers, as unacceptable, adequate but below average, average, definitely acceptable, and excellent; also, the ratings may be made relative to the supervisees, as first-year trainees, experienced clinicians, etc. To provide the most accurate picture, we believe the SRS should be accompanied by a narrative description, elaborating on the areas and providing any additional pertinent information as well as making recommendations for the supervisee's future training and progress.

THE SUPERVISOR'S RATING SCHEDULE

1. *Presentation of material.* Is the material appropriately recorded by the supervisee, is it organized properly, is it presented in a lucid manner, is it sufficiently detailed, etc.?
2. *Theory.* Does the supervisee understand and conceptually articulate a theoretical picture of the patient's difficulties and the therapeutic techniques necessary for their resolution?
3. *Diagnosis.* Is an accurate diagnosis made according to current DSM criteria, as well as in terms of the theory of psychotherapy and problem development being used by the supervisee?
4. *Therapeutic attitudes.* Sensitivity, warmth, empathy, capacity for

critical thinking, ability to deal with patient's feelings, particularly dependency and hostility.

5. *Theory–practice integrating.* Ability to translate theory into technical maneuvers in the therapeutic process, such as giving explanations, appropriate timing, and dealing with patient maneuvers.

6. *Self-understanding.* Supervisee's awareness of a personal role in the therapy, recognition of possible intrusive personal factors, and willingness to do something to remedy any such problems.

7. *Supervisor–supervisee relationship.* Type of relationship with the supervisor, use of supervision sessions.

8. *Learning ability.* General willingness to learn, ability to do so, progress made over time.

9. *Overall competence.* Considering all factors involved, a general rating of effectiveness as a therapist.

This is designed as a general schema with overlap in some of the categories and with the last two as the most general. An accompanying narrative provides the possibility for detailing the more global ratings. These areas should be discussed with the supervisee both as the supervision is in progress and at its completion, when the final ratings are determined. The supervisor can also benefit from this by encouraging comments from the supervisee about the supervisory process and the work of the supervisor.

There are a number of aspects of the supervisory relationship that we want to discuss further. The first is the value of providing a choice on the part of both supervisor and supervisee about working together. In many training situations the choice is quite limited and the result can be either or both of the parties enduring a designated number of sessions to complete a requirement. In connection with making this choice, each party would do well to gain whatever preliminary information about each other that he or she can. For example, potential supervisees may have opportunities to take courses from the potential supervisors, hear lectures, read books or articles, and/or hear accounts from other supervisees about the possible supervisors. Supervisors have less opportunity to gain advance information, but they may also get some chances to observe possible supervisees. Prior to making a formal agreement about supervision, it probably would benefit both supervisor and supervisee to use a few sessions to "screen" each other in an attempt to assure a good fit.

In addition to the desirability of as much mutual choice as the situation allows, an openness on the supervisee's part is very helpful in setting a tone for the supervision that encourages exploration. Specifically, we find it easier to work with supervisees who seem genuinely interested in the "why" of their behavior with patients. The more guarded person restricts the exploratory nature of supervision and emphasizes the need to build trust rather than being able to start with a relative alliance. Since supervision is usually time-limited, the quicker development of the learning alliance is definitely advantageous.

Not surprisingly, we also enjoy supervisees who appear to share our views on how to work with patients. The similarity in general viewpoints is appealing and provides a general trust that opens paths to the development of personal supervisee styles. Such styles are desired but developed cooperatively rather than out of opposition to the supervisor. Our general approach is that when the supervisees are having trouble, we will make suggestions, but we also make it clear that the supervisees can, and probably should, try their own solutions. Of course if we considered these harmful to the patient, we would be more insistent on the supervisee following our directives. However, we have learned that if the supervisee is really opposed to a procedure we are proposing, the supervisee will not do it correctly.

Thus, we try to provide for as much personal freedom as possible, and try to work out difficulties between ourselves and supervisees when they come to our notice. Perhaps the easiest problem is the presence of parallel process because then the style with the patient is a visible model for the repetition with the supervisor. More complex are transferential problems arising in the relationship where one or both parties may be replaying old issues stimulated by the supervisory situation itself, such as relationships to authority figures. Sensitivity to problems in supervision of course is at the essence of really listening to what is happening and then deciding what to do about it.

We see the supervisory process as highly personal and akin to therapy, although the teaching and evaluative aspects of it create more of an authoritative tilt in favor of the superior status and knowledge of the supervisor. Lesser (1984) has described one of the illusions in supervision as "the supervisor knows best." Although it is true that the supervisor does not always know best, nor certainly everything, nonetheless the supervisor ought to at least "know better," and the supervisee ought to be willing to accept that. We are not interested in slavish adherence, establishing constricted disciples, or duplicitous patronizing. However, we believe students ought to want to learn from us and expect us to know more then they do, and be interested and willing to teach them.

Since we see this as a personal relationship, we are more willing to share aspects of ourselves than in a therapy session. We are also attuned to the personal needs and problems of our supervisees and willing to spend time discussing them. We also see as the ultimate referent the supervisee's therapist, or if the supervisee is not in therapy at the time of supervision, we feel that a therapeutic issue be discussed and resolved in detail in a formal therapy situation, not in supervision. We believe that supervisors may become effective therapists for supervisees, but prefer supervision and therapy not to be occurring at the same time with the same person. We use the word "prefer" because as every therapist knows who has therapists as patients, their practices do get discussed. It is not formal supervision, just as formal supervision is not therapy, but it is an artificiality to see supervision and therapy as completely distinct.

We would also like to put in a plea for more formal training for supervisors. Current methods of supervisory selection are based more on experience as a therapist and knowing somebody than on any supervisory credentials. Much of this is the result of the lack of training available, which ought to be altered, and some of it is caused by the narcissistic assumption that being a therapist makes one an effective supervisor, which is by no means the case because supervision is primarily teaching. It was the good fortune of one of us that as part of the psychiatric nursing graduate education, a supervised learning experience as a therapy supervisor was provided. But this is rare.

Finally, we like to stress the need for more interest in supervision at the discipline level, which is really the introduction to a possible career as a therapist. Bad starts are notorious at this level, and psychoanalysis has been neglectful in this regard, relegating most of its focus to supervision at the training-institute level where the trainees already have a relatively strong commitment to psychoanalytic approaches. However, the interest needs to begin earlier and is dependent on creation in people training to be psychologists, psychiatrists, psychiatric nurses, social workers, etc. If we fail as models at this level, we limit the students' future development. It is not as appealing, or easy, for the supervisor to be "selling" as well as teaching, but in an appropriate fashion interest has to be stimulated in what we believe is a valuable way to do psychotherapy.

Our aim in this chapter has been to stress the need for good listening in the supervisory process for both supervisor and supervisee. Research is limited in the area, and it is a process in development, so our comments are given in such a spirit. Definitive words would hardly be that, but opinions are becoming more apparent and useful, so we have attempted to expand the learning possibilities with the hope of increased and continued examination of supervision.

III

The Patient's Contribution

*A*ctually, any number of phenomena occurring within patients
and in their relationships might threaten the therapist's narcissism. We have selected four from the many possible phenomena to
explore as contributors to the therapist's already ongoing narcissism.

The first is the patient's resistance, often taken both as a professional and personal affront and surely, after a "respectable" albeit arbitrary time, considered by most therapists to be a nuisance, an obstacle to
their ministrations, and an offense to their self-image. Rationally the
resistance is seen as preventing treatment, but the real narcissistic assault
is that irrationally it undermines the therapist's narcissistic need to help.
We examine resistance as obstacle, symbol, and vehicle—an unconscious
patient tool for therapy rather than a weapon against it. To this end, we
explore the use of resistance in the service of therapy, showing how it
requires observation and exploration of the threat to the therapist's
narcissistic conception of the therapy process and his or her place in it.

Next we look at loneliness, having early mentioned it as an occupational hazard. But what if the therapist comes to the profession vulnerable to loneliness in others or in the self or defended against the experience? We propose a unique conception of how loneliness emerges
developmentally, how it becomes a problem, and how it works in the
service of the person. All this is important because loneliness can be a
threat to the therapist's image as a model of a "relator" of interpersonal
skills and demands and is therefore a narcissistic threat.

Envy is another phenomenon we explore. It has powerful dynamics
and has the potential of threatening therapists in ways they would rather
ignore. The therapist may envy the patient and feel inadequate, perhaps
trying to act aggressively or brilliantly as a reaction to the envy and the
felt deficiency. Any number of narcissistic moves prompted by envy

essentially limit the therapist's ability to deal with envy in the self and in the patient. The patient who has chronic problems with envy might not attend to a sense of personal accomplishment, envying instead whatever the therapist is or does positively in the therapy, thereby diminishing the self and the relationship. A therapist's narcissistic response could reinforce such pathology. Our unique microscopic look at the psychodynamics of envy is designed to facilitate understanding of how developmental processes contribute to its evolution so that envy does not get caught in the crossfire of the therapist's narcissism.

Passive–aggressiveness, the fourth phenomenon we discuss, is perhaps the most irritating frequently encountered behavioral phenomenon in and out of therapy, yet it is barely discussed in the literature. Passive–aggressive patients wear down the stamina of the healthiest therapists and assault the authority and control of the narcissistic ones. Our exploration of the phenomenon is unique in that we move beyond the usual description to suggest dynamics and link those to developmental aggression that has been frustrated. Thus, there are phase-related narcissistic links to passive–aggressive problems as well as therapist narcissistic responses to this universal phenomenon.

10

The Value
of Resistance

It can happen in a variety of ways. The patient changes the subject, misinterprets the therapist, is antagonistic or unusually reasonable, forgets a session, or prematurely terminates therapy. The patient talks incessantly or apparently irrelevantly, is insistently silent, or relentlessly struggles with or questions the therapist. The patient suddenly forgets or loses track of a thought or cannot remember past experiences, refuses to note the present or remember current dreams; and when dreams are remembered, he or she insists on their literal rather than symbolic meaning.

Resistance refers to the unconscious process whereby the patient acts out a reluctance to "know" anxiety-provoking experiences. Fenichel (1953) notes, "It is impossible to tabulate the various ways in which resistance can be expressed" (p. 325). Although resistance originally (Freud, 1895/1964) referred to the patient's inability to remember, the concept was extended to include all obstacles to the aims and process of psychotherapeutic treatment (Greenson, 1967). It is as if the acting out of resistances in the outer world of therapy serves the purpose of protecting the patient from crucial problems in the inner world of the self.

Classically then, resistance is seen as a counterforce operating against therapeutic progress (Freud, 1895/1964). It is an automatic, unconscious phenomenon called out when there is a perceived, though not necessarily conscious, threat to some dimension of the self-system. As such, resistance itself is unconscious and implies a motherlode of anxiety that is defended against, as Sullivan (1954) says, a "four-square collision" with the threat. Resistance serves as a security operation outside the patient's awareness (Fromm-Reichmann, 1950), expressed through thoughts, feelings, actions, attitudes, impulses, and fantasies (Greenson, 1967).

Such behaviors serve as symbolic representations of unacceptable inner experiences. Since the symbol, resistance, becomes observable through behavior, it serves as an opening wedge into the patient's inner world, only indirectly accessible. Does this mean that resistance then is both obstacle and vehicle? The answer is yes, implying that resistance moves beyond opposition, at once representing unwitting movement toward cure and movement gathered to oppose it (Freud, 1905/1964). Although Freud first labeled resistance as opposition alone, he came to see it as a useful tool as well (Freud, 1905/1964, 1917/1964). In fact, he saw it as a clue to one's original need to forget pathogenic experiences (Freud, 1910/1964), an unconscious tool to assist therapist and patient in learning about the patient's inner life. His thought was that in skillful hands resistance can become some of the best support available in treatment (Freud, 1917/1964). As Singer (1965) says, resistance "seemingly" impedes therapeutic discovery.

We agree and indeed move beyond the position to suggest that behavior classified as resistance is at once obstacle, symbol, and vehicle, and indispensable tool to move the therapy forward. Resistance is disguised communication, telling us something that would otherwise not be discernible. In other words, in the guise of inhibiting communication, resistance unwittingly facilitates and enhances understanding if the therapist is there to get the message, to recognize and decode the communication, or as Freud (1917/1964) might say, to give it the "right turn" (p. 291). Thus, although resistance is a defensive operation, it is also a facilitating device having therapeutic value as a communication vehicle if recognized and utilized as such by the therapist. In this sense, we are in agreement with the communications approach to psychotherapy à la the Palo Alto school (Haley, 1963; Jackson, 1971), whose thesis is that resistance can be utilized for the sake of therapeutic progress. In addition, our view is compatible with Langs's (1981) use of empirical observations of the communication context of resistances as well as their intrapsychic sources. Further, we see the interpersonal context as a clue to the intrapersonal experience.

The benefit derived from the resistance experience is contingent on the therapist's cognitive receptivity and clinical handling of the patient's behavior. As we note elsewhere in the book and as Parsons (1986) says, "There is a parallel between the patient's need to give up . . . established ways of coping and the analyst's need not to cling on to . . . familiar ways of understanding" (p. 487). The issue is that although resistance may evolve from defensive reluctance, its course and outcome and disruptive ability depend a good deal on the therapist's response (Blatt & Erlich, 1982). It is important to realize that, if the therapist is free to listen to the disguised communication called resistance, it becomes clear that on one level the patient is signalling to the difficulty, whereas on another, he is covering it up. The task is to "listen with the right ear" while having little investment in foisting the sounds on the patient. The therapist ". . . must learn to discover and decipher the oncoming messages, without [necessarily] making them public" (Gaddini, 1982, p. 60).

THE FUNCTION OF RESISTANCE

The way resistance manifests itself has a profound effect on the process of therapy and on a given therapy session. Studying its communication microscopically yields clues as to how it arises, where it comes from, and how it is utilized as defense and as opportunity.

A patient's daughter was getting married at the same time he found out his insurance was not going to cover his therapy. Until this point he had always seemed supermotivated, not obviously resistant, but unusually altruistic and compliant. Having had a long-standing problem with repression of anger, he was now able, however, to feel annoyed at the exorbitant wedding expenses and angry about the insurance plan. Consequently, he was certain he needed to cut down on his therapy. After he made the decision, with clearly no discussion allowed, he seemed relieved—ostensibly angry that he felt forced to cut down, but relieved nevertheless. Then the telephone rang, and the therapist interrupted the session to answer, speaking for no more than 30 seconds. Seemingly buoyed by anger, now displaced onto the therapist, he said, "You know, I don't like when you answer the phone. I want my money's worth. I don't want you on that phone during my time."

In fact, the frustration and anger he had experienced was indeed displaced onto the therapist, but the experience ran even deeper. On another level, the money problems were fortuitous. Without them, resistance would have been more difficult, but with them, the resistance moved forward. In effect he said, "I'm coming less, I'm telling you who's boss, and while I'm at it and in the safety of my resistance, there's something I don't like about you, so there! It's nearly the end of the session and I won't see you next week either." It is fascinating because, without the manifest resistance, the patient was heretofore unable to be critical of the therapist, the same problem he had with most people. By arranging to not come, he could in fact move closer to the therapist and to a more authentic self. The resistance made possible the initiation of a move from the defensively altruistic false self to a more human one.

After years of standing by, waiting for a patient to become "motivated toward introspection," a therapist finally made an interpretation that ran something like, "It certainly sounds as if you have grave reservations about marriage. All you want to do is titillate and capture this guy and all the others and in the process collect data on what jerks they are." The patient was very angry, protesting the content and the felt intrusion. So the next session, through her resistance she proved the therapist correct. For a half-hour, she titillated him with sexual details of her latest exploit, and just as he was about to give up hope, she blurted out that she had been very angry that he had been right. The resistance in the session was indeed a defense, in function similar to the one she used in everyday life to avoid interpersonal contact and emotional closeness. At the same time, it allowed her entry to the relationship on her terms. The resistance showed the character of her interpersonal relationships, including that with her therapist. It was the therapist's task to recognize the unconscious desire for entry and to help the patient negotiate the tentative contact through the resistance, a tricky business indeed.

Starting with Freud (1926/1964), theorists have identified categories of resistance. Freud's categories number five: resistances due to repression; to secondary gains from symptoms; to transference where repeating early patterns with the therapist takes place, where acting out replaces remembering; to id impulses; and to superego needs impelling guilt and punishment, perhaps related to the death instinct (Freud, 1937/1964). Later (Freud, 1937/1964), he added bisexuality and a metaresistance, that is, resistance to noting any resistances, which is actually quite similar to Abraham's (1919/1927) concept about resistance to the whole analytic process.

Whereas Freud's categories identify the source, others classify the degree of ego syntonicity (Greenson, 1967), or the presenting behavior (Glover, 1955; Langs, 1981), or the style of the resistance (Horney, 1942), or level of personality functioning as shown through the sequence of the clinical process (Spotnitz, 1969). Our clinical experience shows that many of the suggested categories or classifications have merit, and several books present excellent reviews and original presentations of various theorists' work on the subject (Marshall, 1982; Milman & Goldman, 1987; Wachtel, 1982). It is not our intention to present, compare, assess, or come up with new categories. It is our aim, however, to show how resistance occurs in the therapy process and how the therapist can utilize the resistance for the good of the patient.

The reader might think we are saying there is something to be said for "going with resistance" (Applebaum, 1979; Spotnitz, 1969), that is, not interpreting it, and we are, but we are careful. Whereas not interpreting does avoid the patient's negativism and struggles for control, it can go too far if the therapist inattends to the possibility resistance presents for understanding the patient's past and present experiences and the patient's unconscious desire to experience and communicate that which he or she is defending against. Not interpreting can deteriorate into therapist acting-out if contrived interventions such as mirroring the patient's self-objectionable behaviors characterize the noninterpretative intervention. Such "ego-dystonic joining" (Spotnitz, 1969) is likely to promote anger because of implicit therapist control.

Our object is not to say when or when not to interpret resistance. To conceptualize those principles from observation and intuitive clinical judgments is certainly necessary in our field, but we leave that task for another work and time. Our aim is to look at the defensive motivation for interpretation, the narcissistic function served by unnecessary and defensive use of interpretation mainly to bolster the therapist's narcissism, and the fueling of the therapist's narcissism in the guise of therapeutic intervention.

THE THERAPIST'S PARTICIPATION

The original formulation of resistance was based on the focus of instincts, drives, and consequent defense formation. It later expanded to include a focus on ego functions and processes, namely on the object-relations role in development and the interpersonal therapy context at hand. This implies that resistance is not simply a unitary experience in the patient, a defense against access to the unconscious to be circumvented or conquered, but a process ultimately involving patient and therapist. Thus, although it disrupts, it also educates and elucidates; although it advances repression, it expresses through distortion and symbol. Resistance presents an opportunity to process facets of experience heretofore unnoticed. It is opportunity for communication and intervention up to the limits of the patient's participation balanced by the therapist's skill, stamina, and lack of narcissistic need.

Let us take, for example, the patient who came to sessions with prepared lists of topics to "discuss." In the patient's mind, the therapist was included in an exchange, but indeed there was none. If the therapist deigned to say anything, it was considered an interruption. The patient looked up disdainfully from his notes and magnanimously waited for the therapist to finish her comment before returning to his list. Obviously, this avoidance behavior represented "character armor" (Reich, 1949) from daily life emerging as resistance in therapy. There was a steel wall between patient and therapist. Indeed, on the list one day (after about 2 years) was a dream in which the patient was surrounded by a gigantically tall gray steel door, "like for a giant," a door familiar to him the patient reported. But he noticed for the first time there was a little window on the top that he could hardly reach, but he knew it was there.

The patient was at once defending against and seeking relatedness. The orders were clear: Both patient and therapist were privately to note his receptivity to and avoidance of interpersonal contact; the observation was not to be discussed. In fact, the therapist must barely exist lest she intrude on the patient.

Obviously, resistance is nothing new created by the therapy (Greenson, 1967). Therapy becomes the arena wherein the difficulties manifest themselves. Whereas resistance is often episodic (Blatt & Erlich, 1982), with some patients it is a constant, thorough experience. Abraham (1919/1927) describes this kind of patient well. The patient adds "interesting contributions to the autobiography" (p. 306). Curing takes a back seat to narcissistic interests, although on the surface such patients seem to be eager and ready to be analyzed. They begrudge the therapist any remark, which they see as deprecating to their own powers for "auto-analysis" (p. 307). In the process, the patient stays in control, the therapist is inferred to be weak yet an authority to be revolted against, and the patient thinks he or she is compliant, doing the work that needs to be done.

In the case described above, it would seem as if the patient should not have bothered to come to treatment, for little could take place in any active sense. The therapist was to fit in with the patient's narcissism, on one level barely breathing so as not to disturb the patient, while at the same time being the object whose intentions the patient could thwart. On the other hand, the patient came to treatment regularly, indeed relentlessly, and periodically the therapist indulged herself by making a comment or raising a mild but crucial question. She admittedly did this to keep awake, to feel that her presence was not simply gratuitous, to feel less fraudulent, and for therapeutic reasons to plant a seed that another person existed independent and apart from the patient, one who might contribute to a relationship without taking him over. Had the therapist's narcissistic need predominated she could not have operated this way. Instead, she would have early interpreted the resistance, "the list," and then the content, as represented here by the dream.

Although these are classic steps (Greenson, 1967) in the analysis of resistance, in our estimation, such interpretation could have been a costly error, reinforcing the patient's worst fears and his defensive armor. It would seem that the need for interpretation at this phase would be premature, motivated more by therapist narcissism than therapeutic indication. It was this sort of patient that likely drove Freud to the point of pessimism, where he looked for biological and neurological etiology (Freud, 1913/1964, 1937/1964). Freud surely had an authoritarian view of the world and the analytic process, and although he indeed expressed his understanding of the need to move slowly with resistance, studying its clues until the patient was ready to move (Freud, 1905/1964), the sooner this happened the better. By today's standards he was in a big hurry to battle and wrest resistances from the patient through interpretation. It would appear that ultimately his narcissism required patients not to oppose his interventions and, at the very least, to make his ministrations possible by presenting the data through recall and free association.

Patients like the one just discussed are reluctant to get into the whole relationship and process of therapy. Although most patients' resistance appears and disappears, theirs infers an unconsciously programmed defiance, often concealed in the guise of eagerness to comply, at least initially. Another patient, after coming to therapy for a year, her attachment to the therapist and the process apparently strong, started coming late and then missed a session. Later, it became clear that as she was on the verge of consciously acknowledging the attachment, she had an inner need to show that the therapist was not important to her. At that time, it was crucial for the therapist: to recognize, silently, the positive transference; to realize the separation implications of the patient's attachment to her, namely, that attachment to another mother would bring real trouble, perhaps abandonment fears, from her internalized and living mother; to realize that at this point, although her behavior represented some negative transference and a defiance of her regularly scheduled mother and therapist, a latent purpose of the acting out was to protect the attachment to the therapist by not coming; to sit with it, hold it, get used to it, and now, only secondarily, to protect the attachment to her mother.

With such patients, the therapist must accept a "clandestine therapeutic alliance" (Gaddini, 1982, p. 60) in which the therapist is available and reliable for that unconscious part of the patient that is working to keep the experience secret in order to have it as long as the patient needs it that way. As Semrad (1983), an early supervisor of one of us, said, "The only time people leave their mothers is when they're ready to go" (p. 53), just as he aptly said, "All defenses are forms of self-deception . . ." (p. 151). So the object is to recognize the defense and the process and let the patient be. The same injunction applies with many patients who make a big case for not doing something in order to allow themselves to do it.

For years, one patient started her weekly sessions saying either, "I don't know why I'm here," or "I'm thinking about leaving." By about the 10th year, the therapist was allowed to laugh and even comment. Many of these patients are obsessionals who know intuitively about resistance. One patient comes to his sessions begrudgingly so that he might come.

Obviously, the defensive quality provides a hedge against involvement, against having too good a time, against thinking he might want to come (as opposed to coming because his wife sent him). The value of the resistance is simply that it allows him to come. Without the paradox he could not do that. And with power struggles about his general resistance to the process and to specific issues in a session or forced analysis of the resistances (tantamount to a power struggle), he would bolt. And the therapist would be left alone with his or her own narcissism.

Often, resistance arises before the therapist or patient sees it coming. A patient left a message on a therapist's answering machine that she was not coming to group that day, giving no reason for her cancellation. The next day in her individual session she said she did not really know the reason. She had just felt the urgency to cancel and did not feel bad about it. What she did realize was that she did not want to call and hear the therapist's voice, so she timed the call when she figured the therapist would not be around. The patient made it clear there was nothing more to explore, since what she said was all she knew. The therapist paid attention.

During the session, the patient talked of not having close friends, of being whatever anybody wanted her to be, and of her need to "read" people to meet that internal demand. In group the patient had gone through several phases. During the first, she was isolated and detached, damned if she would associate with these plebians, a multiple transference resistance reenacting one level of her relationships. This level then gave way to the next, where she felt herself slipping into the clutches of the group, being what she was supposed to be, talking about what she was supposed to, reacting, interacting, feeling susceptible to being whatever anybody wanted her to be. This was yet another level of transference at which she was not really uncomfortable until she unconsciously noticed her resentment and anger. Then she felt compelled to cancel group and to avoid the therapist's anticipated anger about it.

In this case, the resistance was truly the vehicle for projection of her anger and for playing out ways she had related her entire life. It was the tip of the iceberg, representing a whole dimension of her inner response to relationships. Although the patient spoke in her individual session on issues that just came to mind, consciously unknown to her, the content of the session provided clues to what was going on in group. What to the patient appeared as a new topic and to the therapist as *resistance, was thematically the same issue as in group. So in the process of resisting analysis of the cancellation, she actually laid the groundwork, the data, for analyzing it. The connection was obviously there, but was unconscious, arising through the process of the session. The therapist saw the connection, but not until the "resistance" was played out did she comment that perhaps the patient's experience in group was "getting too close to home."

To a patient such as this, one with a highly private self, vulnerable to criticism, one whose powerful parental expectations and demands mitigated against a relationship with "outsiders" and against transferential "insiders," little about resistance needs to be interpreted until the patient takes the lead in doing so. On the other hand, such a "good" compliant patient needs leeway to maneuver some acting out, which will be the window of opportunity for both patient and therapist to see what is going on.

The literature notes that resistance is inevitable, but therapists often have a hard time living with it. They go into this business demanding to help, and when the patient refuses, or makes it difficult, they feel diminished. In fact, Rank (1972) thought the therapist resented the patient for not performing in expected ways. Unlike Freud, he came to believe that resistance was an indication of the patient's will, a sign of progress and independence. Nevertheless, although eventually he softened his approach, initially, he, like Freud, was quite controlling with the patient in forcing explanations of the resistance. It did not work then, and it still does not. As Wolberg (1973) says, "The aim of treatment is to help the patient let up on the creation of defenses rather than force him by premature confrontations to increase his defenses" (p. 207).

Patients need space to determine the direction their therapy will take. The therapist may facilitate from the data at hand and guide as an expert on human behavior, but the guidance is only on cue from the patient. This is not to say patients should run roughshod over therapists and therapists say, "Great, you're expressing yourself," or that therapists in exasperation and in wise therapeutic endeavor should not say, "Look, at some point, if you're ever going to move, you've got to look at some of this," and, removing the self from the nonresistance investment, say, "Whether you do or not, it's nothing to me personally. My life isn't going to change one way or the other, but sometime you have to take notice." It is truly difficult, on the other hand, not to be invested if the therapist's view of self is at stake needing the patient's progress for self-affirmation and needing the mother/patient to come around.

One such therapist got into a power struggle with a patient, lost the patient, and later heard that the patient left triumphant but paid with rage and depression. The problem started when the patient "forgot" to come for a regularly scheduled session. When asked why that might have been, the patient said probably because things were going fine. Instead of not commenting, thinking the question had been comment enough and waiting for explanatory "unconscious data" to come up through the process of the session, the therapist immediately confronted the patient with the idea that the patient and therapist were surely not so stupid as to think wellness could be the reason. This provocative tactic simply incited anger. But because the unconscious desire for understanding is relentless, in the process of the session, the reason for the resistance weedled its way through supposedly unrelated data. But because the therapist had been so relentless and single-minded, he missed the clue and cue.

It seems that early in the day of the forgotten session the patient and her mother had talked on the telephone. The patient's mother, a powerful university academic and a controlling woman, was chagrined at her daughter's reluctance to do her thesis. The patient explained that although a thesis was necessary for her graduate degree, it was unnecessary for a job in graphic design; in fact, the degree was not even necessary. This traditionally oriented academic mother failed to understand such a distinction, so mother and daughter became locked in a familiar struggle. The patient later said to her therapist that during the time she was supposed to be at her session she was thinking that it was her mother's relentless pushing that made her dig her heels in and not ever want to do anything but watch television. Besides, she had only gone to graduate school to appease her mother. Obviously, the patient was acting out transferentially with the therapist by not coming to the regularly scheduled session, but doing so allowed her to observe a pattern that heretofore had eluded her: wanting to do something, her mother wanting her to do it the mother's way or to do something else, losing the struggle, doing nothing, thereby retaliating. Well, this time, she quit therapy. She did nothing but repeat the pattern, and the therapist helped her do that, concluding she was untreatable anyhow. Difficult yes, but definitely treatable if the therapist's narcissism had not interfered.

MANIFESTATIONS OF THE THERAPIST'S NARCISSISM

Resistance is built into the process of therapy on both sides of the couch. Certainly the patient comes with it, so might the therapist, and certainly the therapist responds to it. Some has little or nothing to do with the therapist or content but is a kind of developmental resistance to change (Blatt & Erlich, 1982). Virtually all the literature on resistance acknowledges the effect of countertransference on the arousal, continuance, and aggravation of resistance. In particular, we focus on the therapist's narcissism, how the patient's resistance inflicts its wounds, and how the therapist's response reinforces the resistance. We discuss five therapist responses: overidentification, competition, overconcern about the patient's productions, the need to manage behavior, and intrusiveness.

Overidentification with the patient often results from personal therapist resistance to dealing with the same characteristic, experience, or phenomenon that the patient resists. The therapist is too nice and too careful and builds a case for supportive treatment rather than investigative work. Eventually, the patient feels cheated and angry about the inhibition and control, and of course, the resistance not only remains untouched, but has been reinforced. A patient of one of our supervisees finally quit treatment because no therapy was taking place. The patient was a good girl nurse, taking care of the world. She was totally unappreciated by those in her care and her superiors, not noticing that through all her altruism she demanded love and honor. The therapist, strikingly similar to the patient, though more sophisticated, did not notice either. So instead of identifying the pattern or listening to the supervisor, she simply cherished the patient, thinking she was fragile and in need of a corrective experience. This tactic was simultaneously resistance caused by overidentification and a hostile gesture toward the patient, consonant with the narcissistic needs of the therapist and sacrificing the therapeutic needs of the patient. The experience was a transferential one replicating the mother–daughter relationship of the patient rather than a potentially corrective transferential relationship of therapist and patient.

Competition with the patient can occur in a variety of ways. Often, it manifests itself through power struggles about the patient's acting out or the meaning of a behavior or pattern, or through a therapist's relentless search for the true truth. The therapist needs to be right and may even try to control the direction of the session or the vehicle through which the patient expresses behavior. This is rationalized by those therapists who, by their goal-oriented approach, keep the patient on the topic. Sometimes, the competition only becomes clear to the therapist when he or she suddenly notices making one interpretation after another or sharing "learned opinions" unnecessarily. Although therapist competition engages the patient, the patient cannot move beyond it, thereby fueling their mutual resistance and the therapist's narcissism.

The therapist's inordinate need to be a good parent yields *overconcern about the patient's productions.* If the patient is silent or rambles or goes off on what appears to be a tangent, the therapist acts as if the patient had not had a proper potty session. Such a therapist misses the opportunity to join the patient in his or her own unwitting route to the expression and analysis of the situation. If the therapist can delay gratification enough to be led by the patient, the ultimate production is usually rewarding. The following is an example:

A patient called to say he could not come to his appointment because he was anxious and depressed about an imminent weekend visit from his new lady friend. With urging, however, he came and indeed talked about his anxiety and lack of control of the situation. In the process, however, he abruptly switched topics, inadvertently communicating concerns otherwise obscured. The patient, himself a therapist, talked in detail of the seeming helplessness of a competent patient he was seeing. Unknown consciously to this therapist, bringing up his patient was significant. With patients, he felt competent because he knew the parameters of the relationship, whereas in a personal relationship, especially one just developing, where boundaries are less rigid, he felt totally incompetent, like the patient. Until he "resisted," however, with the clinical case material, he had not identified the problem. Furthermore, on another level, by bringing up the clinical data he was also suggesting to himself that maybe he, like the patient, was not so helpless and incompetent. Also, perhaps he could just let the new relationship develop the way he could with a patient, and then he would feel better.

When the patient/therapist noticed his digression, he was annoyed, saying, "Why did I do that? I didn't mean to waste time like that." He had not wasted any time, however, Indeed, he digressed to allow material to come into consciousness unhampered by anxiety and unconscious editing, like a dream, a symbol used as a route to or implying unconscious content. The task for the therapist is to allow the production to occur, digressive as it might seem, in order to decipher or decode the symbolic communication. If the therapist does this, the patient takes the lead, and the therapist facilitates enlargement of the patient's perception on the basis of data before the eyes of both, an excellent learning experience unhampered by preconceived notions about quality and quantity of patient production.

Without realizing it, many analytic therapists have a *behavioral management focus* by their overconcern about the patient's acting out. In a distortion of analytic doctrine and concern, they may even rationalize the focus by saying that all acting out should be *in* therapy rather than *outside* of it. Although acting out ultimately needs to be explored, if the therapist tries to manage the behavior, the patient will either be compliant and in the therapist's lap forever, which obviously brings its own problems, or the patient will act out more. Either way resistance is fueled that, under ordinary circumstances, simply needs to take its course. An interesting example follows.

Years of sexual acting out in the external world served the purpose of obscuring inner anxiety about closeness for one patient; that is, until one day, after years of analysis and years of liaisons, when a young man's words touched the patient's inner life. She had known him casually for some time, and one day when she was bored, she finally responded to his advances. He would not leave her apartment after having sex, insisting on staying the night. She agreed but fabricated a story about her sister arriving at 7 a.m. so he would have to leave very early.

In the morning, the man, whom she always thought of as sort of simple, suddenly acquired stature when he said, "You don't care anything about me, do you?" Her arm near his began to ache incredibly as it occurred to her that he was right, that she did not care about any of her men and that the sexual acting out was used as a defense against interpersonal contact on an emotional level; it was a defense, a resistance. On the other hand, the resistance allowed her to take on relationships in small doses, building up to the point of noticing the thought that she cared little about the men, and at that moment allowing herself to be reached emotionally, although with discomfort.

Prior to this, had the therapist tried to manage the behavior by forcing interpretation, he would have fostered the patient's resistance because the patient simply had not been ready for such "contact" with the therapist either. A therapist's need to bring the patient into line is a reflection of therapist anxiety about loss of control and is itself a resistance against noting the source of the anxiety. Surely it is reminiscent of the narcissistic need to straighten out the mother, to make the mother into the nurturer she was not.

Intrusiveness in the usual sense denotes that the therapist is in there pitching verbally or nonverbally with and for the patient when there is no need for a partner, helper, or advocate. Such behavior is more an indicator of therapist narcissism than patient need. Although intrusiveness is often noticeable through direct observation, sometimes it is quite subtle, especially when it involves unconscious therapist personality characteristics that impinge on patients. Such was the case when a patient broke the ostensible rules of conduct in group therapy as set by a therapist who unconsciously flaunted his sexuality around patients. His patients always seemed to hint about possibly acting out with one another outside group. This time, a patient actually went out on a date with someone from group, a prohibited move.

As the patient was telling her individual therapist what happened with this great date, she slid off the track with endless tangential examples of "men as shits." Thus, in the process of the resistance the patient got to the point. The individual therapist, silently noting the thematic relationship, said, "So in other words, if Jim (the group therapist) is a tease you can be too, and if he is a jerk and doesn't know what mixed message he's sending, you can legitimately drive him crazy with it." The individual therapist brought the patient back to the original focus but only because the patient had brought herself back first.

On the other hand, the group therapist's intrusion was so unconscious that, when discussing the situation with his supervisor, he failed to understand why his patients always taunted him with possible extra-group contacts. His resistance was so great, no hard data seemed to intrude on his narcissism.

FINAL NOTES

Resistance provides both obstacle and opportunity. As symbol it is a necessary ingredient for communication in disguise. It is the human being's way of simultaneously keeping the door shut while opening it a crack. As such, it is part of every therapy experience. Internalized inter-personal relationships representing conceptualizations of the world will always impinge on or interfere with the corrective relationship. There-fore, there is always a "pull" on the corrective experience, a resistance to decrease the dissonance between old and new concepts. Therapy assures there will be a collision of existing concepts (Peplau, 1989) of self and other, and self in relation to other, and changing self–other concepts. The collision implies dissonance, which in turn implies anxiety, defended against yet represented by the subtleties of resistant maneuvers. We as therapists must grasp the subtleties and grapple with them as they are presented to us by our patients. Resistances constitute as much problem-atic subject matter as that which is expressed directly. As Sullivan (1954) says, "They are data" and ". . . it is of such things that the practice of [therapy] is composed" (p. 208).

11

Developmental Roots of Loneliness

Loneliness is a dreadfully uncomfortable experience. A manifestation of the need for human intimacy, often the phenomenon of loneliness is neither expressed openly nor experienced in awareness, and it is not observed directly. Consequently, loneliness may be difficult to notice and more difficult still to decipher, for the defenses against it are complex. Patterns of relationships inferring loneliness and defenses against it start early and emerge throughout life. They can be detected through the psychotherapeutic process when the need for others is exaggerated, retarded, or distorted. The particular relational pattern depends on the dynamics of early interpersonal relations. This chapter focuses on those relationships and how they influence the phenomenon of loneliness. To this end, we address the problem of loneliness from the standpoint of emotional isolation (Weiss, 1973) that develops in an interpersonal context, and as that incredibly uncomfortable yearning for intimacy (Sullivan, 1953b).

To understand the origins of loneliness and the defenses against it, we explore a particular class of developmental antecedents: interpersonal antecedents. In deciphering the roots of chronic loneliness, we suggest a relationship between aloneness and loneliness that occurs in the attachment to a parent. We distinguish between healthy aloneness, premature aloneness, and defensive aloneness and suggest a pattern of cognition and behavior that develops to defend against the feeling and perception of loneliness, which ultimately interferes with a viable search for intimacy.

This chapter was originally published in *Archives of Psychiatric Nursing* (1, 25–32, 1987) and is reprinted with permission of Grune & Stratton.

The idea that loneliness is an early developmental problem is not new. In 1930 Freud (1930/1961) mentioned defenses against loneliness, which implies a developmental process, and Karl Menninger (1930) skimmed the surface of loneliness when discussing failures in guiding children toward reality. In 1938, Zilboorg suggested that pathological loneliness was attributable to the damage or loss of narcissism, surely a developmental concept. If a child is not apprised of the reality of not being omnipotent, says he, the external world does not respond favorably to the child's self-centered approach to the world, responding instead with hostility and isolation and thereby evoking loneliness. Suttie (1952) postulated that if needs for tenderness and intimacy in early life were unsatisfied, the ground was fertile for loneliness. Sullivan (1953b) extended this postulate by delineating motivational systems that enter into the experience of loneliness. In infancy there is the need for contact, for tenderness; in childhood, the need for adult participation in activities; in the juvenile era and beyond, the need for peers and acceptance; and in the preadolescent era, the need for intimate exchange.

As early as 1955, Peplau proposed that the lonely patient is unable to discriminate the boundaries of his or her environment, a developmental problem indeed. Just as the infant sees the mother as part of the self, the lonely person distorts others as part of the self, maintaining this infant-like illusion. Unable to see themselves as separate, they cannot observe themselves in action.

Loneliness then, has clearly been tracked to early development for some time now. Peplau was the first theorist to actually make a connection between boundary discrimination and loneliness, using the term "emptiness" as one way of showing the relationships, although other psychodynamic theorists did not credit her work on loneliness. She was the first theorist to describe loneliness as inferred through its defenses. She connected loneliness to an individual's inability to see the self as separate from the environment, and from the mothering-one—what later was to be seen as an essential ingredient in schizophrenia. Fromm-Reichmann (1959) did make the connection to schizophrenia that Peplau implied through her description and clinical examples, as did Searles in 1967 (1979a) and Arieti (1974). Klein (1963/1980) linked loneliness to the loss of the earliest preverbal need to be understood by the mothering-one.

Peplau (1955) was also one of the first theorists clearly to distinguish between loneliness and aloneness, saying being alone may be pleasant or unpleasant, but loneliness is a dreadful, desperate experience. In agreement with Sullivan (1953b), she determined that the roots of loneliness were sustained, repeated experiences or patterns in early life where remoteness, indifference, and emptiness in interpersonal relations resulted in loneliness. Peplau (1955) pointed out that, because it is unbearable, loneliness is defended against; that is, not consciously experienced but experienced in other forms.

Today, social psychologists (Weiss, 1982) would say that such defenses against loneliness would teach us something about certain deficiencies in "relational provisions," about the consequences of living with certain attachment figures, with a certain attachment process, and in a certain attachment system.

ATTACHMENT AND THE CAPACITY TO BE ALONE

Healthy Aloneness

The need for human intimacy, for interpersonal intimacy, is something all human beings have (Sullivan, 1953b). Loneliness can be seen as a hunger for intimacy (Rubenstein & Shaver, 1982). Without intimacy, psychological stability falters and erodes and so does development. We first learned of this with Spitz's (1945) work with infants in institutions and the now-so-popular Harlow and Harlow (1965) experiments where monkeys, deprived of their mothers, suffered in their ability to grow, to relate, and to mate and reproduce. This implies that there are complementary behaviors (Bowlby, 1973a): attachment behaviors (proximity exhibited by the young toward another older member of the same species) and caretaking behaviors on the part of the parents toward the young. Together, these behaviors are the substance of the strong ties that children develop even without rewards (Bowlby, 1973a).

The quality of attachment, however, is linked to the quality of the caretaking. For example, in "anxious attachment," (Bowlby, 1969, 1973b) the child clings to the parent, feels anxious when separated, and lacks confidence in the self and others. This implies a lack of accessibility or responsiveness, a lack of emotional resource in the caretaker.

Recent research (Rubenstein & Shaver, 1982) now tells us that loneliness in adults is significantly related to the perceived quality of the child–parent relationship. Developmentally, it is clear that the child needs the mothering-one early on for contact and tenderness, and later for active participation in the child's world of play when interpersonal skills start to be acquired and the world actively investigated. At that point, particularly in early childhood, the mothering-one is, in a sense, an emotional resource, reliably physically and emotionally present. This consistent relationship, along with confidence, promotes a sense of "sufficiency of living" (Winnicott, 1965a). The child's immaturity is balanced by the mothering-one's support.

Indeed, it is Winnicott's (1965a) contention that development of the capacity to be alone is contingent on the child having had the opportunity to be alone in the presence of a benevolent, good parent. For initially, it is only when alone (in the sense of being self-absorbed) in the presence of a reliable other that the infant can have no orientation, can flounder, and can become unintegrated, without crippling anxiety.

The infant discovers the precarious, personal life experience while securely balanced by the support of the mothering-one as an emotional resource person. Throughout exploration, the mothering-one is near. Satisfaction and confidence result when there is assurance that the mothering-one is available when needed: to "check in" or "check back" with, for "refueling" (Bowlby, 1973a). The contact of a caretaker temporarily identified with and interested solely in the infant, who is primed for self-discovery, sets the stage for the infant to believe in a benign environment and to proceed into it alone, armed with an internalized presence of the mothering-one (object constancy) and the relationship.

Healthy aloneness, then, requires that an essentially faithful, predictable, nonanxious, nonintrusive, non-needs-competitive mothering-one is internalized, a mothering-one who has the capacity to be a genuinely concerned caretaker, but one who, in effect, does not need the child for emotional completion as advocate or adversary, one who also has the capacity to be alone. Healthy aloneness, therefore, is the capacity to not require another for a sense of protection or completion; it implies that one can withstand the vicissitudes of internal and external disequilibrium in everyday living without disintegrating or requiring a rescuer. In internalizing the relationship, the child comes to identify with a caretaker who can withstand psychic disequilibrium in another, thereby holding the memory of the child's own disequilibrium that did not spell disaster (Herron & Rouslin, 1982/1984). Developmentally, then, under such conditions, aloneness is not equated with lack of assistance. Rather, it is equated with a good someone, a benevolent, helpful resource person the memory of whom becomes part of self-sustenance.

Premature Aloneness

On the other hand, there are those persons who can develop no such concept of aloneness because the emotional resource, the mothering-one, has not been accessible and responsive. At the time the child needs the parent most, the parent is simply not available. It is not surprising to hear reports in the research surveys on loneliness of bodily feelings of "emptiness," a "hole," a "space" (Rubenstein & Shaver, 1982). For when the infant is in the presence of another, the other must be able to meet the infant's need to explore the self, the environment, and the self in relation to the environment, and be able to withstand the infant's psychic disequilibrium. If these abilities are not present in the caretaker, then something is indeed missing in the contribution to the attachment system. There is an emptiness, a hole, a space. It may mean that the mostly ungratifying mothering-one and the relationship are not internalized for need of further searching, or it may mean the internalization denotes that in experience with another human being the necessary ingredients for sustenance are missing.

To whom then, must the young child turn? Well, there's always the self. The problem is, of course, that the self is being formed, and with little favorable assistance. The child is thrust into a position of meeting his or her own needs without the necessary antecedents that would make the task possible. Further, such a task is beyond the emotional and interpersonal capacity of the child. The child has been catapulted into a state of premature aloneness.

Premature aloneness occurs, then, as a response to the existence of the child's needs for protection, exploration, and encouragement that are perpetually unheeded, unresponded to, or thwarted. Not only is the child unprepared for the aloneness because something really is missing externally, an adequate caretaker concept is missing internally. In our estimation these are the "children who learn to equate being alone with being lonely and rejected" (Rubin, 1982, p. 267).

THE COGNITIVE PICTURE

Cognitively, an idiosyncratic concept of being alone comes to be determined by the early blueprint of interaction in relation to the meeting of needs. Let's take the so-called experiential nontransformational rule (Kagan, 1971; Mussen, Conger, & Kagan, 1974) that governs static relations between concepts by giving an example in "Kaganesque" format: "A mothering-one is need-meeting." The two concepts are "mothering-one" and "need-meeting." The relation between the two concepts is a description of at least one dimension of the concepts. For instance, "A mothering-one is need-meeting" states a relationship between the concept "mothering-one" and the concept "need-meeting." Mothering-ones have many characteristics, among them that they are need-meeting. The quality of need-meeting is characteristic of many objects, among them a mothering-one. So then, it becomes clear that the relation of the concepts is determined by the meaning of the concepts. Given what has come to be seen as experiences with good mothering, therefore, a basic concept of mothering-one would form, and inherent in its meaning would be the concept of needs being met.

But what if the example were the following: "A mothering-one is need-ignoring or need-frustrating." Applying the same rules, we see that early and repeated observation and participation in a relationship with such a mothering-one would result in a concept of mothering-one that would have inherent in its meaning "need-ignoring" or "need-frustrating."

Since we know that, without intervention, the way we see the world and our place in it is a generalization or reflection of the way originally we came to see our parents, ourselves, and ourselves in relation to our parents, this means that the child whose concept of parent is need-ignoring or need-frustrating will associate that concept with other significant persons later in life. Instead of being able to equate aloneness with the inner resource of strength that comes from having been alone in the presence of a need-gratifying caretaker, the child will equate aloneness with a sense of something missing; as indeed it was, first from without, then from within.

The absence of a sustaining object is not, as some psychodynamic theorists would have it (Adler & Buie, 1979), simply a problem because of the lack or because there is no affective memory of it. The problem is so great because there is no cognition of a sustaining figure, not one formed, not one remembered. The cognition and the affective memory are linked instead to the original perception that the mothering-one was need-ignoring or need-frustrating. So the problem is not one of a lost memory, but that the memory evoked of so unsustaining a figure would be so painful, so rage-filled, that the likelihood of dissociation is very great. Indeed, there can be a sustained mental representation of the object even in its absence from the child's perceptual field (Piaget, 1954). The problem, then, is not one of ability. It is one of quality, and the quality is what influences whether the memory can be evoked.

It has been noted (Peplau & Perlman, 1982) that in the study of loneliness, "the needs approach emphasizes the affective aspects of loneliness; cognitive approaches emphasize the perception and evaluation of social relations and relational deficits" (p. 5). From clinical work, this dichotomy would appear to be artificial, for in real life it is not possible to separate affect from cognition (Lazarus, 1982; Solley, 1966).

The problem with the formation of the concepts "mothering-one" and "need-meeting" is that the meaning is crucial to development. Furthermore, because the mothering one's actual or inferred appraisal of the child is that the child is unworthy or impossible to gratify, the child's appraisal of himself or herself becomes the same (Sullivan's concept of reflected appraisals [1953b]). Now the package: The mothering-one's concept of the child is internalized, articulating with the child's concept of the mother and the relationship pattern. So, if the mothering-one will not gratify and the child feels ungratifiable and is not prepared anyway, what happens?

From a research standpoint, this process of internalization of appraisals and how they are repeatedly lived out is incredibly important because "available evidence suggests that people conceptualize the causes of loneliness on the basis of whether they reflect something about the self versus the setting, and whether they are relatively permanent or changeable" (Peplau, Miceli, & Morasch, 1982, p. 141), and further, how much control they have over the situation. Obviously, a child has little control, and since the process of reflected appraisals in the way the self system is laid down is automatic, the original appraisals of self, others, and the relationship between the two is lived out repeatedly, out of one's conscious control.

Peplau and her colleagues (1982) suggest that what lonely people attribute their feeling to is of crucial importance in determining explanations of why their relationships have failed and why they are lonely. It is thought that the most problematic attributions are those that are internal, stable, and uncontrollable. Now, let us keep in mind that their research concerns itself with consciously perceived loneliness and is conducted with "normals." What we are talking about here is loneliness that is largely dissociated, inferred only through behavior, or loneliness that emerges through therapy when it is no longer so strongly defended against.

If it is true that the most problematic attributions are internal, stable, and uncontrollable, then indeed the self system that has chronic loneliness as an integral component may be in big trouble. For we know the self system to be an internal system reflecting external interaction attitudes and patterns that are internalized to be lived out interpersonally. Without intervention, the self system is relatively stable as opposed to changeable; and the self system, again without intervention, operates out of one's conscious knowledge or control. This means that, in a psychodynamic sense, chronic loneliness as part of the self system fulfills all the criteria for the most problematic attributions.

LONGING FOR ANOTHER

It seems to us that in the state of premature aloneness the child works incredibly hard to hold up, trying repeatedly to repair the concept "mothering-one": to make a change in that which is nontransformational, to change the cognition by changing the interpersonal facts and images that make up the concept "mothering-one." Failing that, the child tries to enlarge the concept of self, rudimentary though it is, to include a definition of mothering that is gratifying. The self becomes mother.

This state of "do-it-yourself" gratification initially carries with it frustration, then anger, perhaps rage, and longing too, before despair and hopelessness set in. It would seem that not even a fantasy of a soothing, sustaining figure from the past would be possible (Adler & Buie, 1979). The longing for a gratifying other (Leiderman, 1969/1980) to meet needs and to mentor, if you will, we see as a primitive form of loneliness arising out of the state of premature aloneness. As social psychologists have found in their research of adults (Perlman & Peplau, 1982), being alone and being lonely are not synonymous. However, being alone is a key antecedent that can lead to loneliness. The chances seem all the more likely with a premature state of aloneness as an antecedent.

In the longing for another, there is a desired image based on felt needs. As the longing proceeds, it becomes clearer that there is a collision of the desired image with the actual image; and with that, the distressing feelings of loneliness surface, or, in the words of social psychologists Peplau and Perlman (1982), cognitively "loneliness is a response to a discrepancy between desired and achieved levels of social contact" (p. 5).

Such dissonance, producing extreme anxiety, panic, and rage, would readily result in dissociation. But whereas many theorists (Fromm-Reichmann, 1959; Peplau, 1955; Sullivan, 1953b) note that the dreadful experience of loneliness itself is dissociated, inferred only through behavior, theorists have not said more. It seems to be that not only is the loneliness dissociated—that is, the resultant felt component of a horrendous interpersonal experience—but the activity and accompanying thoughts and feelings of the original nonresponsive, need-ignoring, need-frustrating interpersonal experience are dissociated. Since cognition and affect are always related (Lazarus, 1982), it is not simply that the loneliness is shunted aside. The original perception of unavailability and the child's affective response to it that underlie the loneliness are also put out of awareness. This means we must look to current behavior to infer the original interpersonal dynamics and cognition.

ACTIVE SEARCH VERSUS DEFENSIVE ALONENESS

It would appear that what had been a prematurely alone infant and young child, then a longing, lonely child and adolescent is a person now either actively searching for an accessible, responsive attachment figure or is defensively alone. Although the active searching assuredly takes place throughout all phases, it can develop insidiously as a way of life. It would seem that early on, active searching for a physically accessible, emotionally responsive caretaker would precede the protest behavior posited by

Bowlby (1973b) in his study of responses to absence of the attachment figure. We would speculate that the longer the active search goes on with the actual mothering-one to the exclusion of others, the more disturbed the searcher and the mothering-one, the more the need for merger (to make the mothering-one whole so a self could develop), and the less the ability to discriminate boundaries. In later life, with the physical absence of the mothering-one, the indiscriminate "anyone" would take the place of this elusive attachment figure. Or, as Bowlby (1973a) would say, "Were a child to exhibit no behavior other than attachment behavior, he would, of course, remain tied to his mother's apron strings" (p. 44).

Thus, we see persons who insinuate themselves with strangers, with unlikely characters, with anybody who happens to come their way. Although ostensibly what they seek is a need-gratifying other, what they get or what they drive another to be is what they always had, a need-ignoring, need-frustrating other. So the loneliness and the cognition or the originally perceived factors that cause loneliness (known as *attributions*, Peplau & Perlman, 1982), continue. Although such persons feel the pangs of premature aloneness and longing, they do not seem to be able to leave the attachment figure long enough to feel the incredible despair that comes with the recognition that one will never get from such an attachment figure that which one wants and needs.

There are those, however, who do feel the despair. Such persons are more likely to leave the mothering-one earlier, that is, to turn to others as sources for gratification. The problem, though, is that the choice of "other" remains contingent on the original cognition so the original set of observations and appraisals is lived out repeatedly.

Bowlby's (1969, 1973b) work tells us that despair does not go on indefinitely; a state of detachment results. Others (Adler & Buie, 1979) suggest that when detachment persists, a fundamental long-standing aloneness develops. And still others (Leiderman, 1969/1980) write that the person has an "urge to independence" to counteract the need for closeness. We postulate that when premature aloneness and longing occur, and it becomes clear that gratification from another remains elusive, the person is filled with despair. With what is now experienced as intolerable loneliness within, the person despairs of finding an external source of gratification, and instead chooses to do the gratifying alone.

This position of defensive aloneness is a defense against the despair, the loneliness and longing, and the anxiety and memory of the premature aloneness (although that is its progenitor). Too, it is a defense against the cognition of the mothering-one as need-ignoring and need-frustrating as an attachment figure, and it is a defense against the corresponding cognition of the self as a person unfit for gratification or unable to be gratified. In short, defensive aloneness is a defense against the human need for intimacy. The defense is incredibly strong, barring self and others from seeing any needs and any deep feelings.

Just how strong this defense is came to our attention when such a defensively alone patient called for an emergency session. It was quite unlike her to be noticeably anxious and quite unlike her to ask anything of anybody, including the therapist. An executive in a large corporation, she had been alone, away from her ungratifying husband and needy children, at, as she put it, "the solitude of a meeting" in another city. While she was there, she started thinking about what she did not have in her life: "tenderness and sensitivity" as she put it, that had always been missing, that she now remembered as a yearning she had turned off. At the meeting she became very anxious, feeling she would fall apart, but fearing more that everybody at the meeting, especially those responding favorably, would see, as she said, "what I want, who I am, my neediness, my longing," feelings that had long been obscured from herself and others by anger and control on one level, and on a deeper level by dissociation and the not-so-free choice that she do everything herself, meet her own needs.

There is repeated evidence from clinical practice that, with therapy, the need for human intimacy does eventually emerge, often inferred at first, later seen through anger, and then through anxiety that feels totally disorganizing; this is the kind of disequilibrium that in early life is desirable to experience in the presence of a sustaining caretaker before one feels capable of experiencing it alone. As with this patient, the need for human intimacy emerges with a great expression of loneliness, but also with a feeling of shame. The shame is defended against by doubt, a sense as she said that, "Maybe I'm wrong, maybe I don't see the situation right," as if blame lay in the lap of the one who needs another. Here it would seem that the patient defends against the original perception of where the blame lay by attributing it to the self. Not only does this defense help protect the self by obscuring feelings of rage, it gives latitude to the attachment figure to change, a pathological hope that the attachment figure will come around (Herron & Rouslin, 1982/1984).

A patient, who through many years of therapy held this pathological hope about a totally self-centered mother and every other such person he encountered, was going to attend a class reunion in his home town. In making the plans, he was filled with an anxiety that was not his usual anxiety and anger at the prospect of seeing his mother in his home town. The day before leaving he was anxious; he felt incompetent and unable to get everything done, although he was competent, always completing the task at hand. At work his thoughts vacillated between the idea of his boss really being a jerk after all and the desire to focus on the boss' good points. On the way home from work, the patient's attention seemed expanded; indeed, he was drawn to the perpetually drunk men in the neighborhood that he usually ignored. On passing, he heard one say to another: "I'm so lonely," and he could not stop thinking about it. When he got home, still preoccupied but newly anxious, he thought suddenly, "I'm all alone, I have no one." Until this time he had seemed not to notice his lifetime of detachment and defensive aloneness. With this awareness, he felt overwhelming sadness, recalling, he related to the therapist, the endless experience of despair at failing repeatedly with his parents to elicit the response he needed.

What we see here is a condensed version of this person's life, a developmental sequence influenced by premature aloneness: a longing for a desired image based on felt needs; a collision of the desired image with the actual image; the despair, with the search to have needs met given up and defended against by defensive aloneness, only to arise again briefly when the mothering-one or another authority figure intruded.

Surely persons who can reach the point of experiencing their loneliness are in a better position than they were when defending against it, even though they do not necessarily feel better at the time. It does feel terrible and the defenses against it are intricate and formidable. It is up to clinicians to understand the many components of chronic loneliness, and how the antecedents become obscured by defenses against loneliness, and yet how the same defenses infer something about the antecedents. Such professional, theory-based practice will ultimately yield greater knowledge of the phenomenon of loneliness and how it works for and against the need for human intimacy.

12

Envy and Its Consequences

When one of us (S.R.W.) was still a graduate student, a paranoid patient she was treating railed often at her about "enviness" in the world and sometimes about "enviness and jealousy." With intimidated interest the therapist listened, thinking the preoccupation peculiar and the distinction somehow noteworthy, both likely part of her pathology because she had difficulty explaining the particulars of her experience with each phenomenon along with their similarities and differences. When she tried, she experienced something of a surge of incredible anxiety, immediately followed by uncontrollable rage as she hurled invectives the therapist's way. Humbled, the therapist thought possibly she was premature in asking and so read Sullivan (1953b, 1965).

Unlike some theorists, Sullivan (1953b, 1956) is clear but leaves one wanting to know more. Indeed, although envy is a universal phenomenon experienced by all persons at one time or another, it has not been written about in a universally understandable way. Freud (1908/1959, 1923/1961, 1925/1961) was anatomically focused on penis envy and Jones (1927/1948, 1935/1948) with maternal power of giving birth. So too were Boehm (1930) with womb envy and Klein (1957/1975) with breast envy, which is virtually a constitutional given in her theories, attributing much criticized/questioned ability (Joffee, 1969), that is, the ability of secondary process thinking, a more advanced developmental competence, to an infant. Interestingly though, if one is not put off by the concreteness or by the absurdity, all these theorists have enormously useful things to say about envy and its interpersonal origins, although, for most of the early theorists, envy was considered instinctually based

This chapter was originally published in *Archives of Psychiatric Nursing* (1, 322–333, 1987) and is reprinted with permission of Grune & Stratton.

rather than interpersonally inspired. In this chapter, we share some decoded abstractions from major theorists that are combined with our own conceptions of envy.

PATHOLOGICAL ENVY

The recognition and study of envy have moved from later eras of development, that is, oedipal and genital in Freud's terminology, to earlier eras of development, preoedipal, because through the years, it has become obvious that life begins with mother. We now know that a good deal of health and pathology results from that beginning, early, mother–child relationship, how one "uses" it, how one separates and individuates from it, and how one conceives and fashions subsequent relationships because of it.

Envy is one of those universal, highly uncomfortable phenomena that is automatic and that is not always consciously recognized by its holder. By others, it is observed through behavior, often indirectly inferred only through defenses against it (Klein, 1957/1975). Envy refers to an inner sense of deficiency (Jones, 1927/1948) triggered by anything that is seen to undermine one's estimation of oneself. It pertains to personal attachments or attributes that someone else has what one does not have but what one wants. It is a feeling that something is missing, "an active realization," according to Sullivan (1953b), "that one is not good enough, compared with someone else" (p. 348). It involves self-devaluation accompanied by resentment and sadness (Neubauer, 1982). Envy, then, is an intrapersonal and interpersonal concept. It is felt within the self, but it arises through a process originally involving relationships with significant others, an interpersonal relationship principally with the mothering one. Envy manifests itself later through relationships with others. Thought of in this way, without another for comparison, envy could not exist.

Pathological envy has several characteristics not addressed in the literature but ones implied, characteristics certainly observed by the "student" of envy. One is that *envy is pervasive*; it affects the whole personality and all relationships eventually. Not only is envy pervasive, it is *enslaving* (Bank & Kahn, 1982). Every relationship is ultimately contaminated. Every contact becomes an arena for comparison. Consequently, all relationships are guided not by desire for closeness or communication but by discontent about the self. Relationships are responded to or acquired according to and derailed by vigilant concern about how one is doing when compared with the other; indeed, any other person and certainly a relationship is of secondary concern to what we call this "comparison preoccupation." In effect, a project, a goal, a relationship, even what would appear to be a significant relationship, takes a back seat to the comparison preoccupation. The other person may be selected or responded to favorably because he or she is admired, the better to feel about oneself through attaching oneself to the other's attributes. Or the other person may be selected or responded to favorably because he or she is devalued, the better to feel about oneself through contrast. In either case, the comparison preoccupation, based on the experience of self-unworthiness, guides the selection of the other and ultimately destroys any potential for closeness or communication.

Envy, therefore, is enduring, always ready to spring forth, an important point to remember for those misguided persons who try to woo or fix the envious person through acts of kindness and generosity of spirit or through playing "footsies" to appease. Obviously then, *envy is an automatic experience.* In other words, one does not consciously think, "My goodness, I am envious; therefore I will act despicably to this person whose qualities or objects I want so much to have." Instead, the behavior simply shows itself spontaneously, falls out of the person as it were. The behavior that is observed by another is an external manifestation of envy; it is the end product of a process involving the way one sees oneself and oneself in relation to others that is largely internal, that is unwittingly repeated over and over again without conscious, formulated thought, permission, or consideration of the effects on the current situation or future consequences for that matter.

All this said, it becomes clear that the pathologically envious person does not make for a good, loyal, predictable friend, except when one is having a bad time. Often, then, the envious so-called friend, whose self feeling is boosted by the other's misfortune and, thus, feels better by comparison, does a heroic job of helping the other person out, only to lay low again or do the person in once the crisis has passed. As far back as 1921, Abraham (1921/1927) warned that "the envious . . . person shows not only a desire for the possessions of others, but connects with that desire spiteful impulses against the privileged proprietor" (p. 382).

Such impulses poured forth from an envious older sister whose one claim to fame over her younger sister in her estimation was that she had a husband and children and her "maiden aunt" sister did not. So when the now-engaged younger sister called excitedly to say a date was finally set for her wedding, the older sister, who ostensibly had been ecstatic for her sister, responded by deciding that the cherished adult nephew, her emotionally cuckolded son, would not be there. Spite, signifying envy; not being good enough as compared with someone else, had soared forth quickly, in fact automatically, without conscious, formulated thought, and without consideration of the effects on the current situation or future consequences. It is rather like toddlers of 1½ or ? who, when they feel envy, simply act (Frankel & Sherick, 1977) without regard to anything but the possession, without regard for the future and without anticipation, plan, or delay.

In this case the envy response had a long history, however. The older sister had always felt inferior. First, she had felt like a disappointment to her quietly grandiose but depressed, inferior-feeling mother. She had been born a physically unattractive, difficult, cranky baby of a physically beautiful but emotionally hateful, unworthy-feeling mother. In a way, she did not have a chance, even before her sister came along about 4 years later. Dynamically, the mother saw in this child the "ugly" dimensions of herself, which were also dimensions of her own hateful, hated mother. In the mother's eyes, the older child seemed to have had no redeeming features. Any that might have been, like her energy and her intelligence, the mother demeaned or ignored, a reminder of either what she, the mother, was not or feared she was not, or a reminder of her own mother. The view the child developed of herself was as someone never filling the bill, never being "right" for her mother, never having the "right fit" with the mother; never was she pleasing to the mother. By her "being," she never supported the mother's need to see herself as a lovely, gentle, nice person that she appeared to be but was not.

Also, because as Sullivan (1956) notes, such a child does not rate with the parent who set goals that the child can never attain, she feels deficient no matter what. So when the sister came along, envy of this lovely, placid child was not simply a transient experience that we come to expect at this time and throughout life (Abraham, 1920/1927; Bank & Kahn, 1982). Instead, already beset by the woes of feeling unworthy and helpless to be pleasing, she was at risk for experiencing intense chronic envy, which had already started with envying the power and beauty of this difficult mother and envying the image of what she herself could never quite be.

ENVY AND JEALOUSY

Although the genesis of envy involves two people, the way is set for jealousy, which involves at least three people. The nub of jealousy is that an interloper, a third party, somehow "makes it" with the parent or, later in life, with the parental stand in. Enormous resentment develops (Neubauer, 1982) because of the love, respect, or regard this third party receives from the mothering one. So, added to the resentment, self-devaluation, and sadness (Neubauer, 1982) of the already envious child who has failed to be good enough for the mother is someone who comes along who is good enough and who apparently has something the other one does not have and, with that attribute then, has what it takes to capture the interest, favor, and love of the mothering one.

Jealousy, then, is actually an outgrowth of envy, (Klein, 1957/1975) in that, developmentally, the jealous person first feels terribly deficient and then later feels envy, which predisposes him or her to concern that love, regard, or respect that is felt to be due him or her is taken away or threatened to be taken away or achieved by a rival. What starts out as "wounded narcissistic expectation and injustice" (Meissner, 1978) predisposes the person to displace the blame for the lack in self-esteem or respect to a third party. In the process, the self is protected, and ironically so is the parent to some degree. Hope remains that if only something would happen to this third party, some punishment, banishment, something destructive, then the parent would bestow the love, regard, and respect onto oneself.

So, although envy, which originates in a two-person situation, includes "a desire to have what someone else has" (Spielman, 1971), and, perhaps, although not always, not wanting the other person to have it, especially if there's little chance of acquiring the attribute or its equivalent. Jealousy is that plus the notion that the person has somehow been bested by a third party for the admiration of the parental figure. Envy is a precursor to jealousy (Spielman, 1971). Jealousy is a more complex interpersonal phenomenon (Sullivan, 1956) subsuming envy. Interestingly, jealousy is also somehow more socially acceptable. Its almost compulsive focus on the third party belies both a longing for the desired attribute and, importantly, shifts the focus and attention from the intense need for continual external (parental) supplies to regulate self-esteem, which, if experienced, would fill the person with shame.

Fifty years ago, Fenichel (1935/1953) discussed envy to explain the jealous person's problems with a loss of love. Although envy is a precursor to jealousy (Jones, 1929/1948; Klein, 1957/1975; Riviere, 1932), jealousy may be a defense against envy (Klein, 1957/1975; Riviere, 1932) in that by focusing on a third party, jealousy dissipates intense feelings such as hatred and rage against the mothering one, often displacing them onto the father or sibling. So too, it happens later in life when the original figures are represented through other relationships. We are reminded of the patient who came into treatment because for over a year she noticed that her husband had been withdrawing from her. She was upset but, noticeably, not angry. What did emerge, however, was that she had observed herself becoming what she identified as "jealous" of her daughter because, from her, the husband was not withdrawing his attention. Although jealousy certainly applied in this three-person situation and was certainly something to be reckoned with, it obscured an underlying envy that permeated the relationship with the daughter, an envy based on the mother's yearning for a father she had lost as a young child. The primary problem was one of envy of the daughter who had a father. The patient yearned for a father–daughter relationship like the one her daughter had. She did not see the daughter simply as a third-party interloper taking away the husband's interest and affection. Rather, a father–daughter relationship was a long-held desire that she had tried not to notice throughout her life, but now she could not ignore it.

To return to the example that prompted the discussion of the relationship betwen envy and jealousy, namely, the older sister who had such a strong reaction to the imminent marriage of her younger sister, here also both envy and jealousy operated. Although the envy dimension has already been discussed, what about the jealousy? Why did this particular circumstance provoke jealousy in addition to the ever-present envy? Jealousy was provoked, not because the younger sister got the man the older sister wanted. On its face that would be the reasonable answer, but it is much too simplistic an explanation and, anyhow, not accurate. It is certainly possible that on one level the younger sister's man represented the mother who frustrated and deprived the older sister and chose instead to cherish the younger child. On another level, the younger sister actually had been distorted as a "mother" to the older one even though, ostensibly, the older one seemed to do the mothering. So when this little "mother" chose somebody else to be "family," the older sister relived the original experience of feeling inferior, disregarded, unloved, and replaced. In addition, the status achieved and nourished for the world to see—the wife and adoring sister to her maiden aunt sister—was crumbling. So, closer to the surface, the older sister had been bested once again by the younger sister who was now to be judged equal in status.

In jealousy, however, there is no such thing as equality. The change in the younger sister's status meant that because the older sister could not feel superior she would feel the underlying sense of unworthiness with its accompanying envy. And what better punishment for the younger sister than to take away her son, the nephew her sister adored. She would take away her son from his aunt the way the younger sister had taken the mother away from her: automatic, unwitting reliving of the original situation plus sweet revenge. And besides, she never did like that this interloper sister had enjoyed a close relationship with the son, again a replication of the disruption of the original relationship with the mother. But of course, with all the retribution, revenge, and taking away, the envy remains. A pleasurable internal state is no closer at hand than it ever was.

CIRCUMSCRIBED ENVY

It is well to bring attention to a kind of envy not described in the literature, envy that we call circumscribed envy. It is pathological in that it is not transient—it stays with the person—and it comes about predictably but only in certain situations. It is circumscribed, then, in that it is confined to these certain situations, does not pervade all aspects of the self-concept or view, or seep into all relationships. In other words, the envy is limited to specific troublesome dimensions of the self and the self in relationship to others. Definitively, one could not say, "Now, there's an envious person."

We realized that such a variation as circumscribed envy existed some time ago when we saw the patient mentioned earlier who was troubled about her 7-year-old daughter. Before there was a problem between the husband and wife, she noted that the daughter tugged on her; she whined, did not want to go to school, did not want to go to parties, felt sick a lot, in general wanted to be around her mother. Now, this mother was not so inclined. She had had a good deal of trouble making a commitment to marriage and even more to motherhood. Although she was highly responsible and would have appeared to have been physically available, that is, involved with her daughter and activities related to her daughter (e.g., PTA, Brownies, swimming), she was not emotionally responsive or available to her, and she always found herself noticing and carefully controlling her physical availability. In fact, she could not understand why the child would want to be with her, to the point of being phobic about leaving her, because she was rather grouchy to her. Bowlby (1969) would say there was certainly an "anxious attachment" on the part of the child, worrying, as the patient said, that maybe the mother would not be there when she got back if the child actually left the mother's side. The patient was rather preoccupied, then, with this tug and with the child's use of anxiety to make the mother pay. It had seemed enough that the child was too emotionally demanding on someone highly sensitive to that sort of thing; surely that was this patient's problem. But there was more.

In describing what happened when the child was to go to a party, the mother explained how her husband, the child's father, dealt with her successfully when the mother was simply frustrated with the child's phobic response. Now, at that point, the therapist was not sure what she was responding to because this was an early session with the patient. Obviously, the therapist knew very little about her background, certainly not enough consciously to make any connections between the patient's early life and her reaction to her daughter. Maybe it was because the therapist was immersed in envy because of her interest in the phenomenon, or maybe it was her nonverbal way of describing the father's success. The therapist does remember that the patient had such a warm, almost serene look, neither competitive nor envious, when she said how good her husband had been with the daughter that day. In retrospect, it would seem that the therapist was responding intuitively to her observations of the patient that were not yet consciously noticed at the time when she asked, "Are you envious of your daughter?" The patient burst into tears, saying, "Oh, yes," and volunteered that her father had been ill for most of her childhood and had died when she was still a young child. She had so envied that her daughter had something this special with her daddy, something the patient spent years yearning for with a father of her own.

In no other area but this was envy to prove to be a problem. Indeed, the patient had a big problem with commitment, but that actual problem obscured the problem with envy, feeling a lack, a void, something missing in one dimension of her life, wanting what was missing, and envying her daughter who had it. The envy was confined to this one area, but it certainly affected the relationship with her daughter and in fact turned out to be related to the problem of commitment. Because of the father's long illness and early death, she had had to grow up too fast. The emotional demands she experienced beyond her years, a demand for premature maturity, made her very anxious about involvement with anyone lest there be too great a demand or lest she show any needs that, as a child, she would have been in trouble for having and frustrated in getting met by either of her parents.

Circumscribed envy is noticeable in everyday situations, an envy confined to one area of living. It is a prevalent reaction in losing a child for instance. How often can women who have lost a child look at pregnant women or babies without experiencing excruciating envy? Yet the rest of their lives do not wreak of envy.

NORMAL ENVY

Envy, then, is not always chronic and pathological. In fact, researchers (Frankel & Sherick, 1977) have observed the development of normative envy over time, as occurring in increasingly controlled, varied, and sophisticated ways in toddlers and young children, and have noted that evidence of envy indicates "the child must have developed some capacity to fantasy a desired endstate which would occur if his wishes were to be fulfilled" (Joffee, 1969, p. 540). Further, "When the envy response does not include the need to destroy the admired or idealized object, it can act as a motive for further development" (Spielman, 1971, p. 62).

The precursors of normal envy start when the child begins to separate but sees others still in the service of the self. At this early point (1 to 1½ years) there is a sense of entitlement, actually for the possessions of others rather than related to or directed at the other because the other is not terribly distinguished as separate from the possessions that define or represent him or her. During the next era (1½ to 2 years) when there is anxiety about separation and a need for refueling, the toddler is watchful of the mothering-one's response. Losing something to another evokes envy; losing mother's attention to another provokes a rudimentary jealousy. Yet before the envy, there is curiosity, interest, and anger and with the envy, attempts to gain something of value, which is certainly healthy.

A colleague brought to the therapist's attention how many of her patients, who otherwise had been reluctant to do so, started buying houses after seeing her do so while managing to survive and thrive. It seems that as she came into her newly renovated office in her home when the group was starting she heard several patients say how they would like to have a similar room. She said she did feel a little jolt, for being envied certainly can cause anxiety. But quite automatically she said, "Why shouldn't you have one?" So five patients in the last 2 years have bought houses.

We have certainly noticed similar sorts of things. Some time ago a patient who has spent years talking about being unable to choose wallpaper sat in a corner of a demolished therapy office that was being redone and said that she had gone out and chosen some wallpaper and found a person to hang it, to boot. Yes, the literature does certainly say that emulation (Spielman, 1971) is part of or based on envy; there certainly is clinical evidence to that effect, and it would seem to be healthy.

The danger, of course, would come if the therapist were so encouraging of the patient as to control the patient, that is, if the therapist needed the patient to be the same as oneself, almost demanding that he or she do the same things. Then, of course, the therapist would just encourage the patient's being a narcissistic extension of the therapist. Another possible pathological reason for encouraging the patient would be that the therapist might be defending against his or her own envy and so need to present the self as loving and supportive, the grand person bestowing approval on the lesser being. Behaviorally, this would eventually manifest itself in a spiraling pattern of competition, one-upsmanship. Lots of wallpaper and paste! If the therapist's envy were not disguised, obviously the case would be clearer, the therapist either openly or "clinically intentioned" discouraging, disparaging, or confronting about their obvious differences in status and station.

Normal envy, we have observed, may also manifest itself through a transitional object. A transitional object (Winnicott, 1951/1975), it will be recalled, is that inanimate object that stands for the relationship between the self and the mothering one. It provides comfort when the relationship is not available to the child and before the mothering-one and the relationship are fully internalized. But residuals of it last beyond the "blankie" stage for most of us, with our favorite inanimate objects we use to comfort ourselves.

Often the therapist's house (if the office is in the house) or office is seen that way, one patient saying, for instance, "I was thinking of your house all week." And another, who was in her late 60s, on first seeing the house but having been in treatment for many years, said nostalgically, "This is the kind of house I had always wanted." When she left that particular session, the therapist felt uncomfortable, thinking perhaps that she had "showed off." But when the patient came for her next session, she said she had been telling everybody about it. She felt about the house just as she felt about her grandson whom she adored. In effect, the house, as a transitional object standing for the relationship, was a concrete representation of a good, significant relationship that had become part of her identity. And envy was definitely involved. But there was a normative, healthy display of envy.

Furthermore, as observed in 2- to 3-year-olds (Frankel & Sherick, 1977), differentiation between the self and other is enhanced by envy. It is inevitable that the child begin to see similarities and differences between others and between the self and other. Although earlier the objective may have been to "get" the possession without regard for the possessor, a sense of entitlement with no room for delay, later envy is characterized not by wanting to deprive the other but to have an equivalent thing and does require some ability to delay gratification. The focus of what is envied is still on the possession, activity, or recognition rather than on the holder of the attribute or object (Frankel & Sherick, 1977). After age 3, however, there is a shift in the envy field from home to peers where the characteristic need is to gain admiration and possess what will encourage it. "The aim is . . . to feel more competent . . . to make oneself worthy of admiration" (Frankel & Sherick, 1977).

As the child gets older, there develops a wider range of possibilities for dealing with envy, envy that now includes envy of adult prerogatives and capabilities. Frankel and Sherick (1977) have observed ways of dealing with envy: First, the child attempts to gain recognition by pleading, emulating, or compromising; then, the child attempts to gain recognition by being bossy and demanding, anticipating a lack of recognition or deprivation and, in defense, taking an active and controlling stance.

As children get older still, 4 or 5, the peer group becomes a second major arena for envy and concern, especially regarding the issue of social exclusion. It also becomes the milieu in which family issues are relived and mastered (Frankel & Sherick, 1977) at the same time that family issues are being worked out with the family. And fantasy is used now to repair injury and to help tolerate discomfort. Let us consider the situation of the little boy whose mother would not let him play with trucks in the house because it would be messed up and other children might even join him in that endeavor and did not let him play with trucks outside because it was dirty out there and the trucks were too good to mess up and be played with by other dirty children. This little boy envied other boys whose mothers had regard for their needs. Surely he envied the power of that kind of reasoning and the power of that mother to control his play and his pleasure. His fantasy was to have a big house someday, away from other houses looking in on him, and, incidentally, one where he could put anything he wanted and with a big yard where he could play with trucks and friends. That fantasy kept him company, gave him pleasure, and at least partially repaired the injury to his self-regard.

This is also the time when what is envied are parental prerogatives and capabilities, especially those of the same-sex parent and when children take on admired, envied characteristics of the parent and others and start excluding others, thereby reenacting parental exclusion.

Normal envy, then, serves as an impetus to action, to attainment and repair of deficits or injury to self-esteem. It becomes a motive for emulation, a means for seeing similarities and differences, an incentive for comparisons (Jacobson, 1964), a way to start to come to grips with realistic differences between the self and others (Jacobson, 1964; Neubauer, 1982). Fantasy of a desired end state that is based on envy not only requires the ability to tolerate discomfort (Frankel & Sherick, 1977), it helps the child begin to live with the disequilibrium of anxiety. Some authors (Smith & Whitfield, 1983) even think that, when it is impossible to possess the envied attribute, the person can use the feeling as a rational explanation that the world needs both the haves and the have-nots (of the attribute) and that's life. An interesting idea proposed by Smith and Whitfield (1983) is that the envy potential in others can be used for the promotion of closeness, a "display" to make friends. But one might also choose friends to share in attributes to experience them vicariously or for a balance.

Furthermore, aggression concerning envy can certainly be used for development of the self, that is, to differentiate or distinguish attributes of the self from others' and to individuate, to develop a self to call one's own, to learn that there are loving and hostile components of the self and in others (Jacobson, 1964). An interesting point in thinking about envy is that actually there is a bit of health "potential" in envy because through admiration of the other, there is a hopefulness. As Meissner (1978) points out, the person does not simply accept or become resigned to the felt deprivation. The coveting and desire for what is not possessed drives one to close the discrepancy between how one is and how one wants to be or thinks one should be, to use one's aggression to do the job.

AGGRESSION IN ENVY

Speaking of aggression leads to the next portion of the discussion of envy, that is, the place of aggression in envy. Most theorists who have talked about envy have talked about aggression that occurs as an outcome of it. For example, Abraham (1920/1927) writes of aggression against the envied person and the desire to deprive that person of what is envied. He writes of the envious person having spiteful impulses against the so-called privileged proprietor (Abraham, 1921/1927, p. 382). Klein (1957/1975) writes of anger, with the impulse to take away or destroy what the other possesses and enjoys, to scoop out the breast that has and enjoys all the supplies. And intense aggression is consistently seen alongside envy in borderline and narcissistic patients (Kernberg, 1975) and in paranoid patients (Meissner, 1978).

Although Sullivan (1953b, 1956) does not actually say that the envious person has a problem with aggression in general (aggression is not in his vocabulary) and anger in particular, it is certainly a natural conclusion to the events he describes. If there is a deficiency in the self-system, surely the person is made uncomfortable by realizing that another has more prestige or ability. Now if one has been appraised as unsatisfactory and inadequate to the task of being satisfactory, one cannot use aggression for further development or to get someplace. Instead, one uses it to feel pretty angry at the appraiser. If the appraiser sets excessively high goals that the person could never attain, healthy aggression would be for naught and turn instead to anger at the appraiser. Or, as Joffee (1969) points out, early disturbances in the regulation of one's well-being may promote the turning of aggression against the self.

But what does aggression mean? Previously, (Rouslin, 1975b, p. 171) one of us (S.R.W.) summarized,

> Aggression can be viewed as a useful, productive activity, having its roots in primitive-life feeling states. Aggression is necessary for the child to separate from his parents and to achieve independence. However, if aggression leading to individuation is obstructed in its development, anger, rage, hostility, and hate become intricately

bound up with it, leading to distortion. When this occurs, aggression goes beyond self-preservation and mastery and often becomes
self-destructive.

Healthy developmental aggression is destructive only in the
sense that it is the primary force in the gradual dissolution of
parent–child fusion and the symbiotic bond. Aggression progres-
sively becomes a vehicle for development and preservation of the
self.

[On the other hand] defensive aggression is actually a drive
toward maintaining a level of fusion or early symbiotic bond and is
not the independence it would appear to be. Though defensive
aggression can take many forms, it is always unconsciously designed
as a disguise against the desire to remain attached to the parent [or
parent representative in later life].

All of this becomes uncommonly clear when we deal with envious
people. The aggression that would otherwise be used to aid separation
and individuation is inverted instead. That is, it is used as a vehicle to
maintain the symbiotic bond rather than advance from it.

If one looks at the pathological envy relationship, one sees aggression on the face of it, but aggression associated with anger, rage, hostility,
and hate. The envious person is angry at not having what the other has,
maybe even wants to destroy the other or at least take away the valued
attribute if it cannot be acquired. But in any event, through the desired
attribute and the anger, rage, hostility, and hate, the person remains
attached to the other. In pathological envy this defensive aggression
unwittingly binds the person to the envied other, so the person is not free
to acquire the attribute or envied possession or live with the reality of the
unfavorable comparison. Indeed, we cannot understand envy unless we
look at the envious person's relationship to the other by way of defensive
aggression, that is, the aggression that is used to maintain the symbiotic
bond rather than break away from it. Developmentally, this means that
trouble seems to come in the later phases of separation, which requires
the use of aggression for going out into the world.

Exploring the meaning of the film *Amadeus* (Shaffer, 1984) is
educational regarding the place of aggression in chronic pathological
envy. To summarize the essence of the film: The story is about Mozart,
whose middle name was Amadeus, and a self-appointed musician rival,
Salieri. Salieri spends his life in awe and admiration of Mozart's genius,
which repeatedly fuels his envy by pointing up the differences between
the two musicians, with Salieri always coming out on the losing end.
There is an inherent discrepancy between the way Salieri is (the self-
representation) and the way he needs desperately to be (the ideal self-
representation). Such a discrepancy (Meissner, 1978) is the material

envy is built on. Salieri devotes his energy to being better than Mozart, but he simply is no genius. Because he cannot emulate or compete with Mozart and cannot live with Mozart's genius, he becomes obsessed with rage, hatred, and spite (while mixed with awe), aggression that eventually is used to destroy Mozart.

The fascinating part of the story is how Salieri's aggression is not healthy aggression leading him to develop his own way, his own route, coming to grips with his own capabilities and limitations. Defensive aggression is Salieri's driving force, which, if it is recalled, helps reinforce a parental bond rather than facilitate separation and individuation. His aggression actually has very little to do with Mozart directly. Mozart is simply an instrument used in the service of the parent–child symbiotic problem. There is much evidence in the story of that parental bond. Early on, it is obvious that Salieri wants his uninterested father to be as helpful to him musically as Mozart's father was to his son. When his father was unresponsive and actually died, Salieri thought God had arranged it because he had already turned to Him in his quest to be made famous and immortal by this external, all-powerful force.

Everything goes well for a while, but, again, enter Mozart. To quote Salieri, "Everybody liked me; [as court music master] I liked myself—until he came." Now he is angry, not simply at Mozart, but at the new authority figure, God, and once again is filled with longing and rage at what he considers to be God's choice to be His instrument. He actively competes with Mozart—to best him—not for his own self-development, but to prove that God had chosen him, not Mozart. This is jealousy that is used to obscure and defend against envy, to explain his sense of inferiority, his lack. The issue is that the parent, the authority, did not give him what he greatly needed. Such a deficiency promotes envy, which in turn promotes jealousy of those who have the attribute.

When Salieri does well he thanks God; when he does poorly or Mozart does well, he asks why God implanted the desire in him yet denies him the talent. He can only wonder what the authority was up to. In admiration and reverence he sees in Mozart "the very voice of God," with himself "staring through the cage . . . at absolute beauty." Finally, because God gave him only the ability to recognize, he declares God his enemy and vows to "hinder and ruin" His incarnation, Mozart. And after he does that (interestingly through driving Mozart mad by becoming the ghost of Mozart's own demanding father), in his own demented state all is not over. It is not Mozart he hears laughing at him, but God. This untenable yet tenacious bond with the authority figure remains.

In thinking carefully about this example, Salieri starts off feeling that he does not rate or that he is second rate, that he desperately wants that attribute possessed by Mozart. So the basis of the problem is envy.

He admires Mozart to the point of destruction because the better Mozart is, the worse he is by comparison. His aggression is used against Mozart, of course, but in the process his aggression is used to continue the bond with Mozart, who stands for his idealized self and the authority figure, God, whom he sees as withholding an attribute he desparately needs. Moreover, jealously now starts to be noticeable.

THE RELATIONSHIP BETWEEN CHRONIC PATHOLOGICAL ENVY AND JEALOUSY

Although envy and jealousy are distinct phenomena, envy is a precursor of jealousy, and jealousy can be used as a defense against envy, we have observed and concluded that, clinically, jealousy is always a part of chronic pathological envy. The reason is not as obscure as it may appear, for there is always an authority figure lurking unconsciously, so the third party is always present in an internalized sense. When the envious person is threatened by someone holding superior cherished attributes, not only is this admired/envied person seen as an idealized self in contrast to the self, and perhaps as the superior parent, but on another level, in one's mind there is competition between this person and the self for the approval of the parent. This person who is better than the self will get the approval and regard, the goodies, from the parent. We need only look at Salieri and his struggle to be pleasing, more pleasing than Mozart, to the illusory authority figure. In the earlier example of the older sister when envy was definitely a terrible problem, so too was jealousy. Her every act in life was to show the best people in the world, obviously representing the parents, that she was good and better than her sister.

So long as pathological envy originates in the context of parental appraisal, that parent will hang around, hovering in the unconscious to be summoned up with every threat to one's sense of self-view and regard. So, although jealousy is not a necessary ingredient in the original formation of pathological envy, jealousy is present as a motivating force in envy ever after. Furthermore, there is virtually no healthy aggression turned on to work out the current relationship, the one out in the world. Instead, the aggression is automatically directed backward, trying to impress the hovering parent while preventing the interloper from doing so. The pathologically envious person, in interactions with the admired envied one, is forever trying to acquire an attribute through that person or in competition with the person for the approval of the internalized significant other. Thus, there is the constant presence of the other. Aggression used is always in relation to this other, never simply to help one "freely" develop in this or that direction.

The aggression, then, consistently helps maintain a symbiotic union reflective of the original parent–child relationship where not only was there enormous frustration of needs but, as a consequence, frustration of the healthy ability to separate. The aggression ties one to the object instead of releasing one from it to get what one needs in the world. The child, now an envious adult, relives the original relationship, always trying to get the goodies, the supplies, from or through another and for the love from another. But the very getting fed, so to speak, by the other points up that (1) one needed it, so there is a lack, (2) the other then would be seen to hold the goods, therefore to be admired and envied, and (3) the original parent–child relationship would move into awareness or at least be touched off unconsciously, thereby inciting resentment and rage. So, in order to not feel the rage and not feel envy, such people devalue whatever they receive. Actually, they need and want an inordinate amount from others, but by not acknowledging the so-called gift, "they always wind up empty" (Kernberg, 1975, p. 237) and often, depressed.

This is illustrated by the case of a depressively inclined patient who always talks about how much his friends give to him, emotionally, that is. They sound like the best people in the whole world, almost too good to be true, "idealized" the envy literature would say (Kernberg, 1975; Klein, 1957/1975). This is in sharp contrast to his former wife who had given him nothing, literally and figuratively, and a totally narcissistic mother who gave only to herself. For years, this patient had secretly depreciated and treated with contempt those from whom he supposedly expected nothing (Kernberg, 1975). Underneath a charming, engaging manner lay a cold and ruthless attitude, as Kernberg (1975) would say of the narcissistic personality, and intense envy. And for good reason, life had been emotionally bleak.

For many years this patient used his aggression to try to get blood from a stone, a detached, empty, schizoid wife, by sealing off his envy of the world around him. The wife looked different from his mother; she was a calm, nice person, whereas the mother was rather nasty and explosive, but the incredible self-absorption was the same. The patient had chosen carefully, according to his original concept of significant other. Once he was ready for some really giving people, he actually started to choose some but got depressed. Dynamically, what happened was that as soon as he got something from somebody, it touched off the memory of having received so little from his mother. It was a reminder of deficiencies in a crucial relationship and resultant deficiencies, emptiness, and hunger in the self, which filled him with rage and envy, whereupon he would become depressed. He would find himself wanting more and more, to deplete the breast, as Klein (1957/1975) would say. Indeed, it was never enough, but not for the present; the present was simply a reminder of what he did not have in the past.

The implication here is that the patient's aggression could not be used to successfully, at least completely, go after and appreciate what he wanted, needed, and got. The aggression (in this case seen as depression) was defensive in that it bound him to the mother who could not give what was needed. He said in effect, "Okay, I get something now, but where were the goods when I needed them?" Subsequently, when his aggression was freed up, not only did the patient become ruthless, that is, showed a lack of consideration of the other, a healthy characteristic of children during early phases of separation by the way (Winnicott, 1975), but slowly he showed considerable envy.

FINAL NOTES

Many questions remain, awaiting further qualitative data. For instance, who is a pathologically envious person? That is, who is at risk for chronic, pathological envy; is there a single profile, or are there many? Is there a pattern of early, significant relationships promoting envy? And what happens to envy in the therapist–patient relationship? Although we have begun to answer some of these questions, psychological envy literature *per se* falls down in these areas. However, if one thinks carefully about characteristics of paranoid persons, borderline personalities, and narcissistic personalities, one can get an idea of who the pathologically envious are. All this pathology is rooted in the latter part of the separation–individuation phase of development where what happens with aggression is of paramount importance in determining in which direction the person will head: to or from the mothering-one. Envy is, of course, noticeable first in this phase (Spielman, 1971) because it is then that cognitive ability to discriminate self from other takes a leap in development. Further, some theorists suggest that extreme frustration and spiteful aggression from a callous, indifferent mothering-one causes dependency to become equivalent to hate, mistreatment, frustration, or exploitation (Kernberg, 1975). Envy in such a situation would be of so powerful a mother and other "regular" people and might, in addition, be from identification with a mother who herself was pathologically envious.

Therefore, in treatment, envy of the therapist becomes of paramount importance, as does dependency. Because dependency is equivalent to all that spells envy and frustration, such patients want terribly to avoid it even though it looks as though they are dependent (Kernberg,

1975). Actually, the admired therapist is not depended on; he or she is merely seen as an extension of an idealized self that underneath knows the discrepancy between that and the realistic appraisal. As a consequence, envy might erupt at any time. The therapist is idealized (Kernberg, 1975; Klein, 1957/1975) as a defense against the destructive impulses of envy, but interestingly, such an idealization does imply (Klein, 1957/1975) that good exists somewhere and leads to a longing for the good object and the capacity to love it.

If this admired therapist is dethroned (Kernberg, 1975), how little real involvement there is will soon be evident. There is no real closeness in the sense of a separate person relying on and using the knowledge and emotional resources of the other. The tendency is to drop the relationship at the slightest provocation or offense (Kernberg, 1975) and to devalue whatever is received at the first sign of closeness (Abraham, 1919/1927; Klein, 1957/1975), closeness even meaning a meeting of the minds, as in realizing the significance of an interpretation or comment that really rings a bell. The patient almost immediately must devalue what the therapist has said to indicate that there has been no impact, for it will be unconsciously recalled that, cognitively and affectively, closeness is equated with badness in the parent–child relationship. Also, in the patient's scheme of haves and have-nots, if the therapist is smart, the patient must be dumb.

As a result, several implications for the therapist are as follows:

1. Do not be flattered by the idealization, and do not encourage it by doing nice things, saying nice things, or avoiding making uncomfortable comments or interpretations or raising crucial questions in the hope the patient will think you are a good person. The patient will devalue you eventually and will ultimately feel controlled by you.

2. Realize you will be devalued, say what you have to say, and do not be distressed when the patient becomes grandiose, saying he or she said it, unable to attribute the gem to you lest envy show itself. This quasi-independence on the patient's part is a defense against internal dependence on the object (Klein, 1957/1975), now the therapist.

3. In turn, recognize that when the patient devalues the self he or she denies envy while unconsciously punishing the self for it (Klein, 1957/1975). Therefore, it is not helpful to encourage devaluation by showing off with fancy clothes or fancy interpretations or simply to make a fetish of "valuing" this devalued patient. First, that does not work because it does not fit with the way the person sees the self or the self in relation to others. Second, it is obviously a ploy, unconscious or otherwise, to avoid dealing with the patient's rage and envy, which will inevitably come your way.

4. Keep in mind that defenses against envy interfere with the patient's capacity to take what the therapist has to offer (Klein, 1957/1975) and that the defenses represent defensive aggression, that aggression fostering symbiosis rather than separation–individuation. Defensive aggression will occur in the therapist–patient relationship as in all others. Expect it, live with it, analyze it, and let it go, in that order.

5. Expect that envy of you, realistic and distorted, will be part of every patient's therapy. Therapists are obliged to become aware of the envious dimensions of themselves and certainly to become knowledgeable about the phenomenon. One way to do this is to become familiar with the literature, difficult and dense as it might be.

The substance of what the early writers had to say is theoretically illuminating and clinically helpful, especially those rare formulations not encumbered by obsessionally thick concrete language. For example, when Klein (1957/1975) talks about breast envy, the important thing to pay attention to is what the giving or withholding breast represents so far as the relationship is concerned. Klein does talk most cogently about that, even if she does not say in her theory description itself that to the child the breast is important because it represents the mother, the mother's emotional nourishment, and the mother's power. With Freud (1908/1959, 1923/1961, 1925/1961) it is important to pay attention to what the penis represents in nongenital terms, although it is not conceptualized in that way in either the theory presentation or subsequent discussion. Perhaps it represents a curiosity (Moulton, 1970) that the little girl wants and can never get, the beginnings of living with injustice. Maybe it is early a toy to play with and later, perhaps, a source of power.

The important task is to decode the symbols breast, penis, and womb by realizing that, although one might think the theorist starts off with a misguided premise in what is identified as the motivating force in envy, the symbol is a concrete representation of an abstraction occurring in an interpersonal context. Interpersonal relationships are, after all, the arena for the development and manifestation of envy, and, additionally, in the therapist–patient relationship, an opportunity for a corrective interpersonal experience.

13

Passive Aggressiveness

Everybody knows such a person, *only* one if lucky. If not lucky, it is one's partner or best friend or child or patient. The passive–aggressive phenomenon is perhaps the most enraging characteristic in a relationship at the same time that it is perhaps the least studied interpersonal and intrapersonal phenomenon. Although the literature contains articles on test results identifying the passive–aggressive characteristic in personality (Small, Small, Alig, & Moore, 1970; Whitman, Trosman, & Koenig, 1954), it includes few works describing the phenomenon and even fewer exploring its dynamics. It would appear that no major theorist (or even minor one for that matter) has studied passive aggressiveness as an independent phenomenon (Stricker, 1983).

Passive aggressiveness is probably a misnomer. Anyone who has been involved with a passive–aggressive person knows that nothing passive has gone on. Passive aggressiveness may be a trait, or it may be a state, or a clinical entity. It is the more or less passive or covert expression of aggression. Therefore, there is no conscious awareness of the aggression on the part of the passive–aggressive person. Passive aggressiveness refers to ways of being, behaving, and experiencing (Mahrer, 1983). According to the existential, experiential view, the person behaves in ways that are helpless and needy, from passively infuriating others with thinly disguised anger to "apparently helpful cooperativeness" (p. 100) and aggression clothed in innocence. The person may be negativistic, obstructionist, uncooperative, and stubborn; yet he or she manifests these traits all indirectly, by dawdling, inefficiency, and procrastination. "The person behaves in ways which are superficially compliant and acquiescent, with undertones of whining, complaining and grumbling"

This chapter was originally presented as a lecture by Sheila Rouslin Welt at the Medical College of Pennsylvania, Psychiatric Nursing Update, April 1988. It was revised for publication in this book.

(p. 100), heard or recognized only perhaps by the person who knows him or her well, or one who has a similar parent. How many times has the partner of the passive–aggressive person said, "everybody thinks he's great. He is until you get really close to him and then need something from him. You only hate him once you get to know him."

Passive–aggressive behavior is controlling and provocative, although the perpetrator genuinely feels like an innocent victim, a benign alleged perpetrator, falsely accused of having hostile intent. Being passive–aggressive is risky business. Life, as one patient put it, is "lived on the edge." A frustrated partner said this about her passive–aggressive lover:

> It's always having something on the back burner to screw up his life. For example, his son runs around the restaurant, he doesn't stop him and then complains how terrible the kid is and what an embarrassment he is to him. But he asks for it by sitting still!

The passive–aggressive person often lives on the brink of disaster, not paying taxes, not noticing that his lover is angry at him until, in shock and consternation, he finds she has moved out with all of her belongings and only an angry note remains.

Passive aggressiveness may be a diagnostic category in itself (part of personality disorders) or a pattern of behavior seen within other diagnostic categories. In this chapter, passive–aggressive behavior is explored as an enduring characteristic independent of broader diagnosis, for the operations are the same whether or not it is seen as a distinct category. Although anyone is capable of a passive–aggressive act, the dynamics presented in this chapter refer to those persons whose lives reek of the behavior, those whose interactions are often characterized by it. As Stricker (1983) suggests, since motivation is inferred from the interpersonal impact of the behavior, the task of clarifying the concept is difficult. Empirical literature is sparse, and diagnostic reliability a problem. Psychodynamic formulation is either so sophomoric or simplistic that data are difficult to apply, or formulation is so murky that clinical data cannot be ordered or categorized except to say that yes, indeed, passive aggressiveness is an unconscious process expressing hostility indirectly.

But why the anger, and why the indirectness? The explanations to date seem facile and certainly incomplete, which accounts for our interest in clarifying the phenomenon. According to Stricker (1983), anger results from failure to have early dependency needs met. In this formulation, the child does not dare express the angry feelings directly, because to do so would risk further frustration and consequences from restrictive, demanding parents. Initially, bedwetting, bowel retention, stuttering, or eating poorly elicit parental suffering but do exact a toll on the child's sense of competence, success, and self-esteem. As adults, their passive–aggressive behaviors become more sophisticated, more complex, and disguised. When they are adults, anxiety and then depression (Whitman et al., 1954) bring these people into treatment, although in the course of treatment for other more general interpersonal problems, the pattern often emerges.

PSYCHODYNAMIC PATHWAYS

The psychodynamics of passive–aggressive behavior are best understood by examining the way the self-system (Sullivan, 1953a) is laid down, for the sequence of operations in passive–aggressive behavior follows the same route, and then some. The self-system develops by way of reflected appraisals (Sullivan, 1953a). The child behaves in a certain way, parental approval or disapproval (the appraisal) is given, and the child observes the appraisal, later to internalize the whole experience, namely, the act, the response, and all accompanying thoughts and feelings. Thereafter, the child lives out the original appraisal. Obviously then, the route to passive–aggressive behavior starts as soon as there is some discrimination between the self and other.

Psychodynamically, the passive–aggressive phenomenon can take two pathways. The expert uses both. In one, the person indeed lives out the appraisal but exaggerates it in such a way as to make the parent look absurd. Since this lived-out appraisal is a reflection of the original, the parent is enraged to see now what is a caricature of the original appraisal. So, in living out the appraisal, the person bests the parent with his or her own medicine. The person does this quite automatically and quite unconsciously, which is why it works so well to infuriate the parent. Although the passive–aggressive person is surely conscious of the other's anger, neither the process nor his or her contribution to it is in awareness, although it may be close by.

Recently, a patient who had a psychotic episode was thrown back into the arms of her waiting parents. The parents alternately held her, held her down, kept her locked in their house, bathed her, slept with her, read her nursery rhymes. Later, when she was no longer psychotic and was standing up for herself, they said that, unlike the present when the patient returned to her willful self, the past episode had been the best time they had ever had with her in all her 29 years.

While the patient was still psychotic she did various passive–aggressive things, which ultimately rankled the parents but which at first they did not notice. Conscious awareness of the process, however, is unnecessary for neurotic pleasure. The person on the receiving end does not have to notice, testifying to how narcissistic an experience this whole operation is. As some enlightened patients have said, "it is as if unconsciously I know, and God knows, so the whole world knows how foolish and foul they are." What matters is that although the parents may not know what the child is doing, they react anyhow. Furthermore, although the child may not consciously instigate the process, the results are carefully heeded.

In the above case, when lunchtime arrived, suddenly baby-voiced, the daughter would say to her mother, "Should I eat? Am I hungry? Is it okay to eat now? Should I have a sandwich?" To the observer, the daughter was making a mockery of the mother's need to infantilize her. In the high-pitched voice of a reassuring nursery school teacher, the mother would say, "You're a big girl, you can decide." On other occasions, the patient did such things as run for the door when it was momentarily unlocked, thereby living out and reinforcing the original appraisal that she was willful yet incompetent and lacking in judgment, while at the same time showing her parents to be jailers. Thus, the patient took the original appraisal that she was a good girl if she did what her parents said, showing no autonomy, and carried it to such an extreme that her parents looked ridiculous. In a single operation she accomplished two tasks: She complied with the appraisal and retaliated against her parents, the appraisers. On the occasions when she tried to "escape," she lived out the original appraisals that she was willful and not ready to be independent. At the same time she made the parents pay for their control, reinforcing to herself the notion that they were jailers and making them look like jailers to the neighbors, a sorry, shameful fate to these secretive, socially self-conscious parents.

Sometimes, passive–aggressive behavior is experienced by those on the receiving end as a hostile set-up, because it is, albeit an unconscious one. A young girl of 11 had a mother who herself had had a thoroughly malevolent mother. The child's mother had spent a good part of her life trying to please and appease her own mother, of course to no avail. So, one facet of her self-concept was that if she did something for someone, she would get kicked in the face, as she did by her mother, who turned all tender advances into malevolent experiences.

Through genetics and interpersonal response, this 11-year-old was turning into her malevolent grandmother. The genetics are a given, but the interpersonal development we can try to decipher. The child was definitely hostile and, approaching puberty, was in a state of hormonal turmoil. She liked to use her mother's hair dryer but never returned it, leaving it anywhere she wandered. When the mother wanted it for herself, of course, it was nowhere to be found. Sometimes, when she did find it, it was broken. The question is, why did she never learn from her experience and refuse to lend her daughter the dryer? Well, if you are living out an appraisal that you are good if you try to do something for somebody regardless of how badly your good intentions are received, or more to the point, you are good if you do something for somebody who responds to the tender gesture with hostility, thereby creating the opportunity for a hostile exchange where you can feel superior to an ungrateful, nasty child, you keep trying. That is exactly what happened with this mother.

Unconsciously knowing that this daughter could not be nice to her or considerate of her, she tried on a conscious level to appease her. Unsolicited, she asked the daughter in fact, if she wanted to use the dryer. When the daughter did refuse, at such times trying to control her hostile behavior and avoid wrenching scenes, the mother insisted, or left it handy for the daughter, impossible to resist. On one level, the mother was consciously enraged at her daughter's disrespect. Nevertheless, the mother created and chose as unlikely a character as her own mother to be the recipient of a tender gesture, thereby living out and reinforcing the original appraisal and relationship. Now, the gesture was ostensibly tender, a hostile daughter could not respond favorably, and unconsciously the mother knew how predictable the reaction was. The mother's act of kindness was hostile; she was so good as to offer herself for martyrdom, and the daughter helped her. The daughter unconsciously knew it was a hostile gesture and, when she could not escape the field, was enraged at being set up to show her colors. The mother of course was actually making a fool of her own mother through the transference with the daughter. But she certainly paid a big price for it emotionally and interpersonally.

Earlier it was mentioned that the passive–aggressive phenomenon can take two pathways. The following is an example of the second. In this pathway, the person uses two sets of appraisals simultaneously; one set justifies or rationalizes the use of the other. For example, recently, a patient was going to Virginia during his vacation. Having gone many times, he collected much information from his trips and generously offered the material to a colleague who was considering travel to the area. He told his wife, who always liked to have all her data at hand even if she did not need it. Although she said nothing in response, during a fight about a particular injustice while on the trip, the wife yelled at her husband for always considering others before he did her, which indeed was the case. The patient had no idea what his wife was talking about. She had all but accused him of being passive–aggressive toward her, and he truly felt maligned. (Incidentally, not catching on is often a passive–aggressive maneuver.) He had no idea he had been passive–aggressive by giving the materials to his colleague because he knew that he and his wife did not need the maps or materials. The hitch was, he knew his wife, and he knew how they usually traveled, loaded with boxes of materials, for security lest they need something, and for easy access should they add new materials.

Dynamically, this is what happened. One set of appraisals involved being rewarded for generosity. On one level, the patient thought he had done a great thing; someone had a need, to which this priest turned social worker responded, and he felt he had performed an act of charity. He used this act and this appraisal to rationalize another set of appraisals, namely, that he was a bad boy if he did anything he really wanted to do. As a child his mother or her agents (his four sisters) had controlled his every move. He got away, though, once in a while to do some grocery shopping for his mother, after which he would get distracted on the way home so that he was always late, holding up supper for everyone. Under such circumstances he would explain that there had been a sick dog he had to tend to or saw some guys playing ball. Since he knew he was supposed to be kind to animals and also that his mother had a fetish about wanting her scrawny son to learn to play baseball, unconsciously he had reasoned that surely it would be all right to do such things even if it meant he were late. Unconsciously, he also knew that such reasoning, pitting one appraisal against the other, would drive the mother crazy, which of course it did. In the current situation, the patient really did not feel like carting around all the materials, but he feared taking on his wife. If, in an act of generosity, he gave them away, how could this former nun, selfless teacher, deny him this act of charity? Well, it did not work.

Although it seemed inconceivable that the passive–aggressive act was an unconscious operation, in fact it was, as it always is, or it could not work so smoothly. When the patient related what happened on the trip, he had no awareness he had been passive–aggressive. However, when his masterful operation was pointed out, he finally said, "Maybe it's like seeing what I can get away with. I think I always had in mind as a kid how I could squeak by." Maybe he would not get caught, and maybe he could drive his mother crazy with the ambiguity and complexity of his behavior.

MANIFESTATIONS

Examples of passive–aggressive behavior come up all the time, most often reflecting attitudes held toward the original parent–child relationships and attributing the same characteristics to the current person and relationship. That the attributes fit is fortuitous, making it all the more difficult for the passive–aggressive person consciously to recognize the process. A nurse, who in her tasks as a quality assurance reviewer, had to question physicians about their treatment plans and procedures provides a good example. In the interaction with one physician, it became clear that her *magical use of words* was her way of being passive–aggressive.

It so happened that this particular doctor was quite indignant about what appeared to be and was valid criticism regarding his treatment of a certain patient. He said, in his superior way, "I don't want you people questioning my authority; you're trying to practice medicine." The reviewer, in a most condescending way, said, "Of course not, doctor, we're all concerned for the welfare of the patient. I'm not practicing medicine, or questioning your obvious knowledge or skill or your position with the patient. We just need to know why the drug that is standard in treating such a patient wasn't ordered." This physician may have been wrong about a lot of things, but he was correct in assessing that he had just received a mixed message. He exploded from the assault of passive–aggressive behavior. The reviewer thought she had done a masterful job, but her boss did not, saying, "Just ask him why the drug wasn't ordered. Don't say all the other stuff." The reviewer had made the doctor look ridiculous by painting for him the caricature of the authoritarian person he was and by competing with him by her attitude and apparent knowledge. Besides, she had muzzled him with her "niceness."

Dynamically, this trait had developed in childhood. If the right words, soothing, placating words, were used, the reviewer could undermine the authority of her pompous mother, meanwhile calming her down and obscuring the tactic with flattery. She would be appraised as a good girl for appealing to her mother's narcissism, meanwhile gathering data on the mother's sick self-centeredness and need for flattery. Unconsciously, she and God knew that she had shown her mother up for what she was. The words were right, so the narcissistic mother did not notice until later. This physician, however, noticed quickly, for his need for power went beyond even her mother's. This passive–aggressive manipulation was of such second nature to the patient that she had no idea what had gone wrong. She knew she could not stand this guy, but she was truly perplexed as to why he was so angry, since ostensibly she had been so "polite" in her words. In this case, there was an insufficient match or fit with the original situation, so she could not have the quasisatisfaction she had had in the past of quietly seducing the mother with words and making her look like a fool. Consequently, the patient was anxious and perplexed, wanting to know what she should have said instead.

A non-passive–aggressive mother recently became aware of how frequently she was perplexed about the behavior of her daughter. It seems the daughter figured out how to control this very controlling mother in an expertly passive–aggressive way. She simply told the mother just what she knew the mother wanted to hear. She had tuned into what the mother wanted—the image of a happy family and a prom-going,

college-bound daughter. With the magic of words she repeatedly prom-
ised to deliver and then retracted, always to the amazement of a highly
responsible mother who was shocked at her daughter's total irresponsibility. The words of promise were magic also to the mother, consciously
convinced that the daughter would deliver and on another level, unconsciously and pathologically hopeful that her own parents would "come
through," even though neither daughter nor parents ever had.

Although generally loathe to admit error, the passive–aggressive
person eventually learns that maybe life would be better by apologizing
for deeds done or undone. Thus, "I'm sorry" often becomes the magical
phrase that is supposed to fix all offenses. The problem is that the person
on the other end becomes enraged, retorting that just saying the words
can not possibly compensate for obnoxious or otherwise passive–aggressive behavior, at which point the offender feels maligned and angry that
the sentiment is not taken seriously and that the magical words cannot
create inattention and harmony. Although it is hard to believe, the
passive–aggressive person honestly thinks the words will work to right
the situation; and on one level, he or she believes it to be a sincere
sentiment.

Honesty, or so-called honesty, accounts for a good bit of the rage
response we see in passive–aggressive situations. A psychology student
was having a most difficult time in therapy work during her internship.
Her supervisor, whom she thought she admired and respected, touted
being entirely open and honest in supervision about one's reactions
during the course of therapeutic work and supervision. So, after testing
the water and finding it receptive, the intern was indeed honest about
acknowledging that she was repelled by her patient, and explained why
that was. Moreover, she admitted that she had been agitated and depressed lately and terribly anxious about graduation also. Feeling inflated
by the shared confidence, the supervisor went on to read wildly into the
data, making obscure and incorrect connections, going not only beyond
the bounds of good supervision, but of good therapy, which she should
not have been practicing anyhow. The intern, quite upset at the interpretations she heard, now worried that she might lose the internship and that
she had misjudged the receptivity of the supervisor.

In fact, however, in her own therapy, while she was talking about
the situation, the intern looked like the cat who swallowed the canary,
although she was certainly distressed. She had gathered incredible data,
perhaps at her own expense, on what an incompetent the supervisor was.
The intern's honesty was not at all honest but a vehicle to prove the
authority wanting and inferior, not unlike her own pompous father who
was himself wanting, a man who was one of those liberals collecting data
to make the establishment look like fools. The passive–aggressive behav-

ior had surged forward at the prelude to emotional separation from her father, just as she was moving into her career. Little wonder she had been anxious about graduation and not surprising that she scurried back to the authority for both security and retribution.

Provocativeness is a familiar manifestation of passive aggressiveness. A patient described how as a child she had goaded her mother into responding like a lunatic by being headstrong, stubborn, and wearing about what she wanted as opposed to what the mother had wanted. At the time, to her mind, she was just asserting her rights. In retrospect, she now thought that she learned how to be provocative by way of unplanned automatic, provocative attributes that first threatened, then enraged her mother. These "provocations" were simply part of her, such as being bright, attractive, and successful in school. However, they filled her mother with envy and rage. The patient then unconsciously learned that if she wanted to drive her mother wild, she could find other things to threaten her, thereby getting back at the mother for punishing her for inherently admirable but envy-evoking qualities.

Sometimes provocativeness is disguised as a well-meaning gesture. Such was the case with the new father whose mother had been restrictive, controlling, intrusive, and possessive, and whose father had been rarely allowed entry to child care. When he was, he had acted harshly and critically. Presently, when the new father was at home but his wife was caring for the baby, he seemed almost to welcome the cries of the baby. He would dash downstairs, quickly admonishing her for not tending to the baby properly. He did this at precisely those times when the wife probably had been a bit lax in responding to the baby, so his concern had a ring of legitimacy to it. In actuality, it would appear that this man was collecting data on his wife's lapses of judgment, ammunition to prove she was not such a good mother after all, that she did not have such great rapport with the baby, obviously acting out the concerns of his father as well as his gripes with his mother, not to mention ventilating his envy of expertise for which he had had no role model and jealously about this interloper baby son usurping his position as the only man in his wife's life. Aside from that, all was well. He did not actively search for instances of poor judgment. He was satisfied instead to stumble across fortuitous lapses, quickly capitalizing on them. When his wife responded to the provocative behavior, he acted as if she were irrational, obviously evidence of her inadequacy as a mother, obviously a good fit with his own mother.

And then there is *helplessness and pitifulness* that hand-in-hand belie passive–aggressive behavior. A patient had what appeared to be a thyroid problem. She went to a second-rate general practitioner physician at a small community hospital in her town for tests. He sent her to a nearby hospital, since his was not equipped with the necessary facilities. Eventually, a call came from the patient saying that she was going to have a thyroidectomy, a drastic, last-resort procedure one would have thought this nurse would have avoided at all reasonable cost. Unconsciously, of course, she did know better. But she whined that if she went to a specialist it would cost too much money, and if she went to a medical center where doctors did a lot of these procedures or at least where they saw hundreds of such thyroid problems in a week instead of one in a year, she would just be a number. She could not afford to go elsewhere and could not find out whom to see.

Actually, the patient was collecting data at her own expense, maybe at the expense of her future health or her life, on how incompetent this sweet, small-town doctor was. With such data, one can see why Reich (1949) talked about passive aggressiveness as part of masochism. The doctor would be seen as incompetent and as a ne'er do well just as her father had been. So this was not free choice, nor was it the choice of a poor, helpless person; it was the tool for a passive–aggressive collection of data. That she might die in the service of passive aggression was of no consequence; it might even have been worth it! In therapy, such patients provoke rage and hate in the therapist to substantiate their view of the world, thereby impeding if not destroying the therapist's capacity to help them (Kernberg, 1965; Mallsberger & Buie, 1974).

An apparently helpless social worker, new in his fast-paced, demanding job on a medical unit, felt paralyzed when a resident had reprimanded him about a particular patient not being ready for discharge. Instead of standing up to him, he had felt inadequate and defensive because he too had been dissatisfied with his performance. On tap, however, was ammunition. The social worker and God secretly knew that the patient's family disliked this doctor and planned to dump him for their own attending physician shortly. So when the resident demanded, "What's the holdup? What are the issues? Why don't you get the family moving?" the social worker savored that he knew and the resident did not that the family held him in contempt. Therefore, he was a fool for carrying on as if he were respected and held in high regard by the family. The social worker, therefore, collected data on what a fool the resident was and, to boot, had him jumping up and down, confirming his own lowly position of the physician. In the process, he protected himself from his contemptuousness through helplessness and genuine anxiety about not being good enough.

Helplessness is particularly difficult for recipients of passive–aggressive acts to deal with. If one thinks of defenses piled on defenses, it becomes easier to see why helplessness causes such a strong response. In passive–aggressive helplessness, there appear to be three levels operating.

There is a presenting level of helplessness, which is a defense against the next level, that is, manipulation to get people to do what he or she wants. In turn, developmentally, the manipulation was a defense, currently relived, against feeling the helplessness of being up against exceedingly controlling or malevolent parents. The helplessness on the third level down initiates the ladder of defenses, so that on the one hand, the presenting level helplessness rings true. On the other hand, ultimately people are enraged because the presenting level of helplessness feels fraudulent because of the implicit competence required for the middle-level manipulation.

Rather than being helpless, some passive–aggressive persons manifest the problem through *pseudoconsideration*. On his twice-a-year visit to his son, such a father does not let his son carry his suitcase or pay the $2 parking fee at the airport. Furthermore, he explains to him that he wants all his property in joint ownership so that upon his demise the son will not have to come down to Texas from New York; everything will automatically be taken care of. The son, feeling his blood pressure rise from the first encounter at the gate to the trip home, cannot figure out why he is so rankled by this apparently considerate father. In actuality, this kind father is insulting his son. He is saying, "You aren't capable of doing anything for me, certainly nothing nice. Moreover, when I die I'm sure you're not man enough or generous enough of spirit to take time off to come down and straighten things out." The son responds to the unspoken but implicit passive–aggressive dimension and eventually feels enraged and uncaring indeed. Whether or not it happens, he can just hear his father saying, "Can you imagine? He can't even carry a small suitcase for me."

On the face of it, pseudoconsideration would seem contrary to the passive–aggressive phenomenon. Not so, as the person on the other end of the activity can attest. Whether from actual interpersonal observation or from reflection about the relationship, the person on the receiving end of the passive–aggressive behavior starts to feel like an ogre for asking or taking so much, even though there may have been neither urging nor request. Too, the recipient feels increasingly controlled by this too-good-to-be-true person, and may even feel inferior or wanting in goodness by comparison. Therefore, the pseudoconsiderate person is actually making a hostile gesture. But who can point the finger without seeming ungrateful, irrational, irreligious, or hostile oneself? Surely, such dynamics generated the admonition, "Kill them with kindness," and the reflection, "Better to get them with honey than poison," or "You can catch more flies with molasses than with vinegar."

Closely akin to pseudoconsideration is false *stupidity or naiveté*. Often patients will talk about how stupid or naive a parent is, when actually what they are responding to is passive–aggressive behavior. One such patient came into his session feeling absolutely murderous after an encounter with his visiting mother. The mother had just arrived in town, they had lunch, and as the patient was leaving for his therapy session the mother said, "Do you pay your therapist in cash?" The patient felt enraged at what he considered a stupid question. "Who the hell pays in cash? Why would a middle-class person do that? Don't you live in this world or what?" He thought his mother was unquestionably stupid and naive, but his rage was too great for him to feel satisfied with that as the only explanation for his distress. This sweet woman, who was only asking because she did not know about such things, as she informed him, was striking a passive–aggressive blow at both her son and his therapist. She could not know about such things since obviously she was not emotionally disturbed and thus had never seen a therapist. Furthermore, therapists are a bit "sleazy"; if you pay them in cash, they probably do not report the money as earned income, so maybe they give "it" (i.e., render services) to you cheaper. Now that type of communication, over time, could engender rage, and that is exactly the kind of communication mother and son had had through the years. No wonder therapy was in order.

On the other hand, some passive–aggressive behavior has the ring of rationality or *reasonableness* to it, so much as to raise the suspicion of irrationality. A patient in group was criticized by members who said that with needs for approval as he had, he could not possibly be a good teacher. The patient reacted only by explaining with extreme calm and care why he indeed was a good teacher. In fact, he repeatedly explained himself, to the point that everybody responded with increasingly hostile comments and criticism. This brought from him renewed efforts, with more examples, to "straighten out" the members. Compulsively "straightening out" the others' viewpoint actually helped the patient defend against noticing his passive–aggressive behavior. He, after all, looked and sounded reasonable, building his case, yet the others responded with hostility, decisively proving how wrong and irrational their assessment was. What the patient did not realize was that "straightening out" everybody was his brand of hostility, well disguised on one level but stripped bare on another, a true passive–aggressive gesture, made and responded to quite unconsciously.

Another patient thought she was being quite reasonable and thoughtful when, on making initial dinner arrangements, she warned her soon-to-be-lost friend that she might not be able to keep them next week. It seems that recently she had forgotten or changed plans at the last minute, and her friend finally expressed her anger at the inconsideration. Therefore, after much discussion about her past behavior, in all good conscience she thought she was only being reasonable when she warned that her current cold might be worse the next week. The friend was livid at this apparently reasonable but obviously provocative behavior. Who, after all, would think to say that in a week's time one's cold might be worse, warranting a change in plans? Where the patient thought she was waving a white flag, the friend saw red!

Passive aggressiveness sometimes manifests itself through *indecision*. Most often the process of indecision is neither quiet nor private. Often, the indecisiveness is unrelated to the magnitude or ultimate importance of the decision. In other words, the dilemma is felt as strongly whether it is a large or small decision, whether it is about what career to pursue or what shoes to buy. Characteristically, it drives other people crazy for it is difficult to remain untouched by the agitation. Advice offered, even when solicited, is seen as intrusive and controlling. Responding to a request for advice is dangerous because as soon as the advice is forthcoming the passive aggressive person fights it, as if the request were never made.

We have noticed that some patients are so passive–aggressive that they even bristle when the therapist responds to their reported decisions. The patient acts as if the decisions were neither made nor reported. For example, a patient said she thought she would change her major to photography and was going up to school to make the plans. When the therapist asked her what courses she would now have to take she irritably and suspiciously said, "Well, who said I should switch to photography? Do you think that that is the best thing to do?" as if the therapist had made the choice or brought up the subject! Obviously, the patient's object is to not decide. Rather, within one's head, or interpersonally, the object is to struggle with the controlling authority figure, to best the other by enticing him or her into the fray. In the process, the other person becomes enraged and controlling, convincing the passive–aggressive person he or she is being pushed around. Besides, why take advice from such an obviously flawed person?

Sins of omission occur with some frequency by those passive–aggressive persons who martyr themselves for passive–aggressive reasons. Note the scenario: Work needs to be done in the house. A husband does not tell his wife he has pain in his hip when he uses the ladder. Instead, he somehow does not get to the job. The wife assumes it to be his usual passive aggressiveness and becomes enraged. Interestingly, what is passive–aggressive about this instance is not the husband's falling down on the job *per se*. Rather, it is in his not telling his wife the problem, therefore causing her to explode into the secret shrew she harbors, the tyrant his mother was.

In speaking of omissions, it occurs to us that one manifestation we inadvertently omitted was *chronic lateness*. Perhaps the omission is not as unintentional as it might appear; maybe it is a slip of the unconscious, signifying an occupational hazard unlike others we have explored thus far. Certainly there are times, with all patients, where we, as therapists, could use a rest. So a patient arriving late, in time only for a partial session, might be doing us a favor. Aside from chronically thinking maybe we have made a scheduling error, the extra time unabashedly feels good, even if it is a secretly hostile gesture.

FRUSTRATED AGGRESSION

The question as to why passive–aggressive behavior develops and continues remains incompletely answered. We think we have made a good start and will proceed. Stricker's (1983) explanation that early dependency needs are frustrated sounds a bit simplistic, and is a bit overinclusive as well as etiology for probably just about everything. And although it is hard to disagree that restrictive, demanding parents are an etiological factor in determining this underground root for the aggression, there seems more to it than that generalization. It is no surprise that in each developmental era one can see the roots of passive–aggressive behavior, where the need for supplies collides with the need for autonomy. Passive aggressiveness has been dubbed an immature defense (Meissner, Mack, & Semrad, 1975; Valliant, 1971). We see it as early as infancy and childhood, and we see a surge of the behavior during adolescence. And therein lies the clue.

It would appear that passive–aggressive behavior has its origins as early as there are signs of autonomy. Of course, these occur within the first weeks of life, when the baby makes it clear where in the crib he or she wants to sleep and in what position, and in what position to nurse. Long before the formal separation period, seeds of autonomy are planted by how the mothering-one responds to the baby's need for expression of separation and individuality: what clothes the baby prefers, how the baby is seen to help or hinder the feeding process, how the baby schedules sleep time. These are not the classic autonomous functions described in the literature; indeed, they are primitive operations. Nevertheless, they are obvious forerunners to separation itself, and how the mothering-one handles them is probably a good predictor of how actual separation will proceed.

Observable passive–aggressive behavior is likely seen first in the rapprochment subphase of separation, the phase of development where the child certainly needs supplies from the significant other that show emotional responsiveness and physical availability. While autonomy is developing the child needs a push, reassurance from the mothering-one that, once one is on the way, it is all right to go it alone, the beginning of life's many contradictions. At the same time, certain baby-like needs continue, and these too, need to be accepted and met. The implication is that a child has to have pretty nonobsessional, nonrigid, nondemanding, non-will-imposing parents who can live with contradiction, with autonomy, and with exploration imperfectly executed. The young child at that time needs to count on others to gratify needs and satisfy wishes at the same time that he or she struggles to move out of the parental–child orbit to see the self not only as separate from others, but different from others, an individual with some characteristics like the parents, and others on the brink of being realized or formed that are quite distinct from those of the parents. The separation era heralds identifying and accepting the self, seeing one's own wishes in relation to the wishes of others, and recognizing that one has the power to stand alone, if only for a while.

These same tasks, obviously refined and at a higher level, reemerge during adolescence, where we also see a surge of passive–aggressive behavior. A major task of adolescence is learning to become independent. In so doing, one learns to evaluate one's own limitations and powers by examining and anticipating consequences of his or her own decisions and desires while also critically evaluating ideals, beliefs, attitudes, and values of those significant others in one's life. The adolescent is then in a position to establish satisfactory sexual relationships, accepting the self as a sexual object and finding other suitable sexual objects. It is little wonder that in adult life passive aggressiveness flourishes in a sexual relationship.

One can certainly say that with passive–aggressive behavior, first in infancy and then in adolescence, there is a collision between what the child/adolescent needs and what the significant others need. Truly, the adolescent headed toward a passive–aggressive life is in an untenable position at this time of necessary separation and individuation if in the earliest rapprochement subphase of separation there was a problem. Surely the mother and father will withdraw emotional responsiveness and physical availability when the adolescent strives to be separate and different from them. The adolescent's separation and individuation in particular constitute a major threat to the parents' need to control and fit the child into their narcissistic orbit. The parents may withdraw the emotional (if not material) "goods" if the child is too different and does not comply with how they see the world. The adolescent, like the younger child, is placed in a double bind: He or she needs the availability of parental supplies to grow, but if he or she grows differently from the parental picture, the supplies are withdrawn.

This can't-win situation accounts for a good deal of the depression we see in adolescence and in passive–aggressive adolescents in particular.

Although some depression is part of normal adolescence, the depression becomes outright abandonment depression in more disturbed youngsters, who experience parental withdrawal as a loss of part of the self. This is often noticeable around the time such a person is making a career choice. As one patient college student expressed, if she does what her mother wants, namely for her to finish school, she feels incredibly controlled and angry. On the other hand, if she finishes school, then she's on her own and feels abandoned and crippled with separation anxiety. So the patient just stays in school incessantly, going from program to program. As she said, "being in school I'm sheltered from disdain, except from myself." Besides, by her either procrastinating or not completing her work in school, the passive aggressiveness proceeds quietly underground; and so does the tie to her internalized mother. The price she pays, however, is great, for she cannot do or even know what she wants, lest there be disapproval and abandonment.

In those persons who cannot leave and move beyond their parents to a large degree, we see clinging to the parent or, later, to transferential figures as a way simultaneously to work out the struggle, relive the original dilemma, and make the parental figures suffer. Passive aggressiveness fills the bill. Paying the price keeps it unconcsious, keeps active the tie to the parent, and keeps alive the rage about the original appraisal. Aggression is used not for development, not to move ahead in a given situation, not to go after what one wants. Instead, it is used defensively, now to engage the other rather than separate from the other (Rouslin, 1975b). It serves as a vehicle to maintain the parental tie as it was. The healthy aggression needed to separate and individuate is now tainted with anger and abiding hostility toward all those seen to have thwarted its original intent.

Since aggression is a naturally occuring phenomenon in development, it always seeks an outlet. If there can be no overt, forward movement, it will proceed underground; there is no choice. In the process, however, since healthy developmental aggression has been derailed, a now disturbed, distorted, defensive aggression tries to move the self forward. The earlier frustrated aggression, however, impedes forward movement as it is now tinged with the products of frustration: anger, rage, and hostility. Without intervention, aggression can never do what it was originally intended to do. Development of the whole self-system is affected. Thus, passive–aggressive behavior binds the user to another. The user is not free to develop. The "choice" to not produce, to not respond, to be deceptively open and honest, to use verbal operations to control, these choices are not free choices. They are choices that force others into involvement in such a way as to fulfill the original meta-appraisal, that one should not really separate and individuate. Moreover, the person stands still with the self-injunction to tighten the bond by getting even and staying expectantly anxious, continually. As one patient said, "I feel like I leave little time bombs planted in deep cover." The price paid for the deep cover is an imminently anxiety-tinged life on one level, and a life precariously defended against separation anxiety on another.

INTERPERSONAL CONSEQUENCES

Certainly everyone is capable of transient passive–aggressive behavior; surely through the process of reflected appraisals, we all have the capacity to get even. From a countertransferential point of view of course the best way a clinician can get even is to tell on his or her patient, even though nobody knows who the patient is. Perhaps an even better way is to best the patient by figuring out the dynamics of the phenomenon in published form. Benign enough, and even helpful, but now suspiciously passive–aggressive. Yes, passive–aggressive behavior begets passive–aggressive behavior. Direct aggression seems to get nowhere, so in desperation to communicate the rage, passive–aggressive techniques flow automatically. Whether a passive–aggressive message is received by the truly passive–aggressive person is open to question, however.

A fascinating thing about passive–aggressive behavior is how incredibly narcissistic an experience it is. Originally interpersonally inspired and most often interpersonally manifested, passive–aggressive behavior is rarely noticed by the perpetrator. Our experience with such persons has shown excellent but frustrating examples of selective inattention to the phenomenon (Sullivan, 1953a). Indeed, the person observes the exchange or the events of the situation but has no idea of the implications or ramifications of his or her behavior. That dimension of the experience is not in awareness at all. So the passive–aggressive person is truly shocked when the other person is jumping up and down and sideways with rage or retaliation. The passive–aggressive person sees the world through his or her eyes only, the other simply fitting into that system, truly a narcissistic experience. Not only does the recipient object to the particular issue at hand but also to not being acknowledged as a genuine partner in an interpersonal exchange. Instead, he or she is turned into and treated as a disdainful transferential figure. Should the current person "fit" the figure to some degree, the passive–aggressive person uses this as fuel for rationalization and continuous inattention.

As part of the experience, the passive–aggressive person would seem to have no notion that there are consequences to behavior, again testimony to the narcissistic nature of the phenomenon. We all know people who are unconsciously provocative yet who wonder why others respond negatively. In their narcissism, they think they can take a dump; should other people notice, they should compliment the perpetrator. When others respond negatively, well, they're obviously lesser beings. If the recipients are indeed flawed anyhow, then it is reasoned that the act was justified. That there are interpersonal consequences to behavior, that there are cause–effect relationships, that a major dimension of relatedness remains unnoticed, all these are inattended to in a strikingly narcissistic fashion. When the bare bones of the passive–aggressive act are noticed, it is rarely seen as problematic. Rather, it is seen, as one patient said, as "a more reasonable way of voicing my disagreement than carrying on."

That particular patient recently lost her job. A lawyer, this bright, intellectual person, hated the small firm for which she worked, looked down on the partners for their "ham and egg" operation, and, in general, reeked of disdain toward all authority involved. She justified her attitude with the realistic appraisal that indeed this certainly was a penny-pinching, disorganized, inefficient, seat-of-the-pants place, chosen out of desperation only. But it was a job, which she seemed to forget. In fact, it never occurred to her that her attitude was communicated interpersonally and that she might lose the job because of it. So it came as a surprise when she was terminated, not for her work, which was exemplary, but for "not having a good fit" with the partners. She was truly caught "unawares" and was enraged.

With righteous indignation, she told her new therapist that in the days following termination the partners took away cases, leaving little work to be done. "What am I supposed to do for the next 2 months there? Nothing, make telephone calls for my next job, eat sandwiches?" In earnestness, she said, "I'm going to tell them there has to be an orderly transition here. I have to know what I'm supposed to do each day, and what's going to happen to the cases I've worked on." "Now that's passive–aggressive," noted the therapist to herself. She then suggested that the patient's primary intention was not so rational at all, since obviously she knew how erratically the office was run. Besides, the partners actually do not owe anything to someone they want to rid themselves of. Indeed, the intention was to appear rational and reasonable while showing up the partners for the plebians they were. Again, the patient had no awareness of the implications or ramifications of her behavior. But the therapist's interpretation reminded the patient of similar behavior, familiar in retrospect. Had the patient proceeded in the direction she wanted, it is likely she would have been punished further by being booted out immediately, or at the very least, herself be treated with overt contempt by the partners.

In this instance, as in most, the passive–aggressive behavior goes way beyond the current persons and events. In other words, there is a transferential element to it as well. In failing at her job, the patient could accomplish several things. She would disappoint and disgrace her narcissistic lawyer mother, who, unrealized in her own career, sought to live through her daughter's. Through the partners, the mother could look incompetent, and both partners and mother would prove to wield power irrationally. But simple acting out is insufficient as an explanation for passive–aggressive behavior. Through the passive–aggressive process, it became clear that the parental tie was reinforced. The operations proceeded something like this: the message from birth was "be like me, do what I want you to, be successful." So the young lady eventually became a lawyer, reluctantly, failing the bar a few times. The appraisal had been, "if you are like me or do what I want, you will be approved." On the contrary, "if you find and go your own way, you'll be disapproved." So, for years the dilemma had been brewing, normal aggression damning up, distorting itself into rage. Obviously the mother and partners were made to suffer and to look like ogres, although they surely filled the bill. In the process, the disturbed integration was further tightened.

There was yet another level operating here, however, making the situation more complex. On a quite unconscious level, mother to daughter, the appraisal had been, "If you are as contemptuous to people as I am, I'll love you forever." So she was. And she did it so cleverly, she bested this mother and her surrogates. Keep in mind, however, all this was totally unconscious, in thought and deed, for both mother and daughter. The explosive mother saw herself as charitable and considerate of others, when that was but a brittle facade or certainly only a small dimension of her personality. Translated then, there actually were two conflicting appraisals operating within this patient: You are good if you stay with me; and you are good if you are successful. To satisfy the first meant that the daughter would have to be like the mother in form and attitude, certainly not a ticket for success. Theoretically, the second implied a separation–individuation that would indeed be difficult in the face of the infantalizing attitude of the first appraisal. It is not surprising that this patient described herself as feeling caught in a vise, realizing she had felt trapped for years in a box from which she could not escape.

Persons habitually trapped in such situations when growing up eventually learn to remove themselves emotionally, an act that becomes automatic. The detachment often becomes generalized to other interpersonal experiences even when it is not appropriate. The problems go underground, surfacing in passive–aggressive ways. Sometimes, in this state of detachment, the persons even look as if they are wandering through life in a haze, which they are. Passive aggressiveness then, reveals a secret pocket of detachment. The person can proceed in a private world for a while, protected from the anger and from the anxiety that direct aggression would yield. The detachment is also an inevitable outcome of the massive selective inattention that goes on. As a consequence, in adult life, when a passive–aggressive person is faced with confronting an authority such as a boss, he or she feels unexplainably anxious. For example, an experienced school psychologist was continually beaten back by his powerful sociopathic boss. He had a terrible time standing up to her even though a confrontation was legitimate, since she was really not letting him do the job for which he was being paid. Although the boss's superior would have welcomed any data on this woman, he could not take that route for irrational fear of retribution from his transferential mother if he told the world on her. Indeed he said, if he were to "direct aggression" against his mother, she would get him for sure and if she did not, she would get God to do the job.

In fact, his anxiety was so great that his passive aggressiveness had to go so far underground it went all the way to his obsessional wife, who was not as formidable as his boss or mother. On the way to school, he would leave the door of the house open, which drove his wife crazy. So to appease her after one of those incidents, he somehow locked the screen door and front door on his way out, making it impossible for his wife to enter the house on her return. He was not seen as a good boy making amends for past misdeeds.

Finally, passive–aggressive behavior is interpersonally indiscriminate. Although certainly the behavior can be directly related to anger felt in a current situation reflective of past situations or relationships, it also arises with no current external stimulus. It's like boxing on your own, no partner needed, or, any old one will do. This is most graphically seen with chronic lateness. The person does not have to be angry at another to be late; the demons are within, so anyone and everyone is treated the same, independent of person or provocation. The passive–aggressive act is not necessarily always a personal attack, although to the recipient that is little consolation.

Inevitably, passive–aggressive behavior exacts a toll on communication. The person on the receiving end cannot readily communicate the frustration nor can he or she easily confront the perpetrator because talking to the unconscious yields little success in everyday interpersonal situations. The passive–aggressive person becomes defensive, struggling or withdrawing from the experience. Either way, a sense of estrangement seeps into the relationship if such behavior characterizes the contacts.

One patient felt enormous relief when it was pointed out that he was so incredibly passive–aggressive it was probably meant as nothing personal when he acted that way with his wife. The behavior seeped out of him, unrelated to much in the present at all. Unfortunately, he was not simply relieved to hear that he did not genetically hate his wife. He felt a reprieve from relating too closely to someone. For chronically passive–aggressive persons, involvement with their "partners" is in its extreme, a hostile integration that by its nature severely limits involvement; or it is a narcissistic opportunity to live out and "correct" reflected appraisals in interactions that indeed never turn out to be corrective experiences.

IV

Narcissism Revisited

Until now, we have focused on pathological, disruptive, disjunctive manifestations of the therapist's narcissism and its effects on the therapist, patient, and treatment process. The other side of the coin is that, indeed, there is such a concept as healthy narcissism carried over into adult life in general and professional life of the therapist in particular. Now, not only do we look at healthy narcissism as it relates to dimensions of the good enough therapist; we provide an update on the concept of narcissism. Coming to terms with one's narcissism, pathological and healthy, is crucial to professional and personal development and to the growth of our patients. The task is lifelong, but the narcissistic gratification is worthwhile!

14

The Good Enough Therapist

In the preceding chapters we have attempted to show that the issue of therapists' narcissism has been neglected in a variety of ways, some quite overt, others insidious. Since an issue is a matter in dispute, if subject to neglect, it remains as controversy and increases turmoil rather than reaching needed resolution. This situation exists because in many instances the possibility of the "narcissistic effect" has been treated as though its resolution had indeed been accomplished, although it has not. Or, many therapists have related to their narcissism as though its resolution were unimportant in regard to actual practice, which is also erroneous. The latter approach defuses the potential impact of therapists' narcissism through an unrealistic lack of concern. In either case the effect of ignoring such narcissism in the therapist–patient relationship is an unacceptable state of affairs for the field of psychotherapy and requires change.

With the hope of beginning to bring about some change, we have concerned ourselves with a number of instances of therapists' narcissism in action. In particular we have described narcissism in the obsessional therapist, then shifted to the broader concerns of occupational hazards and the many meanings of money, as well as the connections between narcissism, fantasy, and countertransference. Our focus then shifted to the therapy process, especially contracts, theoretical formulations, idiosyncratic responses, and constancy and flexibility in the therapeutic relationship. We have concluded this section with the role of narcissism in psychotherapy supervision. Our last concern has been with particular patients problems that tap into therapists' narcissism, namely resistance, loneliness, envy, and passive aggressiveness.

Throughout, our focus has been on narcissism or self-involvement as a core personality factor of therapists. Our aim has been to note the pathological manifestations of such narcissism and, in response to these, propose the development of a healthy self-relations system that has a far greater chance of producing effective psychotherapists. The result of our explorations heretofore has been to lead to this point of tentative proposals for a good therapist.

In the main our discussion up to now has been concerned with therapists' problems in self-expression and self-satisfaction, particularly the disturbing, disruptive manifestations of narcissism appearing in the therapeutic process as well as in some areas indigenous to it, such as delivery systems. Now we want to move into an emphasis on the positive aspects of narcissism and link these with the effective practice of psychotherapy. In order to do this, we need to elaborate further on the concepts of narcissism and on our idea of the "good" therapist, which is less literal than it may seem.

CONCEPTS OF NARCISSISM

Since the formal introduction of the term "narcissism" by Freud (1914/1957) in 1914, it has been used to describe and explain a number of phenomena. By 1970 Pulver found that narcissism had been considered a stage of libidinal development, a sexual perversion, a type of relationship as well as a lack of relationships, and an aspect of self-esteem. Freud had described it as libidinal cathexis of the ego and essentially preceding object-relations, positioned between autoerotism and object love. The infant began life in a state of primary narcissism, feeling omnipotent with libido directed inward. The infant was the world, the source and recipient of all pleasure. This state was pictured as normally giving way to the demands of reality, but never completely. If narcissism remained as a dominant force, then various pathologies would result.

Thus, in its origination, narcissism was implicated in a variety of behaviors, and this continues to the present. Ego psychology expanded the definition of narcissism to a libidinal investment in the self in one of the earliest and more enduring reformulations. The subsequent proliferation of meanings and uses of narcissism prompted a functional definition: "Mental activity is narcissistic to the degree that its function is to maintain the structural cohesiveness, temporal stability and positive affective coloring of the self-representation" (Stolorow, 1975, p. 179).

Although narcissism continues to be used in various ways, Lachmann (1982) has indicated that a functional definition provides for the narcissistic function of any behavior. For example, it is not necessary to see narcissism as an explanation of sex differences in order to observe such differences in the expression of narcissism. This facilitates a more integrative view in accord with our inclinations in this book. In accord with this, we speak of narcissism from a broad perspective, akin to the description by Tonkin and Fine: "Narcissism is often used as a general term for the feelings a person has for himself" (1985, p. 221).

The reformulations of narcissism offer a number of emphases on therapists' narcissism, which is our concern. The early emphasis on libidinal development implicated narcissism in gender differentiation. The female appeared more narcissistic and masochistic than the male. A contemporary refinement of this distinction appears in the work of O'Leary and Wright (1986). They suggest a relationship between shame, narcissism, and gender. An egotistical type of narcissism appears more often in men where shame is hidden while grandiosity is paramount. A dissociative type of narcissism is more typical of women, where shame dominates and grandiosity is concealed. The authors hypothesize that developmental and societal processes reinforce conscious shame in women, unconscious shame in men.

Lachmann (1982) also notes sex differences in narcissism. His focus is the child's representational world, particularly the content of self-representation as well as defense and compensatory mechanisms. Reconsideration is given to the preoedipal mother–daughter relationship, the role of the father, and the influence of the psychosexual stages. Although theorizing is cast primarily in the language of self-psychology, there is considerable integration of other viewpoints. Narcissism is related to gender identity in terms of the development and maintenance of self and object representations.

Our point here is the presence of sex differences in narcissism. As indicated earlier, the number of women therapists is large and increasing. It is important that these women be attuned to their most probable narcissistic expressions and vulnerabilities, which appear to differ from those of men. For example, relatedness appears as a more frequent interest in women than in men. Men may protect their self-image by appearing cool and detached and have to struggle as therapists for increased sensitivity that at the same time threatens their narcissism. In contrast, women may be more adversely affected by negative reactions to them and want to inhibit aggressive impulses in their patients and themselves. Their narcissism is then vulnerable to attacks on their caregiving abilities.

In making these distinctions, we are not insisting that, for example, women are naturally masochistic or men naturally aggressive. Nor do we insist on any one explanation for narcissistic vulnerabilities, but we are taking notice of different instances that appear gender related, and suggesting that therapists take the same notice. Males may more often expect their self-esteem to be threatened by perceived attacks on their grandiose selves, whereas women will be more exposed in regard to their shame-proneness and sensitivity.

Narcissism may lead anyone to believe that gender-related vulnerabilities are nonexistent, which is untrue. Or, the belief may be that he or she is nonsexist and therefore invulnerable, which is erroneously grandiose because we are all influenced by our sense of being male or female. In essence, the protective component of narcissism can hide an awareness of threats. One way of hiding is the use of ideology to remove possible problems. However, even separating narcissism from sex differences in structuralization, as for example to establish that both sexes are narcissistic, does not eliminate gender-related differences in narcissism.

A second area of emphasis is generated by the Kernberg–Kohut controversy. Kernberg (1975, 1976) presents an intrapsychic conflict view of narcissism that is relatively consistent with instinctual and structural theory preceding it. Narcissism is the result of preoedipal conflict centered on the expression and control of aggression. He emphasizes pathological narcissism, considering it a reaction to excessive aggression, which is also involved in it and which appears to be caused by either constitutional factors or sustained frustration with parents, or some combination of these. Narcissistic pathology is placed within the borderline range where the general etiological factor is an oral conflict based on early maternal deprivation. This fosters aggressive impulses and in turn a variety of characteristic borderline defenses, namely splitting, idealization, projection, denial, omnipotence, and devaluation. Narcissistic manifestations of grandiosity and idealization are part of this defensive procedure. As such, narcissism is part of a pathological developmental sequence with an errant fusion of ego and superego. Assuming that most therapists would not fall within the borderline range, their narcissistic indicators would be similar, but more subtle.

Kernberg's approach reinforces an emphasis on the negative connotations of narcissism, as well as the idea of intense affect being associated with narcissism. In this case it is rage, whereas in our previous notation of the work of O'Leary and Wright (1986), shame was considered the major affect. The case for the involvement of both aggression and shame seems plausible and suggests that narcissistic difficulties for therapists will include expression and control of intense affects. Also, there appear to be different types of narcissism, a point made by Shulman (1986) in reference to the Kernberg–Kohut controversy, and so it appears that narcissism can be displayed in a variety of ways with a variety of underlying and expressed affects connected to the protection and development of self-interest. In all views, the great power of narcissism is reiterated.

The work of Kohut (1971, 1977, 1984) contrasts with the past and with the heavy emphasis on pathology and conflict. In reference to the past, it is probably most connected to an interpersonal point of view. Narcissism appears as a positive developmental line where grandiosity and idealization lead to the formation of a cohesive self. Pathology results from parental empathic failures creating an interpersonal environment insufficiently responsive to the child's needs. This is a deficit theory where aggression is a secondary reaction rather than a causal agent.

Kohut's emphasis is less on pathology and more on the positive aspects of narcissism. In particular, grandiosity and idealization are pictured as normal elements in self-development, and parental roles in furthering this development are specified. The concept of the positive aspects of narcissism is now elaborated and reinforced. Another example of this emphasis appears in Kainer and Gourevitch (1983), who note the similarity between Kohut's narcissism and Rank's (1972) will. In the former, grandiosity and idealization are transformed into appropriate self-esteem and values resulting in a cohesive sense of self. The will begins as opposition to others and is transformed into the capacity for self-developed ideals. Although the concepts of narcissism and will are also different in many ways, they are both depicted as developmental lines with basic origins in what could be construed as libidinal and aggressive strivings and eventuate in creative goal seeking.

A third emphasis is summarized by Mitchell (1988). Narcissism has usually been conceptualized as either primarily pathological or as enhancing growth. Both views have tended to take interpersonal relations into account as an etiological factor. The relational aspects of life are increasingly seen as contributing to as well as being shaped by narcissism. Mitchell emphasizes the role of specific parent–child interactions and the need to promote healthy narcissism by developing relationships that provide a balance between reality and narcissistic illusions. Thus, he feels that

> . . . illusions concerning oneself and others are generated, playfully enjoyed, and relinquished in the face of disappointments. New illusions are continually created and dissolved . . . In pathological narcissism, on the other hand, illusions are taken too seriously . . . reality is sacrificed in order to perpetuate an addictive devotion to self-ennobling, idealizing, or symbiotic fictions. (Mitchell, 1988, pp. 195–196)

Mitchell suggests, then, that narcissism is best understood in relational terms and that the task of the therapist is to enable a patient to foster healthy narcissism through a balance between reality and illusion.

Since our emphasis is on therapists' narcissism in the therapist–patient relationship, our concern is with therapists' ability to develop their own balance. The narcissistic illusions of grandiosity, idealization, and mutual enhancement that may appear in patients may also appear in therapists. So, in addition to working with these narcissistic manifestations in patients, therapists have the personal task of dealing with these internally as they may be activated within the therapeutic relationship.

For example, the therapist whose narcissistic vulnerability lies primarily in grandiosity may be inclined toward admiring patients and away from the more angry, critical, or even noncommittal patients. Or if the therapist is determined to avoid his or her own grandiosity, there may be an identification with patients' grandiosity, or an envy of it. The idealizing therapist has a different version of a similar problem where the patient can be overvalued and thus exploration can be limited, or a patient can defensively be envied or identified with depending on what the therapist is intent on doing with personal idealizing vulnerabilities.

Mitchell (1988) has described in some detail how therapists may work successfully with different types of narcissistic patients in a relational mode that provides for integration of negative and positive aspects of narcissism. He also takes note of the probability of countertransferential narcissistic conflicts. "The analyst's own ease in engaging and disengaging in illusions about himself and others is crucial to this process" (1988, p. 234).

THE GOOD THERAPIST

As discussed earlier, we find ourselves inclining toward an integration in developing and understanding theory, so that our view of narcissism, and the "good" and "bad" therapist, has that flavor. In addition, although these descriptions are in the context of psychoanalytic developmental theory, the ideas can be conceived within other theoretical systems as well.

In regard to the integration of psychoanalytic theory, Pine (1989) describes four primary motivational tendencies that undergo developmental transformation. In the realm of object-relations there are propensities for interpersonal connections and the repetition of past relationships in new relationships. Self-development starts with tendencies to correct self-perceived discomfort and continues with the development and maintenance of self-constancy. Ego psychology stresses a related type of equilibrium of reality testing and adaptation, and drives satisfy urges, gain ties to mental representations and has functions incorporating self, ego, and object-relations.

Certainly narcissism can be construed as a component of any and all of these. They are related, linking personal history and personal expression. In this vein, our understanding of narcissism has a notable relational aspect, although drive components are certainly detectable. The fundamental proposition from our point of view is that early in life the infant–child has divided others, and the self, into all "good" or all "bad." This comes about as a movement from the perception of being rather constantly gratified to being more frequently frustrated by significant others, primarily parents. The gratification, and the gratifiers, are the good, and the frustrators, and the frustrations, are the bad. As psychological development proceeds, the child learns to integrate good and bad into one conception of a person, and of the self, and to love someone despite the frustrations involved in the relationship. There is a constancy of impression that is based on a unified representation in one person's mind of what another person is. In that sense, then, there is no such person as the good therapist, or the bad for that matter, since people usually evolve as being too complex for that type of absolutist categorization. It is true that the possibility that indeed someone is all good or all bad can be conceived, but this is an unlikely happening in more mature individuals. So, our term, the good therapist, is to be understood as a qualified one.

The view of any person as a composite of attractive and unattractive features is a relatively accepted one in most theories of personality development, regardless of the belief about how such perceptions may have developed. Thus, whatever the psychotherapist's theoretical orientation, it appears clear that the concern for the development of the good therapist is not the pursuit of an idealized image or process, but of an adequate, "good-enough" person. The good therapist, then, is one who is considered effective by the majority of people with whom he or she relates as a therapist and one who feels a definite, realistic sense of self-proficiency. There is a consistency of perception by others and by the self that validates this person being a "good" therapist.

Although we have given recognition to the fact that therapists are integrated to various degrees, and so a mixture of "good" and "bad" characteristics, up to this point we have stressed the "bad." We have also mentioned antidotes for therapists' problems and struggles, but our focus has been that therapists have personal needs that at times go unrecognized and take precedence over what is most fitting for the success of the therapeutic process. We have tracked this unfortunate happening through events integral to the practice of psychotherapy. We have indicated our strong belief that a fundamental cause of the problems is the therapist's narcissism, which in a variety of ways is assaulted by the therapist being in the therapeutic situation. The therapist's response to the assault is too often a display of disturbing self-involvement and self-absorption, which has the potential of considerable harm for both therapist and patient.

We have given numerous examples of the problems that occur and the resulting damage, as well as suggestions for rectifying these situations. Inherent in our presentation is the idea that narcissism is to be thought of as a normal developmental personality characteristic, present in all individuals. Thus, feelings and perceptions of self-esteem, self-worth, and personal value are essential to a mature, integrated, functioning person. We consider these also to be the material of narcissism, which can be expressed in healthy and helpful ways by the therapist. Although we frame the conception in terms of psychoanalytic developmental psychology, this orientation is certainly not necessary for all therapists in order for them to use the concept. We are stressing the needs of the self for appreciation, attention, and gratification. These are the needs of therapists from all disciplines and all orientations.

At this point then, our general proposal is that the "good" therapist strives to utilize and display "healthy narcissism." Thus, self-relations are thought of as being intertwined with relating to others, and the love of others is considered empty without love of the self. This view of healthy narcissism as an essential and enduring process has been proposed by others, such as Jacobson (1964) and White (1980), although it has not been applied directly to the psychotherapist and his or her practice of psychotherapy.

White has stated: "It may be that the current interest in narcissism is heralding a wider recognition of the developmental need for healthy self relations and is looking toward a new era in therapeutic technique as well as in therapy" (1980, p. 22). In accord with this hopeful probability, we are going to propose some possibilities for the satisfactory use of the self on the part of the therapist, in contrast to many of the unsatisfactory behaviors we have scrutinized in previous chapters. And although we certainly believe our possibilities can and ought to be realized, it is more prudent to consider them as hypotheses to be tested as to their specific value for therapeutic effectiveness. Also, our proposals are not intended as an exhaustive list of successful therapist behaviors in the therapy situation but as some important, useful suggestions that touch on the less acknowledged difficulties encountered by all therapists. We accept as a given an awareness on the part of therapists that it would be helpful to possess such attributes as concern, intelligence, empathy, and the customary list of fairly obvious behaviors that ought to be useful in practicing psychotherapy. Our proposals are a bit different, going after the influential, yet relatively unrecognized components of the therapist's "healthy narcissism."

PROPOSITIONS FOR THERAPISTS

The Profession of Psychotherapy

The current situation in the delivery of psychotherapy is an appalling example of pathological narcissism. Fortunately there are exceptions to this, but too often it is fad-driven, feeding selectively on the limited and conflicted evidence we have as to what works best. The "ins" savage the "outs," who either try to convert to the philosophy of the "ins," or wait impatiently for the "ins" to fail so they can turn them into "outs." In essence, psychotherapists unduly compete with each other in such a way that patients are poorly served. Instead of collaboration and cooperation, the goal seems to be exclusivity and limitation. It is carried out under the guise of "we know best," the "we" being the major power group of the moment. Such behavior is often discipline related; for example, at this writing many psychiatrists have showed a public urge to eliminate or at least dominate all other disciplines involved, but the medicine men are not the only culprits. In addition there is competition among schools of therapy despite the lack of evidence to support relative superiorities. The situation has become quite a morass of self-interests that is only fueled by the declining dollars coming from third-party payers. This is particularly disturbing because, as we have noted in other parts of the book, therapists are a rather kindly lot with a genuine interest in helping their fellow man or woman.

Of course the situation is a complex one with many facets needing attention and change. We will try for just one of those, although it is major and certainly related to others. At present psychotherapy is a rather subjective, loosely organized profession whose recognized identity is attached in relative degrees of insecurity to its practitioners. We see, instead, the need for a more objective and formalized helping process as a profession called psychotherapy. We envision this profession as a distinct one, with its own training programs involving multidisciplinary content. A similar proposal was made in 1947 by Kubie and reinforced by Henry, Sims, and Spray in 1971, yet little has come of it. The project foundered because of disagreements about training criteria, accreditation, and the essence of the curriculum.

Instead of giving such a possibility top priority, the existing professions concentrate on establishing their independence as psychotherapists, and alternate getting along with attempts to eliminate some of the exclusivity of the other professions. No doubt there is fear that a merger may destroy certain favorable status conditions, or result in less effective training and so more incompetence than already exists. However, the consumer is the one who is being poorly treated by the fears and suspicions of the professionals. We need to come together, not just in a collaborative way, but to form a profession of psychotherapy.

Nearly everyone from the disciplines that currently comprise the body of practicing psychotherapists has an awareness of parts of our training that have not proven to be relevant to the actuality of being a psychotherapist. In addition, there are opinions about the kind of training, both content and type, that would be relevant. No doubt there is disagreement as to the relative value of particular bodies of knowledge. Yet a consensus could and should be developed that could be more appropriate and satisfactory than the current diversity.

Rather than take the apparent next logical step of suggesting a sample program here, the more immediate requirement is getting the disciplines together to discuss and solve the problem. In fact, if at this time a program were proposed, it would probably mitigate the likelihood of the concept coming into being. One program might well be written off by other disciplines as well as by those people who balk at any suggested need to acquire a variety of additional skills. Many current practitioners may feel they can have sufficient practices without the development of a profession of psychotherapy. However, the boat should be rocked because a better job could be done for more people through the development of a distinct profession, one trained exclusively in the practice of the psychotherapies.

The following tentative blueprint begins with a series of official meetings of the various disciplines primarily involved in offering psychotherapeutic services. Out of these meetings might come the development of competency-based training programs that would include all the curricula deemed necessary to practice psychotherapy. Undoubtedly this would cover much of what is now taught in medical school, psychiatric nursing, clinical psychology, and psychiatric social work programs, but it would be taught to *all* psychotherapists. Arrangements would also be made for current practicing psychotherapists, as well as those in training at that time, to acquire skills they might be lacking through the proposed new program. Criteria for competency would be established, and all who would be licensed as psychotherapists would have the training and legal license to practice the variety of procedures comprising the psychotherapies.

Our aim is the relative standardization of practitioners and assurance of uniformly high-quality services for clients. To reiterate, the first step is that those who are now involved in practice and training come together, put aside special interests (and suspicions), and formulate an interdisciplinary plan to train and license psychotherapists. This issue is long overdue for solution, and the time for change is now.

At present, all psychotherapists have some difficulty with integral components of the profession that are not discipline-specific, as the definition of psychotherapy, goals, and what does or does not constitute therapeutic behavior by therapists. Although our proposal would help to solve some of these problems, we realize this may not be that much of a motivator to elicit a significant response to our call for unity in the establishment of a profession of psychotherapy. A further appeal to healthy narcissism is that a conception whereby all psychotherapists could have quite similar competency-based identities also has the potential for reducing the shortage of adequate mental health personnel and providing more discernible criteria for accountability.

We certainly sympathize with the struggles of the current disciplines to gain recognition as independent mental health service providers. We both come from parent disciplines that indeed have had to "wage war" for such recognition, but we also see such an approach as unlikely to bring about egalitarianism among psychotherapists. In fact, we doubt it can alter many of the biases and prejudicial impressions currently existing in regard to different groups of psychotherapists. Thus, it is apparent to us that if the most effective changes are to be made and therefore a profession of psychotherapists created, at least two occurrences are vital. Leadership is necessary, and we believe for it to be the most effective, it should come from psychiatrists because they are really the most powerful of the disciplines involved. Then, once agreement has been reached by all the disciplines as to what competencies are necessary to practice as a psychotherapist, all who wish to be psychotherapists, regardless of discipline, must develop these competencies. An assumption is made here that appropriate avenues will be created for such development. We believe in this approach as a most needed solution to what can conservatively be described as the current "sticky situation."

So far, we regretfully admit, we have been pessimistic about getting our proposal implemented. It is our impression that, unfortunately, too many therapists have their heads stuck in their personal sand. For example, some psychiatrists believe that the granting of independent status to other practitioners will destroy their livelihood, and/or the mental health of the entire society. And some of these "others" have their own image problems, so much so that they hasten to become "as-if" psychiatrists, knowing the name of every drug they cannot prescribe. Although there are hopeful exceptions, the degree of dissension existing about who is, or is not, entitled to practice psychotherapy should mandate a better solution than the field's current state of practice. We believe we have made a clear and simple proposal to start that resolution, and we want the consideration of all psychotherapists as a beginning in making the profession of psychotherapy a viable reality.

Our concern recognizes the variety of threats to basic narcissistic components such as self-involvement, status, security, and self-righteousness. It involves a conception of considerable change, and therapists are too well reminded of the difficulties in that through their everyday contact with patients. Thus, although we believe the need is pressing, we also sense there is value in small beginnings about a charged issue such as establishing a psychotherapy profession. We are asking, therefore, for what might be palatable at the moment, and if this ensues, we can go from there to a more detailed proposal. Our hope is based on the belief that "good enough" therapists are fairly determined optimists with sufficient healthy narcissism to see definite value for all concerned in our desire for a unified, competency-based profession. All we need is enough of these "good-enoughs," and our plan could have real possibilities.

Psychotherapists and Research

What we have just promulgated we see as important, with both political and personal implications. But, the establishing of such an integrated discipline is only the beginning. Another major concern of ours is increasing the integration of research and practice. There are many ways in which practitioners can and do "shake off" research, operating selectively in terms of their own needs as far as what is incorporated into an already existing belief system about how any psychotherapist is practicing. Again, we note resistance to change and the threat to the narcissistic self, for the possibility certainly exists as to the empirical demonstration of the efficacy of something other than what one is already doing. And, more disturbing, the possibility is there that the inefficacy of any therapist's theories or methods may be shown if put to a representative test.

However, our impression is that nothing so simple comes out of the research on psychotherapy. Instead, what it really offers is an opportunity for greater understanding of the complexity of psychotherapy. This understanding can in turn improve the effectiveness of the psychotherapies. Concern with, and comprehension of research about the therapies, present a growth potential for psychotherapists, rather than the specter of nihilism and denigration of therapeutic efforts. Of course change may be involved, but perfection can scarcely be a current claim of the healing professions. Besides, change is the essential goal of most psychotherapies. Also, the changes suggested by the research literature, when its limitations are indeed taken into account, are relatively subtle. They support the diversity, and coordinated difficulty, of successful therapeutic interventions, and they pose the possibility of such strategies. In doing so, however, they consistently reveal what we would term "inevitable complexity."

Greenberg (1986) has indicated that a possible reason for the lack of interest in research by practitioners has been the apparent limited relevance for practice. If such were the case, then a new look is forthcoming because information that applies to practice is now being made available. A general example is provided by change process research (Greenberg, 1986). First, this approach considers three types of outcome: immediate, intermediate, and final. Immediate refers to changes evident in the session. These are related to particular interventions and in turn to intermediate changes measured by session indices of changes in target behaviors. Changes in the targets are tracked over time to assess the resiliency of the intermediate measures and their relationships to final outcomes determined both at the end of a course of therapy and with follow-ups.

Further specification of process is provided using levels of meaning hierarchically arranged as content, speech act, episode, and relationship. Content is literal, whereas speech refers to the mechanics of interaction, as advise, inform, direct, and includes features of these actions, as voice quality and silence. Episodes are units of interaction aimed at an intermediate goal, and relationships refer to qualities attributed to the ongoing interaction by the participants that goes beyond content, act, and episode. The levels are seen as related, providing a context for each other and defining the meaning of any communication.

Thus it becomes possible to identify and describe specific therapist–patient interactions aimed at problem resolution. Rice and Greenberg (1984) propose an events-based method in which an event is a therapeutic episode consisting of a patient problem marker, therapist interventions, patient responses, and the in-session outcome. It is possible to determine what patient problems are ready for intervention, what interventions will facilitate changing them, and what patient responses will lead to the changes. Both theoretical and technical constructs are subject to scrutiny in this type of research, and it has potential utility to the practitioner.

Some specific examples of research of value to psychoanalytic therapists are the works of Frieswyk et al. (1986) on the therapeutic alliance; Luborsky, Crits-Cristoph, and Mellon (1986) on transference; and the exploration of theories of narcissism by Glassman (1988). Frieswyk et al. provide a summary of the work on the therapeutic alliance, attesting to its value and clarifying its meaning as the patient's collaboration. This makes it possible to separate therapist factors, as well as to explore the relationship between the state of the transference and the establishment of the therapeutic alliance. Luborsky et al. provide similar assistance in objectively defining transference and providing for its identification through the core conflictual relationship method (CCRT). Glassman used causal modeling techniques applied to observational data to explore models of narcissism. This provided an indication of how deficit and conflict appear to be implicated in narcissistic disorders. In all these examples, there is an appreciation for the complexity of the psychotherapeutic process that should have an appeal for practitioners.

A practical example is given by Strupp (1989) in citing how he makes use of psychotherapy research, much of which he has also generated. His orientation is psychoanalytic–interpersonal, and his focus is on the characteristics of the therapeutic relationship. He envisions research as providing useful information in a number of practical ways. First, it supports the value of therapists creating an accepting, empathic environment as it illustrates how difficult this can be because of the provocations of transference. Patients can elicit negative complementary reactions from therapists, and these tend to limit the effectiveness of therapy. Strupp emphasizes the importance of being able to work with provocativeness, negativism, and hostility. He suggests that although negative complementarity can often be minimized, it is not possible to avoid at all times. Even experienced therapists make errors through the use of confusing and critical communications, and so this is a concern for all therapists.

The conclusions he draws for practice are an emphasis on current experience and accompanying affects, empathic respectful listening by therapists, clarification of patients' experience, and effective management of patients' enactments. Whereas he downplays transference interpretations and confrontations, views that could be disputed, he makes use of research data for practice guidelines.

There is potential enhancement of therapists' skills in research data, and good therapists should respect that possibility. As previously indicated, the field often operates on "best guesses" that need consistent scrutiny if effectiveness is going to be increased. Research is a possible way to enlighten and improve rather than threaten or confuse practitioners.

Furthermore, in describing the characteristics of good therapists Strupp states:

> Lest the impression is created that this discussion has belabored the obvious, I have reason to believe that therapists who meet the criterion of a "good therapist" are by no means the norm; on the contrary, more or less serious deficiencies are common, even among experienced and respected professionals. (1989, p. 723)

We believe the possibility of narcissistic threats to the practitioner has been developed by previous misconceptions regarding research, some of which were fueled by misleading statements from researchers as well. Although these misconceptions seem to have facilitated the past dismissal of research from serious consideration by large numbers of therapists, such does not have to be the case. If research is viewed as we have suggested, the threat is significantly diminished, and recognition followed by curiosity leading to action is a more likely possibility. We focus primarily on the greater use of empirical research, since therapists have been much more receptive to clinical investigation, such as case studies, and seem to feel relatively comfortable with drawing specific and selective conclusions from such material. But, that is not enough since such investigations lack the power of the scientific method. Thus, as empirical research continues, and, as with clinical practice, gains sophistication, we believe the results will provide continual useful opportunities for greater understanding of the therapist's efforts in action. In turn, such understanding can be translated into more effective practice.

THERAPISTS' INNER SOUNDINGS

Even though the narcissistic struggles regarding the development of a psychotherapy profession and the integration of research and practice are major concerns, they pale compared to our belief in the importance of the therapist's use of his or her "inner voice" in operating as an effective psychotherapist. We have indicated in some fashion in every chapter of this book that the therapist's narcissism is the key to how he or she will practice psychotherapy. Our view is that self-interest needs to be served yet is best served in the therapeutic endeavor by attending to the needs of the patient while attending to the needs of the therapist. Therapist and patient require a "good fit" in regard to both their self-images and self-esteem for therapy to be a positive event for both of them. Our particular concern is with the therapist's use of his or her narcissism, even though this is certainly an interactive operation involving the patient as well. Our strong belief is that the therapist who makes sound use of healthy narcissism stands the best chance of effecting therapeutic change in the patient. This is accomplished by close attendance to the self while listening to the patient. This self-focusing is not a new conception, yet many vital aspects of it have been, and continue to be, neglected in the training and development of therapists.

Even some of the more blatant examples of therapists' narcissism, such as sexual exploitation of patients, had at first been treated by nonrecognition or dogmatic disallowance. Recently, recognition has set in that this is an area encompassing great problems, but there is still a strong tendency to avoid the complexities involved. The magnitude of narcissistic needs symbolized by this problem, and the extent to which they exist in all therapists, remain subjects relatively ignored.

We believe that there are beginning to be some positive signs of increased recognition of the diverse manifestations of therapists' narcissism, although the issue tends not to be addressed directly. We are going to consider these "rumblings of concern" and place them within our schema of the uses and abuses of narcissism. Our aim remains the greater development of the self-as-therapist through increased recognition and activation of healthy narcissism in the process of therapy.

Values

Our first area of concern is a constellation we refer to as therapist values, which includes attitudes and beliefs as well. We consider this grouping an important component of the narcissism of the therapist, and we see values as having a motivational loading indicative of individual goals that may or may not be appropriate for the therapy. That is quite crucial because we also believe that the values of the therapist are often brought into the therapeutic situation.

Beutler (1979) presents a strong case for many instances of the therapist's values and beliefs being transmitted to the patient during the therapy situation. This may be positive or negative in its effects, but either way, the potential power of value transmission appears to be strong. Personal and religious values of patients frequently change during the course of therapy, and often in the direction of the therapist's value system. The "persuasive component" of therapy can be helpful, yet there is limited knowledge as to the specifics of the relationship between therapeutic improvement and particular values, beliefs, and attitudes.

For example, one of us recently was admonished by a patient because the patient had the impression the therapist believed that "homosexuality is an acceptable lifestyle for a person." The person the patient had in mind was himself, who although living a homosexual lifestyle at the time, felt guilty about it. In fact, he had repeatedly condemned homosexuality as "wrong." The therapist had raised the possibility a few times that sexuality did not have to be looked on in that way. The therapist in fact did not consider homosexuality to be "wrong." At least ostensibly then, the therapist and patient held different values. The therapist also had the sense that the acceptance of homosexuality as an equally viable lifestyle to heterosexuality could alleviate the patient's conflicts considerably, yet the therapist did not want to appear to be imposing a personal, and controversial, view upon the patient. Nonetheless the therapist's values were involved on a number of levels, and an apparent value conflict was part of the therapy.

The therapist viewed the "morality" aspect as not the main issue, believing instead that the patient's conflicts about homosexuality really involved areas other than morality, yet the therapist's values were involved. The patient was claiming homosexuality was wrong, whereas the therapist did not share his viewpoint, so a value question appeared to be obvious. The possibility that the patient would either insist it was a moral issue about which the therapist was wrong, or simply refuse to recognize any other issues, could be felt as a narcissistic injury by the therapist. Thus, the patient may disparage both the therapist's personal value and the value of the therapist's interpretation of the patient's conflict.

If the patient would have opted for heterosexuality by disavowing homosexuality solely on the grounds that it was "immoral," the therapist probably would have been uncomfortable. What happened instead is that the therapist questioned whether or not there was a "real" value difference here, or whether the patient was insisting on a difference to remain "stuck." The patient had always claimed the practice was evil, yet kept indulging in it and suffering. The possibility of the value difference being used as a defense was gradually accepted by the patient, and therapy proceeded. Of course there was an imposition of the therapist's values here, but we would see the questioning as appropriate, regardless of how the therapist felt about homosexuality. Nonetheless, the patient did accept the therapist's view that the apparent value difference was a defense and its implication that what looked like a difference would dissolve.

We would like to think that if there were indeed a real value difference the therapist would make it clear that if the patient wanted to give up homosexuality and would feel better for having done this, the therapist would attempt to aid the patient in accomplishing this aim, regardless of the therapist's personal view of the "goodness" or "badness" of homosexuality. The therapist's discomfort would have come about if the homosexuality were to be stopped purely on moral principles, since the probable conflict regarding sexual orientation would not really have been resolved. In essence, the therapist strives to remain open to the patient's professed goal, although he or she reserves the necessary option to question it even if such behavior appears as a value conflict, and, in this case, even if the patient really believes homosexuality is bad for the world, but the therapist does not.

The possible influence of the values of the therapist has traditionally received some mention in the psychotherapy literature (Beutler, Crago, & Arizmendi, 1986). However, the role of therapists' values has had limited exploration, although it is clear that such values are involved in a number of pertinent issues inherent to the practice of psychotherapy, such as religion, politics, and social concerns. Regardless of the emotional and intellectual positions any therapist may have on particular issues, the dominant consideration is the degree of pervasion of the therapeutic endeavor by value-laden processes. Psychotherapists have further to consider the implications of their value systems for their therapeutic efforts, particularly since their values often are different from many of the values of their clients. The therapist's tasks are to acknowledge to the self the actuality of his or her values, to then be aware of their possible impact, and to respect the values of the clients. This is *not* to be equated with the therapist changing personal values to accommodate the client, who is often seeking help for conflicts about values and so is scarcely in a position of certainty about personal values.

The therapist legitimately questions the patient's values, but with an awareness of the therapist's own concerns, which enables a sorting out of the primarily self-serving from the therapeutic in the exploration process. In our view the therapist is an investigator and an integrator, but not a value salesperson, even if the values in question would be considered "good" by many people. There are some values the therapist does need to promulgate, such as client honesty with the therapist, but these are integral to the procedure of therapy rather than more absolute beliefs, such as the value of marriage for the "good life." The therapist aids the patient to make clear, relatively conflict-free decisions about how to live, and in our opinion, that is it. We try to understand ourselves and we try to understand our patients, who have a substantial stake in self-understanding.

Thus, for us, the therapist is limited in his or her "teaching" of values, with the client and the therapeutic process defining these limits. Of course the therapy is not neutral for the therapist, but it is definitely restricted when it comes to the expression of personal values. Of course that is a substantive value of ours, which we happen to believe is usually the most appropriate course. There are some degrees of exception, in consideration of the variability of patients' personality structures, but we generally hold by our view and attempt to act accordingly.

Until now we have been concentrating on the somewhat more abstract aspects of personal concerns of therapists, such as values, attitudes, and beliefs, in regard to overall issues. Now we want to concretize the personal to a greater degree, since we believe we have sufficiently established the general necessity of considering the possible significance of the therapists' concerns on many fronts.

Cognitive Operations

We begin this section by considering the discussion by Heimann (1977) of ways to look at the cognitive processes of the analyst at work. She suggests that therapists have a number of tasks deserving more attention than they have received. Her concern is with psychodynamic psychotherapy, but it appears applicable in many of its particulars to all forms of therapy.

The therapist is pictured at the start of therapy as a receptive listener, which involves a fluid attending, that is a selecting of pertinent material in terms of the therapist's impression of its importance. At the same time, the therapist is in continual internal dialogue, noting the flow of the psychic movement and testing these impressions in a variety of ways. Many of these are remembered for subsequent use, whereas some need to be forgotten. The listening process is one of creative selection, with the therapist developing a functional model of the patient's life: past, present, and future. Whereas the therapist is actively involved in imaging and imagining, the patient's communications are continual stimuli for the therapist's associations and formulations.

Heimann describes the chief operations of this stage in therapy as, "mobile attention, running commentary, and trial interpretations," all of which are not overtly expressed. Instead, they serve as the groundwork for another, subsequent activity of the therapist, namely action in the form of verbalizations to the patient. The attending process is an intense one, with numerous opportunities for narcissistic intrusions that deflect the accuracy of the therapist's understanding. As Heimann puts it: "Reik spoke of the 'analyst's third ear' (1949). I think he needs more than three."

This special and difficult listening process then is changed into a still more complicated overt participatory dialogue. The therapist's part in this is designed to be a fashioned one, customized to what is "therapeutic." The judgment factor looms large here, and there are certainly possibilities for the therapist to be self-serving at the expense of the patient and under the guise of therapeutic work. We suspect all therapists can notice at least a touch of this kind of narcissism at work, be it only in retrospect. The need is to tune into it just before the time of occurrence and to gain a different self-satisfaction by the more effective use of the self.

The dialogue begins with the therapist sorting and organizing the diffuse impressions that have been cognitively, and affectively, recorded within the self of the therapist. A personalized internal discussion is carried out in a search for conceptual clarity, which will result in the translation of these concepts into formal speech. At relatively the same time that these formulations are being made, an assessment of the patient's readiness to receive them also has to occur. The patient's reactions must be anticipated as much as possible since the basic thrust of the therapist's communications is designed to be purposive. Also, it is fruitful to recognize that therapists' responses occur in a variety of ways, many of which are gestures, monosyllabic intonations such as grunts and sighs, incomplete sentences, and other less than "perfect" verbalizations. Yet, all these can be meaningful to the patients, even when they are not intended as such. For example, when one of us during a therapy session shifted our position in a chair, the patient lying on the couch at the time stated that the therapist must be bored. The therapist was not bored, nor did the therapist intend the communication, yet it happened. The reverse is also true. If the timing is missed, the patient does not hear the therapist, and a "misunderstanding" appears to have taken place.

The new role of active participant does entail the probability of some loss of attention to the patient's *immediacy* because the therapist is focusing on his or her carefully crafted interpretation which is about to be presented. There is an inherent narcissistic element to the transformation of the inner processes to outer interactions. Because of this, it becomes especially important for the therapist to keep the patient in focus while interpreting. The formation of words from inner images by the therapist during therapy is a creative action deserving more intensive exploration. It is complex, designed to serve the patient and the self of the therapist, yet it can so insidiously become a selfish, narcissistic exercise.

Finally, after the session, the therapist has the opportunity, responsibility, and need to look at his or her own work. Such scrutiny is admittedly selective, and not purely cognitive, being strongly influenced by emotional components. When we ourselves recall what we did in a session, we are struck by what did or did not prove to be effective. For example, one of us was listening to a patient reproach himself for being "confused." The therapist asked, "what is wrong with being confused?" The patient appeared relieved in response to the question, although he remarked that he thought therapy was designed to clarify matters. The therapist nodded, somewhat ambiguously. The next session the patient said: "That was the greatest thing you said, that it was all right for me to be confused." The question asked by the therapist with the intention of probing intense feelings appearing to surround the patient's self-image of confusion, opened up the analysis of the patient's self-esteem/self-degradation feelings; indeed, it went beyond that to alter a "given" as far as the patient was concerned and facilitated a "new look" for the patient and for the therapist. It was a useful verbalization by the therapist yet had some mysterious components. It is remembered more for its effectiveness than its design. Had the patient not responded as he did, it may well have disappeared from the therapist's self-review of the session.

Self-scrutiny is certainly complicated by the narcissistic need for self-justification, as well as by a host of other self-absorbing factors. The therapist's motivation has a wide range, from highlighting themes deemed important, through the scientific communication of what may appear to be a considerable discovery about behavior, to greater analysis of the self. And although material may be overlooked, or overemphasized, the very process of self-scrutiny raises still another possibility for distortion. Also, narcissism can be fed by self-accusation if it is accompanied by a promise to do better next time and a belief in the accomplishment of the promise. When this approach is used, then a castigating superego would seem to be at work, which can be still another distortion. In defusing these unwarranted concerns, reality testing has to be invoked, not only against errors of omission and self-aggrandizement, but to avoid false errors designed as food for guilt. Therapists can indeed do much of their work correctly, and retrospection should reveal that, as well as genuine mistakes. Healthy narcissism means an appropriate perception of the therapist's work in the session.

Personal Concerns

We have just considered the cognitive/emotional mix in the good therapist, with a direct focus on the therapeutic process. Now we look at the therapist's professional–personal lifestyle, following up on our discussion of occupational hazards in earlier chapters. Some authors who have recently addressed these concerns are Berkowitz (1987), Goldberg (1986), and Zager (1988). They cover a variety of therapist variables, some of which we have already delved into sufficiently, so our emphasis now is on selected material that we believe has not yet been emphasized as much as it should be.

Berkowitz emphasizes the relative burden of stress falling on the more inexperienced therapists so that many types of burnout appear negatively correlated with age. Economic issues can be pressing, competitiveness striking harder at the less well-established. Also, rather high expectations of success with patients has to be modified to the realities of more limited effects. Disappointments have to be adjusted to or it is difficult for the therapist to want to continue in the field.

Berkowitz does see a special problem for more experienced therapists, namely loneliness, a state we explored in some detail in an earlier chapter. In our opinion, many therapists have entered the profession with hopes of dispelling loneliness by constantly working with people. But, because of the "work parameters" of psychotherapy, therapists are instead often left with the loneliness of an extreme type of narcissism that imposes an enforced solitary existence of the self. Becoming a psychotherapist does not resolve the intertwining loneliness–narcissism impairment, and in fact, the profession offers strong potential for exacerbation of the problem. Sometimes everyone in the therapist's life may appear to be a patient, leaving the therapist painfully alone. Patients arrive, stay varying lengths of time, and frequently depart. Even allowing for open-ended therapy with unlimited termination so that separations may not be as inevitable as is often suggested, they are fairly probable and inevitable at some point in time. Furthermore, the degree of therapist self-expression, of being the personal "me," is distinctly limited. The pervasive influence of being a psychotherapist is such that it is often a major task for any therapist to be a truly social person with a distinct, autonomous identity that contains and expresses love and intimacy outside of the therapeutic situation.

Goldberg emphasizes the way in which therapists are drawn to help others and, in turn, neglect themselves. Therapists are particularly at a loss when and if they start to lose interest in their work especially after it has become their "life" for some time. Using himself as an example, Goldberg discusses how he felt pulled into the therapist role to the degree that he was drawn away from what could have been the rest of his life. He ultimately identified what was happening to him as a narcissistic distortion and recognized the need to become a healer to himself.

The practice of psychotherapy taps into unresolved early-life experiences and desires that the actual doing of therapy is not designed to resolve. If anything, the situation may stimulate uncomfortable feelings because therapy is constructed to use the therapist as a target of patient enactments. Thus, therapists' anxiety may be relatively common. In their desire to maintain a professional image, therapists may have considerable difficulty in acknowledging doubts about their own lives and any feelings of inexpertness in dealing with other people. Denial, and its variations and derivatives, are tempting in the hopes of avoiding the anxiety of insecurity about carrying out the work of psychotherapy. Also, despite the intimate involvement in the lives of others, we have noted the frequency of loneliness which can be threatening in its reminder of self-vulnerability.

Finally, we want to mention the special difficulty of duality as it applies to working mothers. We have already indicated the increasing number of women in the field, and many of these women have or will have children. Zager (1988) describes their particular problems, especially trying to cope with seemingly unending demands to give to patients, children, and spouses. She recommends a realistic perspective, the setting of priorities, and a willingness to be flexible, with an emphasis on self-replenishment. All the authors cited, as well as others in the past (Herron & Rouslin, 1982/1984) stress the necessity for psychotherapists to learn to "feed" themselves in a constructive manner. In our view, this is an affirmation of the essential nature of developing healthy narcissism.

FINAL NOTES

As far as we are concerned, this ending could become a beginning for psychotherapists. The role of psychotherapist as it is known today can be conceptualized as containing apparent expectations and covert qualifiers. The expectations are supposedly described openly and are available for public inspection, whereas the qualifiers are essentials that tend to be unspecified and relatively hard for the public to detect. In fact, even within the profession, some of these qualifiers, even though known, are given limited mention. In general the title role serves to mask the qualifiers.

Our interest lies in the closer examination of therapist behavior that has become masked and, so often, a large blind spot out of awareness and under limited control. We believe the origins, development, and perpetuation of such masking in psychotherapists is connected to narcissistic concerns. This can translate into therapist need gratification at the expense of the therapy, which is really not in the therapist's self-interest either. In contrast, immediate, rather irrational satisfactions are to be patiently bypassed in favor of the facilitation of healthy narcissism. This means a strong sense of personal and professional identity enveloped in the giving and receiving of affection to and from others, and therefore, to and from the self. Our belief is that far too little attention has been devoted to this type of development in psychotherapists. In response, we have attempted in this book to facilitate exploration of the topic by discussing important situations that are both open to various types of neglect and have at their core the manifestations of the therapist's narcissism or self relations.

And what about us? Where do we stand in respect to all this? Well, we believe we have been clear about what needs to be examined and about what ought to be carried out in many instances. Still, it is possible that readers of this book might want to know how we actually operate in more, or different, instances than we have already described. In response to that possibility, we can offer a compromise answer. Our task as authors has, in our opinion, required that we be both discerning and discreet, preserving the confidentiality of the patient–therapist relationship and our own sense of what we deemed "appropriate privacy." Yet, at the same time, realizing that we are asking others to unmask themselves, we want to be explicit as to our faith in the value of such a procedure. This involves some concluding specific statements on our part regarding what kind of therapists we believe we have been, are, and ought to be.

Essentially we want to be "good-enough" psychotherapists, defined by the criteria we have already indicated. Most of the time we feel we achieve this goal, but it certainly involves a continual working process that shifts its strains and rewards. Undoubtedly we have learned from experience and continue to do so. Much of what we have learned is hopeful, easing the "task" component of our work and increasing its positive flow. But, some of what we have learned is frightening because it makes explicit our limitations and what may have to be done to overcome them; or, it highlights that these limitations need to be accepted and consequently respected in our practices.

The resurrection of insecurity is one of these kinds of concerns. For example, recently a therapist we both know decided to work exclusively in private practice, despite some fears that there would be less economic security. We were discussing how we envisioned this therapist's situation and in so doing began to talk about our reactions to following a similar course. We have tended to hold other "regular" positions as employees, meaning the financial reward in these situations is to be counted on as always arriving at a particular time and in a set amount, which affords the sense of security. Do we pursue this course primarily because these positions satisfy our interests, such as teaching and research, or because they provide a needed measure of security that we feel we will never have if we are exclusively in private practice? Most probably we operate as we do for both reasons, but our point here is that we notice that, despite all our years of practice as psychotherapists, we are still vulnerable to a variety of anxieties that require effort to ensure that they do not interfere with our performance as therapists.

We are not attempting perfection in the sense of aspiring to be able to treat anyone who has a problem and asks for our help as therapists. We are most skilled at a particular type of psychotherapy, namely psychoanalytic, and we have a sense of the fact that within these parameters there is still a quesiton of how appropriate the personal match is between ourselves and possible clients. Although we do not believe it happens very often, it is nonetheless a reality that our personal concerns can prevent us from working with some people who may do well with other therapists having the same theoretical orientation as we do. In accepting this fact, we believe that we also mitigate competing with other therapists, or even with each other. We like to approach our practices with the idea that their success depends on our individual efforts, and we believe we are fairly adept in that regard. In particular, we consider our existence as therapists a very serious undertaking which, although it contains its share of humor and levity among other things, is never to be taken lightly. We believe we convey our sense of commitment to the therapy to our patients, and in accord with this, they respond positively, to their benefit, and to ours.

Our successes and errors have their share of uniqueness and commonness. Thus, in one sense, neither of us is anybody special, yet in another, because we are ourselves, we are very special. We would like to feel that specialness more often. We believe it augurs well for us and for our patients. Sometimes it comes so easily, whereas at other times it is desperately elusive.

In developing as psychotherapists, we have pursued many of the customary and recommended routes. That is, we gained a professional identity through credentials, namely schooling and licensing in our professional disciplines with specialized training in psychotherapy, particularly psychoanalysis. We followed the usual paths of self-knowledge, namely personal therapy and supervision. We also did some unorthodox things as well, so that we did not progress just in linear fashion. In general we were and are impressed with formal learning, as far as it goes. Yet we also believe it often has too impersonal a cast, including the more focused training. In our schooling, the person of the therapist, ourselves, could have remained relatively invisible, and often did. We would change that, and when we are involved in teaching and training, we do. Our persons become visible, and we expect the same of our students. We want to know who the people are we train, and we want them to know us. This is not a plea for indiscriminate openness, but for greater freedom of discussion in exploration and training.

As we come to the last lines, we obsess a bit about what we did not cover and what we did mention but could have said more about, and we awaken in the night with the perfect sentence that does not get written in the morning because we forgot it. The very procedure of writing this book is analogous to the process of working as a psychotherapist, with the blend of creativity and discipline, the compulsiveness, anxiety, and seemingly inescapable miscues, all so characteristic of the profession. These are the behaviors that got most therapists where they are and keep them going. Finally, we cannot end without mentioning one more key ingredient of being a good therapist. We believe therapists improve through learning to live life fully, just as patients do.

References

Abraham, K. (1927). A particular form of neurotic resistance against the psychoanalytic method. In K. Abraham (Ed.), *Selected papers on psychoanalysis* (pp. 303–311). New York: Brunner/Mazel. (Original work published 1919)

Abraham, K. (1927). Manifestations of the female castration complex. In K. Abraham (Ed.), *Selected papers on psychoanalysis* (pp. 338–369). New York: Brunner/Mazel. (Original work published 1920)

Abraham, K. (1927). Contributions to the theory of the anal character. In K. Abraham (Ed.), *Selected papers on psychoanalysis* (pp. 370–392). New York: Brunner/Mazel. (Original work published 1921)

Adatto, C. P. (1977). Transference phenomena in initial interviews. *International Journal of Psychoanalytic Psychotherapy, 6,* 3–13.

Adler, G., & Buie, D. H. (1979). Aloneness & borderline psychopathology: The possible relevance of child development issues. *International Journal of Psycho-Analysis, 60,* 83–96.

Allen, G. J., Szollos, S. J., & Williams, B. E. (1986). Doctoral students' comparative evaluations of best and worst psychotherapy supervision. *Professional Psychology: Research and Practice, 17,* 91–99.

Angel, E. (1979). The resolution of a countertransference through a dream of the analyst. *The Psychoanalytic Review 66,* 9–18.

Applebaum, S. A. (1979). *Out in inner space: A psychoanalyst explores the new therapies.* New York: Anchor Press/Doubleday.

Arieti, S. (1974). *Interpretation of schizophrenia.* New York: Basic Books.

Arlow, J. A. (1975). Discussion of the paper by Mark Kanzer, 'The therapeutic and working alliances.' *International Journal of Psychoanalytic Psychotherapy, 4,* 69–73.

Arlow, J., & Brenner, C. (1964). *Psychoanalytic concepts and the structural theory.* New York: International Universities Press.

Armony, N. (1975). Countertransference: Obstacle and instrument. *Contemporary Psychoanalysis, 11,* 265–281.

Avery, A. W., D'Augelli, A. R., & Danish, S. J. (1976). An empirical investigation of the construct validity of empathic understanding ratings. *Counselling Education Supervision, 15,* 117–183.

Balint, M. (1968). *The basic fault.* London: Tavistock Publications.

Balint, M., & Balint, A. (1939). On transference and countertransference. *International Journal of Psycho-Analysis, 20,* 223–230.

Bank, S. P., & Kahn, M. D. (1982). *The sibling bond.* New York: Basic Books.

Bellak, L. (1974). The life of a psychotherapist. *Treatment Monographs on Analytic Psychotherapy, 5,* 7–10.

Bellak, L., Hurvich, M., & Gediman, H. K. (1973). *Ego functions in schizophrenics, neurotics, and normals.* New York: Wiley.

Berkowitz, M. (1987). Therapist survival: Maximizing generativity and minimizing burnout. *Psychotherapy in Private Practice, 5,* 85–89.

Berne, E. (1964). *Games people play.* New York: Grove Press.

Beutler, L. E. (1979). Values, beliefs, religion and the persuasive influence of psychotherapy. *Psychotherapy: Theory, Research and Practice, 16,* 432–440.

Beutler, L. E., Crago, M., & Arizmendi, T. G. (1986). Research on therapist variables in psychotherapy. In S. L. Garfield & A. E. Bergin (Eds.), *Handbook of psychotherapy and behavior change* (3rd ed., pp. 257–310). New York: Wiley.

Bion, W. R. (1963). *Elements of psycho-analysis.* New York: Basic Books.

Blanck, G., & Blanck, R. (1974). *Ego psychology: Theory and practice.* New York: Columbia University Press.

Blanck, G., & Blanck, R. (1979). *Ego psychology II. Psychoanalytic developmental psychology.* New York: Columbia University Press.

Blanck, R., & Blanck, G. (1986). *Beyond ego psychology: Developmental object relations theory.* New York: Columbia University Press.

Blatt, S. J., & Erlich, H. S. (1982). Levels of resistance in the psychotherapeutic process. In P. L. Wachtel (Ed.), *Resistance: Psychodynamic & behavioral approaches* (pp. 69–91). New York: Plenum Press.

Bleger, J. (1967). Psycho-analysis of the psycho-analytic frame. *International Journal of Psycho-Analysis, 48,* 511–519.

Boehm, F. (1930). The feminity complex in men. *International Journal of Psychoanalysis, 11,* 444–469.

Boris, H. N. (1986). Interpretation: History and theory. In M. P. Nichols & T. J. Paolino (Eds.), *Basic techniques of psychodynamic psychotherapy* (pp. 287–308). New York: Gardner Press.

Bowlby, J. (1969). *Attachment & loss: Vol. 1. Attachment.* New York: Basic Books.

Bowlby, J. (1973a). Affectional bonds: Their nature & origin. In R. S. Weiss (Ed.), *Loneliness: The experience of emotional & social isolation* (pp. 38–67). Cambridge, MA: MIT Press.

Bowlby, J. (1973b). *Separation.* New York: Basic Books.

Brenner, C. (1982). *The mind in conflict.* New York: International Universities Press.

Brenner, C. (1987). Working through: 1914–1984. *Psychoanalytic Quarterly, LVI,* 88–108.

Breuer, J., & Freud, S. (1964). Studies on hysteria. In *The complete works of Sigmund Freud* (Vol. 2). London: Hogarth Press. (Original work published 1893–95)

Broadbent, D. E. (1958). *Perception and communication*. New York: Pergamon Press.

Bromberg, P. M. (1984). The third ear. In L. Caligor, P. M. Bromberg, & J. D. Meltzer (Eds.), *Clinical perspectives on the supervision of psychoanalysis and psychotherapy* (pp. 29–49). New York: Plenum Press.

Brown, H. N. (1986). Clarification: History and theory. In M. P. Nichols & T. J. Paolino (Eds.), *Basic techniques of psychodynamic psychotherapy* (pp. 237–263). New York: Gardner Press.

Brown, L. J. (1985). On concreteness. *Psychoanalytic Review, 72*, 379–402.

Burnside, M. A. (1986). Fee practices of male and female therapists. In D. W. Krueger (Ed.), *The last taboo. Money as symbol and reality in psychoanalysis and psychotherapy* (pp. 48–54). New York: Brunner/Mazel.

Bursten, B. (1973). Some narcissistic personality types. *International Journal of Psycho-Analysis, 54*, 287–300.

Bursten, B. (1977). The narcissistic course. In M. C. Nelson (Ed.), *The narcissistic condition: A fact of our lives and times* (pp. 100–126). New York: Human Sciences Press.

Caligor, L. (1981). Parallel and reciprocal processes in psychoanalytic supervision. *Contemporary Psychoanalysis, 17*, 1–27.

Caligor, L., Bromberg, P. M., & Meltzer, J. D. (Eds.). (1984). *Clinical perspectives on the supervision of psychoanalysis and psychotherapy*. New York: Plenum Press.

Caper, R. (1988). *Immaterial facts*. Northvale, NJ: Jason Aronson.

Carkhuff, R. R. (1969). *Helping and human relations* (Vols. 1 and 2). New York: Holt, Rinehart & Winston.

Charny, E. J. (1966). Psychosomatic manifestations of rapport in psychotherapy. *Psychosomatic Medicine, 28*, 39–47.

Cohen, M. B. (1952). Countertransference and anxiety. *Psychiatry, 15*, 231–243.

Compton, A., Boesky, D., Sachs, D. M., Rangell, L., Abend, S., & Goldberg, D. (1982). *A re-examination of the concept "object."* New York: American Psychoanalytic Association.

Corwin, H. A. (1972). The scope of therapeutic confrontation from routine to heroic. *International Journal of Psychoanalytic Psychotherapy, 1*, 68–89.

DeBell, D. E. (1981). Supervisory styles and positions. In R. S. Wallerstein (Ed.), *Becoming a psychoanalyst* (pp. 39–60). New York: International Universities Press.

Deutsch, C. J. (1984). Self-reported sources of stress among psychotherapists. *Professional Psychology, 15*, 833–845.

Dickes, R. (1975). Technical considerations of the therapeutic and working alliances. *International Journal of Psychoanalytic Psychotherapy 4*, 1–25.

Dorpat, T. L. (1977). On neutrality. *International Journal of Psychoanalytic Psychotherapy, 6*, 39–64.

Eagle, M. N. (1984). *Recent developments in psychoanalysis*. New York: McGraw-Hill.

Ehrenberg, D. B. (1975). The quest for intimate relatedness. *Contemporary Psychoanalysis*, *11*, 320–331.

Eigen, M. (1979). Female sexual responsiveness and the therapist's feelings. *The Psychoanalytic Review*, *66*, 3–8.

Eisenbud, R. J. (1982). Early and later determinants of lesbian choice. *Psychoanalytic Review*, *69*, 85–109.

Eitingon, M. (1937). Report of the general meeting of the International Training Commission. *International Journal of Psychoanalysis*, *18*, 346–348.

Ekstein, R., & Wallerstein, R. S. (1972). *The teaching and learning of psychotherapy*. New York: Basic Books.

Enright, J. (1975). One step forward: Situational techniques for altering motivation for therapy. *Psychotherapy: Theory, Research and Practice*, *12*, 344–347.

Epstein, L, & Feiner, A. H. (Eds.), (1979a). *Countertransference: The therapist's contribution to the therapeutic situation*. New York: Jason Aronson.

Epstein, L., & Feiner, A. H. (1979b). Countertransference: The therapist's contribution to treatment. *Contemporary Psychoanalysis*, *15*, 489–513.

Erikson, E. H. (1959). *Identity and the life cycle. Psychological issues monograph I*. New York: International Universities Press.

Fairbairn, W. R. D. (1952). *An object relations theory of the personality*. New York: Basic Books.

Farber, B. A. (Ed.). (1983a). *Stress and burnout in the human service professions*. New York: Pergamon Press.

Farber, B. A. (1983b). The effects of psychotherapeutic practice upon psychotherapists. *Psychotherapy: Theory, Research and Practice*, *20*, 174–182.

Farber, B. A., & Heifetz, L. J. (1981). The satisfactions and stresses of psychotherapeutic work: A factor analytic study. *Professional Psychology*, *12*, 621–630.

Farber, B. A., & Heifetz, L. J. (1982). The process and dimensions of burnout in psychotherapists. *Professional Psychology*, *13*, 293–301.

Fast, I. (1984). *Gender identity: A differentiation model*. Hillsdale, NJ: Analytic Press.

Fenichel, O. (1938). The drive to amass wealth. *Psychoanalytic Quarterly*, *III*, 69–95.

Fenichel, O. (1953). *Concerning the theory of psychoanalytic technique*. New York: W. W. Norton.

Fenichel, O. (1953). A contribution to the psychology of jealousy. In O. Fenichel (Ed.), *Collected papers on Otto Fenichel* (pp. 349–362). New York: Norton. (Original work published 1935)

Ferenczi, S. (1955). Child analysis in the analysis of adults. In S. Ferenczi (Ed.), *Final contributions to the problem of psychoanalysis* (pp. 126–142). New York: Dover Press.

Finell, J. S. (1986). The merits and problems with the concept of projective identification. *Psychoanalytic Review*, *73*, 103–120.

Firestein, S. K. (1978). *Termination in psychoanalysis*. New York: International Universities Press.

Fleming, J., & Bendek, T. F. (1983). *Psychoanalytic supervision: A method of clinical teaching*. New York: International Universities Press.

Flugel, Z. O. (1982). Half a century later: Current status of Freud's controversial views on women. *Psychoanalytic Review, 69*, 7-28.

Ford, E. S. (1963). Being and becoming a psychotherapist: The search for identity. *Psychotherapy: Theory, Research, and Practice, 17*, 472-482.

Forman, B. D. (1988). How to be a failure in private practice. *Psychotherapy Bulletin, 23*, 11-14.

Formanek, R. (1982). On the origins of gender identity. In D. Mendell (Ed.), *Early female development: Current psychoanalytic views* (pp. 1-24). New York: Spectrum.

Frank, G. (1987). [Review of *Developmental theory and clinical process*]. *Psychoanalytic Review, 74*, 307-309.

Frankel, S., & Sherick, I. (1977). Observations on the development of normal envy. *Psychoanalytic Study of the Child, 32*, 257-281.

Freedman, D. A. (1984). The origins of motivation. In J. E. Gedo & G. H. Pollock (Eds.), *Psychoanalysis: The vital issues* (Vol. 1, pp. 17-38). New York: International Universities Press.

Freud, A. (1965). *Normality and pathology in childhood*. New York: International Universities Press.

Freud, A. (1976). Changes in psychoanalytic practice and experiences. *International Journal of PsychoAnalysis, 57*, 257-260.

Freud, S. (1913). On beginning the treatment. In *Standard edition of the collected works of Sigmund Freud* (Vol. 5, pp. 126-138). London: Hogarth Press.

Freud, S. (1914). Remembering, repeating and working through (further recommendations on the technique of psychoanalysis). In *The standard edition of the complete psychological works of Sigmund Freud* (Vol. 12, pp. 147-156). London: Hogarth Press.

Freud, S. (1957). Notes upon a case of obsessional neurosis. In *The complete psychological works of Sigmund Freud* (Vol. 10). London: Hogarth Press. (Original work published 1909)

Freud, S. (1957). On narcissism: An introduction. In *The complete psychological works of Sigmund Freud* (Vol. 14, pp. 67-102). London: Hogarth Press. (Original work published 1914)

Freud, S. (1958). Recommendations for physicians practicing psychoanalysis. In *The complete psychological works of Sigmund Freud* (Vol. 12, pp. 210-219). London: Hogarth Press. (Original work published 1912)

Freud, S. (1959). On the sexual theories of children. In J. Strachey (Ed. and Trans.), *The standard edition of the complete psychological works of Sigmund Freud* (Vol. 9, pp. 207-227). London: Hogarth Press. (Original work published 1908)

Freud, S. (1961). The infantile genital organization. In J. Strachey (Ed. and Trans.), *The standard edition of the complete psychological works of Sigmund Freud* (Vol. 19, pp. 141-148). London: Hogarth Press. (Original work published 1923)

Freud, S. (1961). Some psychological consequences of the anatomical differences between the sexes. In J. Strachey (Ed. and Trans.), *The standard edition of the complete psychological works of Sigmund Freud* (Vol. 19, pp. 196–210). London: Hogarth Press. (Original work published 1925)

Freud, S. (1961). *Civilization and its discontents* (standard edition, Vol. 21, pp. 59–145). London: Hogarth Press. (Original work published 1930)

Freud, S. (1964). Studies in hysteria. In *The standard edition of the complete psychological works of Sigmund Freud* (Vol. 2). London: Hogarth Press. (Original work published 1895)

Freud, S. (1964). On psychotherapy. In *The standard edition of the complete psychological works of Sigmund Freud* (Vol. 7, pp. 255–268). London: Hogarth Press. (Original work published 1905)

Freud, S. (1964a). Five lectures on psychoanalysis. In *The standard edition of the complete psychological works of Sigmund Freud* (Vol. 11, pp. 1–55). London: Hogarth Press. (Original work published in 1910)

Freud, S. (1964b). The future prospects of psychoanalytic therapy. In *The complete psychological works of Sigmund Freud* (Vol. 11). London: Hogarth Press. (Original work published 1910)

Freud, S. (1964). The disposition to obsessional neurosis. In *The standard edition of the complete psychological works of Sigmund Freud* (Vol. 12, pp. 311–325). London: Hogarth Press. (Original work published 1913)

Freud, S. (1964). Introductory lectures on psychoanalysis. In *The standard edition of the complete psychological works of Sigmund Freud* (Vol. 16). London: Hogarth Press. (Original work published 1916–17)

Freud, S. (1964). Inhibitions, symptoms, & anxiety. In *The standard edition of the complete psychological works of Sigmund Freud* (Vol. 20, pp. 177–249). London: Hogarth Press. (Original work published 1926)

Freud, S. (1964). Analysis terminable and interminable. In *The complete psychological works of Sigmund Freud* (Vol. 23, pp. 209–253). London: Hogarth Press. (Original work published 1937)

Freud, S. (1964). An outline of psychoanalysis. In *The complete works of Sigmund Freud* (Vol. 23). London: Hogarth Press. (Original work published 1940)

Freudenberger, H. J., & Richelson, G. (1980). *Burnout: The high cost of high achievement*. New York: Anchor Press.

Friedman, L. (1988). *The anatomy of psychotherapy*. Hillsdale, NJ: Analytic Press.

Friedman, R. M. (1986). The psychoanalytic model of male homosexuality: A historical and theoretical critique. *Psychoanalytic Review, 73*, 483–520.

Frieswyk, S. H., Allen, J. G., Colson, D. B., Coyne, L., Gabbard, G. O., Horwitz, L., & Newsom, G. (1986). Therapeutic alliance: Its place as a process and outcome variable in dynamic psychotherapy research. *Journal of Consulting and Clinical Psychology, 54*, 32–38.

Fromm-Reichmann, F. (1950). *Principles of intensive psychotherapy*. Chicago: The University of Chicago Press.

Fromm-Reichmann, F. (1959). Loneliness. *Psychiatry: The Journal of Interpersonal Processes, 22*, 1–15.

Fuqua, P. B. (1986). Classical psychoanalytic views of money. In D. W. Krueger

(Ed.), *The last taboo. Money as symbol and reality in psychoanalysis and psychotherapy* (pp. 17–23). New York: Brunner/Mazel.

Gaddini, E. (1982). Acting out in the psychoanalytic session. *International Journal of Psycho-Analysis, 13,* 57–64.

Galenson, E., & Riophe, H. (1977). Some suggested revisions concerning early female development. In H. P. Blum (Ed.), *Female psychology* (pp. 29–57). New York: International Universities Press.

Gedo, J. E. (1979). *Beyond interpretation. Toward a revised theory of psychoanalysis.* New York: International Universities Press.

Gedo, J. E. (1984). *Psychoanalysis and its discontents.* New York: Guilford Press.

Gedo, J. E. (1986). *Conceptual issues in psychoanalysis. Essays in history and method.* Hillsdale, NJ: Analytic Press.

Gedo, J. E. (1988). *The mind in disorder. Psychoanalytic models of pathology.* Hillsdale, NJ: Analytic Press.

Geist, R. A. (1984). Therapeutic dilemmas in the treatment of anorexia nervosa: A self psychological perspective. *Contemporary Psychotherapy Review, 2,* 115–142.

Giovacchini, P. L. (1977). Alienation: Character neuroses and narcissistic disorders. *International Journal of Psychoanalytic Psychotherapy, 6,* 288–314.

Giovacchini, P. L. (1989). *Countertransference triumphs and catastrophes.* New York: Jason Aronson.

Glassman, M. B. (1988). Intrapsychic conflict versus developmental deficit: A causal modeling approach to examining psychoanalytic theories of narcissism. *Psychoanalytic Psychology, 5,* 23–46.

Glover, E. (1955). *Technique of psychoanalysis.* New York: International Universities Press.

Goldberg, C. (1986). *On being a psychotherapist—The journey of the healer.* New York: Gardner Press.

Goldman, G. D., & Stricker, G. (Eds.). (1981). *Practical problems of a private psychotherapy practice.* New York: Jason Aronson.

Gomes-Schwartz, B. (1978). Effective ingredients in psychotherapy: Prediction of outcome from process variables. *Journal of Consulting and Clinical Psychology, 46,* 1023–1035.

Goz, R. (1975). On knowing the therapist "as a person." *International Journal of Psychoanalytic Psychotherapy, 4,* 437–458.

Greben, S. E. (1975). Some difficulties and satisfactions inherent in the practice of psychoanalysis. *International Journal of Psycho-Analysis, 56,* 427–434.

Greenberg, J. R., & Mitchell, S. A. (1983). *Object relations in psychoanalytic theory.* Cambridge: Harvard University Press.

Greenberg, L. S. (1986). Change process research. *Journal of Consulting and Clinical Psychology, 54,* 4–9.

Greenson, R. R. (1960). Empathy and its vicissitudes. *International Journal of Psycho-Analysis, 41,* 418–424.

Greenson, R. R. (1965). The working alliance and the transference neurosis. *International Journal of Psycho-Analysis, 34,* 155–181.

Greenson, R. (1967). *The technique and practice of psychoanalysis* (Vol. 1). New York: International Universities Press.

Greenson, R. R., & Wexler, M. (1969). The non-transference relationship in the psychoanalytic situation. *International Journal of Psycho-Analysis, 50*, 27–39.

Grinberg, L. (1979). Countertransference and projective counteridentification. *Contemporary Psychoanalysis, 15*, 226–247.

Grinberg, L. (1983). Discussion of Joseph and Widlocker. In D. Joseph & D. Widlocker (Eds.), *The identity of the psychoanalyst* (pp. 51–66). New York: International Universities Press.

Groos, K. (1901). *The play of man.* New York: Appleton-Century-Crofts.

Grotjahn, M. (1955). Problems and techniques of supervision. *Psychiatry, 18*, 9–15.

Grotstein, J. S. (1981). *Splitting and projective identification.* Northvale, NJ: Jason Aronson.

Grunberger, B. (1979). *Narcissism* (J. S. Diamanti, Trans.). New York: International Universities Press. (Original work published 1971)

Guy, J. D. (1987). *The personal life of the psychotherapist.* New York: Wiley.

Guy, J. D., Stark, M. J., Poelstra, P., & Souder, J. K. (1987). Psychotherapist retirement and age related impairment: Results of a national survey. *Psychotherapy, 24*, 816–820.

Haley, J. (1963). *Strategies of psychotherapy.* New York: Grune & Stratton.

Hardy, A. G. (1979). Rescue vs. contract in defining therapist growth. *The Psychoanalytic Review, 66*, 69–78.

Hare-Mustin, R. T., Marecek, J., Kaplan, A. G., & Liss-Levinson, N. (1979). Rights of clients, responsibilities of therapists. *American Psychologist, 34*, 3–16.

Harlow, H. F., & Harlow, M. K. (1965). The affectional systems. In A. M. Shrier, H. F. Harlow, & F. Stollnitz (Eds.), *Behavior of non-human primates* (Vol. 2, pp. 118–131). Orlando, FL: Academic Press.

Hartmann, H. (1939). *Ego psychology and the problem of adaptation.* New York: International Universities Press.

Havens, L. L. (1974). The existential use of the self. *American Journal of Psychiatry, 131*, 1–10.

Hedges, L. E. (1983). *Listening perspectives in psychotherapy.* Northvale, NJ: Jason Aronson.

Heimann, P. H. (1977). Further observations on the analyst's cognitive process. *Journal of the American Psychoanalytic Association, 25*, 313–333.

Heinmann, P. (1950). On countertransference. *International Journal of Psycho-Analysis, 31*, 81–84.

Hellman, I. D., & Morrison, T. L. (1987). Practice setting and type of caseload as factors in psychotherapist stress. *Psychotherapy, 24*, 427–433.

Hellman, I. D., Morrison, T. L., & Abramowitz, S. I. (1986). The stresses of psychotherapeutic work: A replication and extension. *Journal of Clinical Psychology, 42*, 197–205.

Hellman, I. D., Morrison, T. L., & Abramowitz, S. I. (1987a). Therapist experience and the stresses of psychotherapeutic work. *Psychotherapy, 24*, 171–177.

Hellman, I. D., Morrison, T. L., & Abramowitz, S. I. (1987b). Therapist flexibility/rigidity and work stress. *Professional Psychology: Research and Practice, 18,* 21–27.

Henry, W. E., Sims, J. H., & Spray, S. L. (1971). *The fifth profession: Becoming a psychotherapist.* San Francisco: Jossey-Bass.

Herron, W. G. (1988). The value of personal psychotherapy for psychotherapists. *Psychological Reports, 62,* 175–184.

Herron, W. G., & Rouslin, S. (1984). *Issues in psychotherapy* (Vol. 1). Washington, DC: Oryn Publications. (Original work published in 1982)

Herron, W. G., & Sitkowski, S. (1986). Effect of fees on psychotherapy: What is the evidence? *Professional Psychology: Research and Practice, 17,* 347–351.

Herron, W. G., Trubowitz, J., Wolkin, J., Kinter, T., Herron, M. J., & Sollinger, I. (1988). The psychoanalytic treatment of bulimia. *Psychotherapy in Private Practice, 6,* 167–182.

Hess, A. K. (Ed.). (1980). *Psychotherapy supervision. Theory, research and practice.* New York: Wiley.

Hofling, C. K., & Rosenbaum, M. (1986). The extensions of credit to patients in psychoanalysis and psychotherapy. In D. W. Krueger (Ed.), *The last taboo: Money as symbol and reality in psychoanalysis and psychotherapy* (pp. 202–217). New York: Brunner/Mazel.

Holt, R. R. (1985). The current status of psychoanalytic theory. *Psychoanalytic Psychology, 2,* 289–315.

Horney, K. (1942). *Self-analysis.* New York: W. W. Norton.

Isay, R. (1986). Homosexuality in homosexual and heterosexual men: Some distinctions and implications for treatment. In G. Fogel, F. Lane, & R. Liebert (Eds.), *The psychology of men: New psychoanalytic perspectives* (pp. 277–299). New York: Basic Books.

Issacharoff, A. (1982). Countertransference in supervision: Therapeutic consequences for the supervisee. *Contemporary Psychoanalysis, 18,* 1–15.

Issacs, K. S. (1988). Affect theory: Challenge to basic assumptions. *Psychologist Psychoanalyst, 8,* 10–12.

Jackson, D. D. (1971). Conjoint family therapy: Some considerations on theory, technique and results. In J. Haley (Ed.), *Changing families: A family therapy reader* (pp. 329–362). New York: Grune & Stratton.

Jacobson, E. (1964). *The self & the object world.* New York: International Universities Press.

Joffe, W. C. (1969). A critical review of the status of the envy concept. *International Journal of Psycho-Analysis, 50,* 533–545.

Jones, E. (1948). The early development of female sexuality. In E. Jones (Ed.), *Papers on psychoanalysis* (pp. 438–451). London: Maresfield Reprints. (Original work published 1927)

Jones, E. (1948). Jealousy. In E. Jones (Ed.), *Papers on psychoanalysis* (pp. 325–348). London: Maresfield Reprints. (Original work published 1929)

Jones, E. (1948). Early female sexuality. In E. Jones (Ed.), *Papers on psychoanalysis* (pp. 485–495). London: Maresfield Reprints. (Original work published 1935)

Jones, E. (1951). *The God complex essays in applied psychoanalysis.* London: Hogarth Press.

Jung, C. (1968). *Man and his symbols.* New York: Dell.

Juni, S. (1984). Psychosexual development as a process of equilibration. *Psychoanalytic Review, 71,* 619–634.

Kagan, J. (1971). *Understanding children: Behavior, motives, & thought.* New York: Harcourt Brace Jovanovich.

Kainer, R. G., & Gourevitch, S. J. (1983). On the distinction between narcissism and will: Two parts of the self. *Psychoanalytic Review, 70,* 535–552.

Karpf, R. J. (1986). Confrontation: History and theory. In M. P. Nichols & T. J. Paolino (Eds.), *Basic techniques of psychodynamic psychotherapy* (pp. 187–205). New York: Gardner Press.

Katz, R. L. (1963). The effective empathizer. In R. L. Katz (Ed.), *Empathy, its nature and uses* (pp. 23–35). Glencoe, IL: Collier-Macmillan.

Keller, E. F. (1985). *Reflections on gender and science.* New Haven: Yale University Press.

Kennard, B. D., Stewart, S. M., & Gluck, M. R. (1987). The supervision relationship: Variables contributing to positive versus negative experiences. *Professional Psychology: Research and Practice, 18,* 172–175.

Kernberg, O. F. (1965). Notes on countertransference. *Journal of the American Psychoanalytic Association, 13,* 38–56.

Kernberg, O. (1975). *Borderline conditions and pathological narcissism.* New York: Jason Aronson.

Kernberg, O. (1976). *Object relations theory and clinical psychoanalysis.* New York: Jason Aronson.

Kestenberg, J. S. (1980). The three faces of femininity. *Psychoanalytic Review, 67,* 313–335.

Kilburg, R. R., Nathan, P. E., & Thoreson, R. W. (1986). *Professionals in distress.* Washington, DC: American Psychological Association.

Kinter, T., Herron, M. J., Herron, W. G., Sollinger, I., Trubowitz, J., & Wolkin, J. (1987). Personal perspectives on confrontation in a peer supervision group. *Voices, 23,* 87–93.

Klein, G. (1976). *Psychoanalytic theory. An exploration of essentials.* New York: International Universities Press.

Klein, M. (1975). Notes on some schizoid mechanisms. In *Envy and gratitude and other works, 1946–1963.* New York: Delacorte Press/Seymour Laurence. (Original work published 1946)

Klein, M. (1952). The origins of transference. *International Journal of Psycho-Analysis, 33,* 433–438.

Klein, M. (1975). Envy & gratitude. In M. Klein (Ed.), *Envy & gratitude & other works, 1946–1963* (pp. 176–235). New York: Free Press. (Original work published 1957)

Klein, M. (1980). On the sense of loneliness. In J. Hartog, R. Audy, & A. Cohen (Eds.), *The anatomy of loneliness.* New York: International Universities Press. (Original work published 1963)

Klein, M. I. (1983). Freud's drive theory and ego psychology: A critical evaluation of the Blancks. *Psychoanalytic Review*, 70, 505–517

Kohut, H. (1971). *The analysis of the self*. New York: International Universities Press.

Kohut, H. (1977). *The restoration of the self*. New York: International Universities Press.

Kohut, H. (1984). *How does analysis cure?* Chicago: University of Chicago Press.

Krueger, D. W. (Ed.). (1986). *The last taboo. Money as symbol and reality in psychoanalysis and psychotherapy*. New York: Brunner/Mazel.

Kubie, L. S. (1947). *Elements in the medical curriculum which are essential in the training for psychotherapy*. New York: J. Macy Foundation.

Lachmann, F. M. (1982). Narcissistic development. In D. Mendell (Ed.), *Early female development. Current psychoanalytic views* (pp. 227–248). New York: Spectrum.

Lambert, M. J., Shapiro, D. A., & Bergin, A. E. (1986). The effectiveness of psychotherapy. In S. L. Garfield & A. E. Bergin (Eds.), *Handbook of psychotherapy and behavior change* (3rd ed., pp. 157–211). New York: Wiley.

Landers, S. (1989). Brochure: Many factors determine sex orientation. *The APA Monitor*, 20, 33.

Langs, R. (1976a). *The bipersonal field*. New York: Jason Aronson.

Langs, R. (1976b). *The therapeutic interaction* (vol. 2). New York: Jason Aronson.

Langs, R. (1978). *The listening process*. New York: Jason Aronson.

Langs, R. (1981). *Resistances & interventions: The nature of therapeutic work*. New York: Jason Aronson.

Langs, R. (1982). *Psychotherapy. A basic text*. New York: Jason Aronson.

Langs, R. J. (1984). Supervisory crises and dreams from supervisees. *Contemporary Psychoanalysis*, 18, 107–142.

Lasch, D. (1979). *The culture of narcissism*. New York: W. W. Norton.

Lasky, E. (1984). Psychoanalysts' and psychotherapists' conflicts about setting fees. *Psychoanalytic Psychology*, 1, 289–300.

Lax, R. F. (1975). Some comments on the narcissistic aspects of self-righteousness: Defensive and structural considerations. *International Journal of Psycho-Analysis*, 56, 283–292.

Lazarus, R. S. (1982). Thoughts on the relation between emotion & cognition. *American Psychologist*, 37, 1019–1024.

Leary, S. (1985). Male homosexuality reconsidered. *International Journal of Psychoanalytic Psychotherapy*, 11, 155–174.

Leiderman, P. H. (1980). Pathological loneliness: A psychodynamic interpretation. In J. Hartog, R. Audy, & A. Cohen (Eds.), *The anatomy of loneliness*. New York: International Universities Press. (Original work published 1969)

Lesser, R. M. (1984). Supervision: Illusions, anxieties, and questions. In L. Caligor, P. M. Bromberg, & J. D. Meltzer (Eds.), *Clinical perspectives on the supervision of psychoanalysis and psychotherapy* (pp. 143–152). New York: Plenum Press.

Levenson, E. A. (1982). Follow the fox. An inquiry into the vicissitudes of psychoanalytic supervision. *Contemporary Psychoanalysis, 18,* 1–15.

Levenson, E. (1983). *The ambiguity of change.* New York: Basic Books.

Lewin, B. D. (1958). Education and the quest for omniscience. *Journal of the American Psychoanalytic Association, 6,* 389–412.

Lewis, J. M. (1978). *To be a therapist: The teaching and learning.* New York: Brunner/Mazel.

Lichtenberg, J. D. (1983). *Psychoanalysis and infant research.* Hillsdale, NJ: Analytic Press.

Lichtenstein, H. (1964). The role of narcissism in the emergence and maintenance of a primary identity. *International Journal of Psycho-Analysis, 45,* 49–56.

Light, N. (1974). The "chronic helper" in group therapy. *Perspectives in Psychiatric Care, 12,* 129–134.

Lipp, M. R. (1978). What's in it for the therapist? *Hospital and Community Psychiatry, 29,* 40–41.

Little, M. (1951). Countertransference and the patient's response to it. *International Journal of Psycho-Analysis, 33,* 32–40.

Lothane, Z. (1984). Teaching the psychoanalytic method. Procedure and process. In L. Caligor, P. M. Bromberg, & J. D. Meltzer (Eds.), *Clinical perspectives on the supervision of psychoanalysis and psychotherapy* (pp. 169–192). New York: Plenum Press.

Luborsky, L. (1984). *Principles of psychoanalytic psychotherapy. A manual for supportive–expressive treatment.* New York: Basic Books.

Luborsky, L., Crits-Cristoph, P., & Mellon, J. (1986). Advent of objective measures of the transference concept. *Journal of Consulting and Clinical Psychology, 54,* 39–47.

MacDevitt, J. W. (1987). Therapist's personal therapy and professional self-awareness. *Psychotherapy, 24,* 693–703.

Mahler, M. S. (1968). *On human symbiosis and the vicissitudes of individuation.* New York: International Universities Press.

Mahler, M., Pine, F., & Bergman, A. (1975). *The psychological birth of the human infant.* New York: Basic Books.

Mahrer, A. H. (1983). An existential view and operational perspective on passive–aggressiveness. In R. D. Parsons & R. J. Wicks (Eds.), *Passive-aggressiveness: Theory & practice* (pp. 98–133). New York: Brunner/Mazel.

Mallsberger, J. T., & Buie, D. H. (1974). Countertransference hate in the treatment of suicidal patients. *Archives of General Psychiatry, 30,* 625–633.

Marmor, J. (1953). The feeling of superiority—An occupational hazard in the practice of psychiatry. *American Journal of Psychiatry, 110,* 370–376.

Marshall, R. J. (1982). *Resistant interactions: Child, family & psychotherapist.* New York: Human Sciences Press.

McGrath, E. (1988). The hungry, tired psychotherapist: 10 steps on the road to recovery. *Psychotherapy Bulletin, 23,* 8–9.

Mehlman, R. D. (1974). Becoming and being a psychotherapist: The problem of narcissism. *International Journal of Psychoanalytic Psychotherapy 3,* 125–141.

Meissner, W. (1978). *The paranoid process.* New York: Jason Aronson.

Meissner, W. W., Mack, J. E., & Semrad, F. V. (1975). Classical psychoanalysis. In A. Friedman, H. Kaplan, & B. Sadock (Eds.), *Comprehensive textbook of psychiatry* (2nd ed., pp. 482–566). Baltimore: Williams & Wilkins.

Meissner, W. W., Rizzuto, A., Sashin, J. I., & Buie, D. H. (1987). A view of aggression in phobic states. *Psychoanalytic Quarterly, LVI*, 431–451.

Menaker, E. (1982). *Otto Rank. A rediscovered legacy.* New York: Columbia University Press.

Menninger, K. (1930). *The human mind.* New York: Knopf.

Meyers, H. C. (Ed.). (1986). *Between analyst and patient. New dimensions in countertransference and transference.* Hillsdale, NJ: Analytic Press.

Michels, R. (1988). The future of psychoanalysis. *Psychoanalytic Quarterly, LVII*, 167–185.

Miller, A. (1979). The drama of the gifted child and the psychoanalyst's narcissistic disturbance. *International Journal of Psycho-Analysis, 60*, 47.

Milman, D. S., & Goldman, G. D. (1987). *Techniques of working with resistance.* New York: Jason Aronson.

Mitchell, S. A. (1988). *Relational concepts in psychoanalysis. An integration.* Cambridge, MA: Harvard University Press.

Modell, A. H. (1975). A narcissistic defense against affects and the illusion of self-sufficiency. *International Journal of Psycho-Analysis, 56*, 275–282.

Money, J. (1980). Genetic and chromosomal aspects of homosexual etiology. In J. Marmor (Ed.), *Homosexual behavior. A modern reappraisal* (pp. 59–72). New York: Basic Books.

Montgomery, A. G., & Montgomery, D. J. (1975). Contractual psychotherapy: Guidelines and strategies for change. *Psychotherapy: Theory, Research and Practice, 12*, 348–352.

Moore, B. (1976). Freud and female sexuality: A current view. *International Journal of Psychoanalysis, 57*, 287–300.

Moreno, J. (1947). *The theater to spontaneity.* Beacon, NY: Beacon House.

Morrison, J. K. (1979a). A consumer-oriented approach to psychotherapy. *Psychotherapy: Theory, Research and Practice 10*, 381–384.

Morrison, J. K. (1979b). *A consumer approach to community psychology.* Chicago: Nelson-Hall.

Moulton, R. (1970). A survey and re-evaluation of the concept of penis envy. *Contemporary Psychoanalysis, 7*, 84–104.

Mussen, P. H., Conger, J. J., & Kagan, J. (1974). *Child development & personality.* New York: Harper & Row.

Natterson, J. M. (1986). Interpretation: Clinical application. In M. P. Nichols & T. J. Paolino (Eds.), *Basic techniques of psychodynamic psychotherapy* (pp. 309–330). New York: Gardner Press.

Neisser, V. (1967). *Cognitive Psychology.* New York: Appleton-Century-Crofts.

Nelson, G. L. (1978). Psychotherapy supervision from the trainee's point of view: A survey of preferences. *Professional Psychology, 9*, 539–550.

Neubauer, P. B. (1982). Rivalry, envy, & jealousy. *Psychoanalytic Study of the Child, 37*, 121–142.

Nichols, M. P., & Paolino, T. J., Jr. (Eds.). (1986). *Basic techniques of psychodynamic psychotherapy.* New York: Gardner Press.

Norcross, J. C., Strausser-Kirtland, D., & Missar, C. D. (1988). The processes and outcomes of psychotherapists' personal treatment experiences. *Psychotherapy, 25,* 36–43.

Ogden, T. H. (1982). *Projective identification and psychotherapeutic technique.* New York: Jason Aronson.

O'Leary, J., & Wright, F. (1986). Shame and gender issues in pathological narcissism. *Psychoanalytic Psychology, 3,* 327–340.

Paolino, T. J., Jr. (1981). *Psychoanalytic psychotherapy: Theory, technique, therapeutic relationship and treatability.* New York: Brunner/Mazel.

Parens, H. (1984). Toward a reformulation of the theory of aggression and its implications for primary prevention. In J. E. Gedo & G. H. Pollack (Eds.), *Psychoanalysis: The vital issues* (Vol. 1, pp. 87–114). New York: International Universities Press.

Parsons, M. (1986). Suddenly finding it really matters: The paradox of the analyst's non-attachment. *International Journal of Psycho-Analysis, 67,* 475–488.

Paul, N. L. (1967–68). The use of empathy in the resolution of grief. *Perspectives in Biology and Medicine, 11,* 153–169.

Peplau, H. E. (1955). Loneliness. *American Journal of Nursing, 55,* 1481–1576.

Peplau, H. E. (1989). *Theoretical constructs: Anxiety, self, and hallucinations.* In A. W. O'Toole & S. R. Welt (Eds.), *Interpersonal theory in nursing practice: Selected works of Hildegard E. Peplau* (pp. 270–326). New York: Springer.

Peplau, L A., Miceli, M., & Morasch, B. (1982). Loneliness & self-evaluation. In L. A. Peplau & D. Perlman (Eds.), *Loneliness: A sourcebook of current therapy, research & therapy* (pp. 135–151). New York: John Wiley & Sons.

Peplau, L. A., & Perlman, D. (1982). Perspectives on loneliness. In L. A. Peplau & D. Perlman (Eds.), *Loneliness: A sourcebook of current theory, research & therapy* (pp. 1–18). New York: Wiley.

Perlman, D., & Peplau, L. A. (1982). Theoretical approaches to loneliness. In L. A. Peplau & D. Perlman (Eds.), *Loneliness: A sourcebook of current theory, research & therapy.* New York: Wiley.

Perls, F. (1972). *In and out of the garbage pail.* New York: Bantam Books.

Perry, S., Cooper, A. M., & Michels, R. (1987). The psychodynamic formulation: Its purpose, structure, and clinical application. *American Journal of Psychiatry, 144,* 543–550.

Peterfreund, E. (1983). *The process of psychoanalytic therapy. Models and strategies.* Hillsdale, NJ: Analytic Press.

Piaget, J. (1954). *The construction of reality in the child.* New York: Basic Books.

Piaget, J. (1962). *Play, dreams, and imitation in childhood.* New York: W. W. Norton.

Pine, F. (1985). *Developmental theory and clinical process.* New Haven: Yale University Press.

Pine, F. (1988). The four psychologies of psychoanalysis and their place in clinical work. *Journal of the American Psychoanalytic Association, 36,* 571–596.

Pine, F. (1989). Motivation, personality organization, and the four psychologies of psychoanalysis. *Journal of the American Psychoanalytic Association, 37,* 31–64.

Pollak, M. (1989). Economic inequities in a marriage. *Psychologist—Psychoanalysts' Forum,* Spring, 4–5.

Pontalis, J. B. (1983). Reflections. In D. Joseph & D. Widlocker (Eds.), *The identity of the psychoanalyst* (pp. 277–287). New York: International Universities Press.

Pope, K. S. (1987). Preventing therapist–patient sexual intimacy: Therapy for a therapist at risk. *Professional Psychology: Research and Practice, 18,* 624–628.

Pope, K. S., & Bouhoutos, J. (1986). *Sexual intimacy between therapists and patients.* New York: Praeger.

Prochaska, J. O., Nash, J. M., & Norcross, J. C. (1986). Independent psychological practice: A national survey. *Psychotherapy in Private Practice, 2,* 57–66.

Pulver, S. (1970). Narcissism: The term and the concept. *Journal of the American Psychoanalytic Association, 18,* 319–341.

Racker, H. (1953). Contribution to the problem of countertransference. *International Journal of Psycho-Analysis, 34,* 313–324.

Rado, S. (1940). A critical examination of the concept of bisexuality. *Psychosomatic Medicine, 2,* 459–467.

Rank, O. (1972). *Will therapy and truth in reality.* New York: Knopf.

Rapaport, D. (1960). *The structure of psychoanalytic theory. Psychological Issues,* Monograph 6. New York: International Universities Press.

Rawn, M. L. (1987). Transference: Current concepts and controversies. *Psychoanalytic Review, 14,* 107–124.

Reich, A. (1951). On counter-transference. *International Journal of Psycho-Analysis, 32,* 25–31.

Reich, A. (1960). Further remarks on countertransference. *International Journal of Psycho-Analysis, 41,* 389–395.

Reich, W. (1949). *Character analysis.* New York: Orgone Institute Press.

Reik, T. (1949). *Listening with the third ear.* New York: Farrar, Straus.

Rice, L. N., & Greenberg, L. S. (1984). *Patterns of change: Intensive analysis of psychotherapy process.* New York: Guilford Press.

Riviere, J. (1932). Jealousy as a mechanism of defence. *International Journal of Psycho-Analysis, 13,* 414–424.

Robertiello, R. C., & Schoenewolf, G. (1987). *101 common therapeutic blunders. Countertransference and counterresistance in psychotherapy.* Northvale, NJ: Jason Aronson.

Rogers, C. R. (1961). *On becoming a person.* Boston: Houghton Mifflin.

Rogers, C. R., & Truax, C. B. (1967). The therapeutic conditions antecedent to change: A theoretical view. In C. R. Rogers (Ed.), *The therapeutic relationship and its impact* (pp. 88–102). Madison: University of Wisconsin Press.

Rosenfeld, H. (1964). Object relations of the acute schizophrenic patient in the transference situation. In P. Solomon & B. C. Glueck (Eds.), *Recent research on schizophrenia* (pp. 135–152). Washington, DC: American Psychiatric Association.

Rouslin, S. (1961). Coping with chronic helpfulness. *Mental Hospitals*, 12, 10–12.

Rouslin, S. (1963). Chronic helpfulness: Maintenance or intervention. *Perspectives in Psychiatric Care*, 1, 25–28.

Rouslin, S. (1975a). Commentary on the primitive mind of childhood. *Perspectives in Psychiatric Care*, 13(1), 9.

Rouslin, S. (1975b). Developmental aggression & its consequences. *Perspectives in Psychiatric Care*, 13, 170–175.

Rubenstein, C., & Shaver, P. (1982). *In search of intimacy*. New York: Delacorte.

Rubin, Z. (1982). Children without friends. In L. A. Peplau & D. Perlman (Eds.), *Loneliness: A sourcebook of current theory, research, & therapy*. New York: Wiley.

Rubovits-Seitz, P. (1988). Kohut's method of interpretation: A critique. *Journal of the American Psychoanalytic Association*, 36, 933–959.

Salzman, L. (1968). *The obsessive personality*. New York: Science House.

Saretsky, T. (1980). The analyst's narcissistic vulnerability. *Contemporary Psychoanalysis*, 16, 82–89.

Schafer, R. (1983). *The analytic attitude*. New York: Basic Books.

Schlesinger, H. J. (1981). General principles of psychoanalytic supervision. In R. S. Wallerstein (Ed.), *Becoming a psychoanalyst* (pp. 29–38). New York: International Universities Press.

Searles, H. (1955). The informational value of the supervisor's emotional experiences. *Psychiatry*, 18, 135–146.

Searles, H. (1958). The schizophrenic's vulnerability to the therapist's unconscious processes. *Journal of Nervous and Mental Disease*, 127, 247–262.

Searles, H. F. (1965). Transference psychosis in the psychotherapy of chronic schizophrenia. In H. F. Searles (Ed.), *Collected papers on schizophrenia and related subjects* (pp. 654–716). New York: International Universities Press. (Original work published 1963)

Searles, H. F. (1975a). Countertransference and theoretical model. In J. G. Gunderson & L. R. Mosher (Eds.), *Psychotherapy of schizophrenia* New York: Jason Aronson.

Searles, H. F. (1975b). The patient as therapist to his analyst. In P. L. Giovacchini (Ed.), *Tactics and techniques in psychoanalytic therapy: Vol. II. Countertransference* (pp. 95–151). New York: Jason Aronson.

Searles, H. F. (1978). Psychoanalytic therapy with the borderline adult. In J. Masterson (Ed.), *New perspectives on psychotherapy with the borderline adult* (pp. 42–65). New York: Brunner/Mazel.

Searles, H. F. (1979). Feelings of guilt in the psychoanalyst. In H. F. Searles (Ed.), *Countertransference and related subjects* (pp. 28–35). New York: International Universities Press. (Original work published 1966)

Searles, H. F. (1979a). The "dedicated physician" in the field of psychotherapy and psychoanalysis. In H. F. Searles (Ed.), *Countertransference and related subjects* (pp. 71–88). New York: International Universities Press. (Original work published 1967)

Searles, H. F. (1979b). The schizophrenic individual's experience of his world. In H. F. Searles (Ed.), Countertransference and related subjects (pp. 5–27). New York: International Universities Press. (Original work published 1967)

Searles, H. F. (1979). Autism and the phase of transition to therapeutic symbiosis. In H. F. Searles (Ed.), Countertransference and related subjects (pp. 149–171). New York: International Universities Press. (Original work published 1970)

Searles, H. F. (1979). Pathologic symbiosis and autism. In H. F. Searles (Ed.), Countertransference and related subjects (pp. 132–148). New York: International Universities Press. (Original work published 1971)

Searles, H F. (1979). Concerning therapeutic symbiosis: The patient as symbiotic therapist, the phase of ambivalent symbiosis, and the role of jealousy in the fragmented ego. In H. F. Searles (Ed.), Countertransference and related subjects (pp. 172–191). New York: International Universities Press. (Original work published 1973)

Searles, H. F. (1979). The patient as therapist to his analyst. In H. F. Searles (Ed.), Countertransference and related subjects (pp. 380–459). New York: International Universities Press. (Original work published 1975)

Searles, H. F. (1979). The development of mature hope in the patient–therapist relationship. In Countertransference and related subjects (pp. 479–502). New York: International Universities Press. (Original work published 1977)

Segal, H. (1974). Introduction to the work of Melanie Klein (2nd ed.). New York: Basic Books.

Segal, H. (1977). Countertransference. International Journal of Psychoanalytic Psychotherapy, 6, 31–37.

Semrad, E. (1983). Growing, maturing and sadness. In S. Rako & H. Mazer (Eds.), Semrad: The heart of the therapist. New York: Jason Aronson.

Shaffer, P. (1984). Amadeus: A Milos Forman film. New York: Harper & Row.

Sharaf, M. R., & Levinson, D. J. (1964). The quest of omnipotence in professional training. Psychiatry, 27, 135–149.

Shulman, D. G. (1986). Narcissism in two forms: Implications for the practicing psychoanalyst. Psychoanalytic Psychology, 3, 133–148.

Shulman, J. M. (1988). Psychologists must "position" themselves in the market place. Psychotherapy in Private Practice, 6, 115–127.

Silverman, D. K. (1986). A multi-model approach: Looking at clinical data from three clinical perspectives. Psychoanalytic Psychology, 3, 121–132.

Silverman, D. K. (1987). Female bonding: Some supportive findings for Melanie Klein's views. Psychoanalytic Review, 74, 210–216.

Singer, E. (1965). Key concepts in psychotherapy. New York: Random House.

Singer, F. (1980). The opiate of the analyst. Contemporary Psychoanalysis 16, 258–267.

Singer, J. L. (1974). Imagery and daydream methods in psychotherapy and behavior modification. New York: Academic Press.

Singer, J. L. (1975). The inner world of daydreaming. New York: Harper & Row.

Slakter, E. (Ed.). (1987). Countertransference. Northvale, NJ: Jason Aronson.

Small, I. F., Small, J. G., Alig, V. B., & Moore, D. F. (1970). Passive–aggressive personality disorder: Treatment implications of a clinical typology. *American Journal of Psychiatry, 126,* 973–983.

Smith, V., & Whitfield, M. (1983). The constructive use of envy. *Canadian Journal of Psychiatry, 28,* 14–17.

Solley, C. M. (1966). Affective processes in perceptual development. In A. Kidd & J. L. Rivoire (Eds.), *Perceptual development in children* (pp. 275–304). New York: International Universities Press.

Sollinger, I., Herron, W. G., Trubowitz, J., & Herron, M. J. (1985). The replenishment process for psychotherapists. *The Independent Practitioner, 5,* 19–20.

Spielman, P. M. (1971). Envy and jealousy: An attempt at clarification. *Psychoanalytic Quarterly, 40,* 59–82.

Spitz, R. A. (1945). Hospitalism: An inquiry into the genesis of psychiatric conditions in early childhood. In *The psychoanalytic study of the child* (Vol. 1, pp. 53–74). New York: International Universities Press.

Spotnitz, H. (1969). *Modern psychoanalysis of the schizophrenic patient.* New York: Grune & Stratton.

Spotnitz, H. (1979). Narcissistic countertransference. *Contemporary Psychoanalysis 15,* 545–559.

Sternbach, O. (1983). Critical comments on object relations theory. *Psychoanalytic Review, 70,* 403–421.

Sterba, R. F. (1975). The formative activity of the analyst. In P. L. Giovacchini (Ed.), *Tactics and techniques in psychoanalytic therapy. Vol. II: Countertransference* (pp. 229–238). New York: Jason Aronson.

Stern, D. N. (1985). *The interpersonal world of the infant.* New York: Basic Books.

Stoller, J. (1968). *Sex and gender* (Vol. 1). New York: Science House.

Stoller, J. (1976). *Sex and gender* (Vol. 2). New York: Jason Aronson.

Stolorow, R. (1975). Toward a functional definition of narcissism. *International Journal of Psycho-Analysis, 56,* 179–185.

Stone, L. J., Smith, H. T., & Murphy, L. B. (1973). *The competent infant: Research and commentary.* New York: Basic Books.

Strean, H. S. (1979). The unanalyzed "positive transference" and the need for reanalysis. *The Psychoanalytic Review 66,* 493–506.

Strean, H. S. (Ed.). (1982). *Controversy in psychotherapy.* Metuchen, NJ: Scarecrow Press.

Stricker, G. (1983). Passive–aggressiveness: A condition especially suited to the psychodynamic approach. In R. D. Parsons & R. J. Wicks (Eds.), *Passive-aggressiveness: Theory & practice* (pp. 5–24). New York: Brunner/Mazel.

Strupp, H. H. (1975). On failing one's patient. *Psychotherapy: Theory, Research and Practice, 12,* 39–41.

Strupp, H. H. (1980). Success and failure in time-limited psychotherapy. *Archives of General Psychiatry, 37,* 831–841.

Strupp, H. H. (1989). Psychotherapy: Can the practitioner learn from the researcher? *American Psychologist, 44,* 717–724.

Suler, J. K. (1980). Primary process thinking and creativity. *Psychological Bulletin* 88, 144–165.

Sullivan, H. S. (1953a). *Conceptions of modern psychiatry.* New York: W. W. Norton.

Sullivan, H. S. (1953b). *The interpersonal theory of psychiatry.* New York: W. W. Norton.

Sullivan, H. S. (1954). *The psychiatric interview.* New York: W. W. Norton.

Sullivan, H. S. (1956). *Clinical studies in psychiatry.* New York: W. W. Norton.

Suttie, I. D. (1952). *The origins of love and hate.* New York: Julian.

Tonkin, M., & Fine, H. J. (1985). Narcissism and borderline states: Kernberg, Kohut, and psychotherapy. *Psychoanalytic Psychology, 3,* 221–239.

Tulipan, A. B. (1986). Fee policy as an extension of the therapist's style and orientation. In D. W. Krueger (Ed.), *The last taboo: Money as symbol and reality in psychoanalysis and psychotherapy* (pp. 79–87). New York: Brunner/Mazel.

Tyson, P. (1986). Male gender identity: Early developmental roots. *Psychoanalytic Review, 73,* 405–425.

Valliant, G. E. (1971). A theoretical hierarchy of ego mechanisms. *Archives of General Psychiatry, 24,* 107–118.

Wachtel, P. L. (Ed.). (1982). *Resistance: Psychodynamic and behavioral approaches.* New York: Plenum Press.

Wallerstein, R. S. (Ed.). (1981). *Becoming a psychoanalyst: A study of psychoanalytic supervision.* New York: International Universities Press.

Wallerstein, R. S. (1989). The psychotherapy research project of the Menninger Foundation: An overview. *Journal of Consulting and Clinical Psychology, 57,* 195–205.

Weiss, R. S. (1973). The study of loneliness. In R. S. Weiss (Ed.), *Loneliness: The experience of emotional and social isolation* (pp. 7–29). Cambridge, MA: MIT Press.

Weiss, R. S. (1982). Issues in the study of loneliness. In L. A. Peplau & D. Perlman (Eds.), *Loneliness: A sourcebook of current theory, research & therapy* (pp. 71–80). New York: Wiley.

White, M. T. (1980). Self relations, object relations, and pathological narcissism. *Psychoanalytic Review, 67,* 4–24.

Whitman, R., Trosman, H., & Koenig, R. (1954). Clinical assessment of passive-aggressive personality. *Archives of Neurology and Psychiatry, 72,* 540–549.

Winnicott, D. W. (1947). Hate in the countertransference. *International Journal of Psycho-Analysis, 30,* 102–110.

Winnicott, D. W. (1958). *Through pediatrics to psycho-analysis.* London: Hogarth Press.

Winnicott, D. W. (1965a). The capacity to be alone. In D. W. Winnicott (Ed.), *The maturational processes and the facilitating environment* (pp. 29–36). New York: International Universities Press.

Winnicott, D. W. (1965b). *The maturational processes and the facilitating environment.* New York: International Universities Press.

Winnicott, D. W. (1971). *Playing and reality*. New York: Basic Books.

Winnicott, D. W. (1974). The theory of the parent–infant relationship. In D. W. Winnicott (Ed.), *The maturational processes and the facilitating environment* (pp. 37–55). New York: International Universities Press. (Original work published 1960)

Winnicott, D. W. (1974). Psychiatric disorder in terms of infantile maturational processes. In D. W. Winnicott (Ed.), *The maturational processes and the facilitating environment* (pp. 230–241). New York: International Universities Press. (Original work published 1963)

Winnicott, D. W. (1975). Transitional objects and transitional phenomena. In D. W. Winnicott (Ed.), *Through paediatrics to psychoanalysis* (pp. 229–242). London: Hogarth Press. (Original work published 1951)

Wolberg, A. (1973). *The borderline patient*. New York: International Medical Book Corp.

Wolberg, L. R. (1977). *The technique of psychotherapy* (3rd ed.). New York: Grune & Stratton.

Wolpe, J. (1969). *The practice of behavior therapy*. New York: Pergamon Press.

Zager, K. (1988). Women, private practice and the family: Special needs/special problems. *Psychotherapy in Private Practice, 6*, 9–14.

Zetzel, E. R. (1956). Current concepts of transference. *International Journal of Psycho-Analysis, 37*, 369–376.

Zetzel, E. R. (1966). The analytic situation. In R. E. Litman (Ed.), *Psychoanalysis in the Americas* (pp. 86–106). New York: International Universities Press.

Zilboorg, G. (1938). Loneliness. *Atlantic Monthly, 161*, 45–54.

Index

347